GENOMICS AND ENVIRONMENTAL REGULATION

GENOMICS and ENVIRONMENTAL REGULATION

Science, Ethics, and Law

Edited by

RICHARD R. SHARP

GARY E. MARCHANT

JAMIE A. GRODSKY

The Johns Hopkins University Press
Baltimore

© 2008 The Johns Hopkins University Press
All rights reserved. Published 2008
Printed in the United States of America on acid-free paper
9 8 7 6 5 4 3 2 1

The Johns Hopkins University Press
2715 North Charles Street
Baltimore, Maryland 21218-4363
www.press.jhu.edu

Library of Congress Cataloging-in-Publication Data
Genomics and environmental regulation : science, ethics, and law / edited by
Richard R. Sharp, Gary E. Marchant, and Jamie A. Grodsky.
    p. ; cm.
Includes bibliographical references and index.
ISBN-13: 978-0-8018-9022-2 (hardcover : alk. paper)
ISBN-10: 0-8018-9022-5 (hardcover : alk. paper)
    1. Genomics—Moral and ethical aspects. 2. Environmental health. 3. Genetic
toxicology. 4. Genomics—Law and legislation—United States. I. Sharp, Richard R.
(Richard Roy) II. Marchant, Gary Elvin, 1958– III. Grodsky, Jamie A.
    [DNLM: 1. Genomics—ethics—United States. 2. Genomics—legislation &
jurisprudence—United States. 3. Environmental Health—legislation &
jurisprudence—United States. 4. Government Regulation—United States. 5. Public
Policy—United States. QU 58.5 G33521 2008]
    QH438.7.G462 2008
    363.7'0561—dc22   2008007949

A catalog record for this book is available from the British Library.

*Special discounts are available for bulk purchases of this book. For more
information, please contact Special Sales at 410-516-6936 or specialsales
@press.jhu.edu.*

The Johns Hopkins University Press uses environmentally friendly book
materials, including recycled text paper that is composed of at least 30 percent
post-consumer waste, whenever possible. All of our book papers are acid-free,
and our jackets and covers are printed on paper with recycled content.

To my wife and children, Linda, Megan, Michael, and Quentin
—R.S.

To my wife, Dawn
—G.M.

To my father, Dr. Gerold M. Grodsky, and to the
memory of my mother, Kayla Wolfe Grodsky
—J.G.

CONTENTS

PREFACE

Genomics is hardly a modest science. From the early planning of the Human Genome Project, advocates of genomic research have maintained that a comprehensive understanding of genetic contributions to biological processes will explain the many mysteries of human disease and revolutionize the practice of medicine. Yet, while biomedical applications of genomics have garnered much attention, it is perhaps the nonclinical uses of genomics that will generate the most contentious social debates. Examples include applications of genomics in the workplace, in setting dietary recommendations based on an individual's genomic profile (nutrigenomics), and in identifying criminals from crime-scene samples using genetic markers (DNA forensics).

This book is about another major new application of genomics outside medical contexts—the use of genomic data and technologies to inform environmental policy and regulation. There are many potential applications of genomic information in environmental decision making, many of which will raise profound ethical, legal, and policy challenges. For example, whereas in the past environmental regulators have conceptualized the population as a relatively uniform whole, at most characterizing risks for large, biologically heterogeneous groups such as children, genomics holds the promise of understanding biological features of much smaller subpopulations. Recent advances in genomics suggest that certain individuals and groups may have genetic profiles associated with increased susceptibility to the harmful effects of environmental toxins. As those susceptibilities are better understood—and it becomes possible to identify individuals who are at risk of developing significant health problems when exposed to pollutant levels below levels deemed "safe" for the general population—regulators will be confronted with a dilemma. Do they provide a level of protection that is greater than that necessary for other citizens—a goal that may be economically burdensome, if not altogether impossible? Or, as genetically susceptible individuals and sub-populations are identified, do regulators exclude such individuals and groups from the guarantee of environmental protection and face a trou-blesome, if not untenable, political and ethical situation?

Another important application of genomic data in the environmen-tal context will be identifying genetic changes that may be markers of early toxicity in exposed individuals. Although this potentially more precise and sensitive information may hold promise for crafting more effective regulatory interventions, it will also raise enormously chal-lenging scientific, legal, and policy questions. One such question is whether or when the detection of molecular genetic changes from ex-posure to toxic substances, unaccompanied by any detectable clinical effects, should trigger legal liabilities or regulatory requirements for re-ducing such exposures.

As we gain greater knowledge of genetic susceptibilities and markers relating to the harmful effects of environmental exposures, genomic in-formation may create public expectations of environmental protection that cannot be delivered under existing laws and regulations. Yet if laws are modified, who should bear the enhanced costs of maintaining envi-ronmental quality, particularly where the risks fall disproportionately on a limited subset of the population? And will a shifting focus on subclin-ical genetic changes rather than subsequent toxic injuries lead to more effective and targeted environmental regulations, or will it simply inflate the costs and burdens of environmental protection without correspon-ding improvements in environmental health?

This book addresses these and other related issues of social justice and public policy raised by the application of genomics to environmental reg-ulation. The chapters that follow are organized into four parts. The first examines the manner in which genomic technologies may shape envi-ronmental-policy debates. In chapter 1, Gary Marchant surveys how one important type of toxicogenomic data, that generated by gene expression assays, are likely to be applied in environmental regulation and the pol-icy opportunities and challenges such data present. More rapid screen-ing of environment chemicals, a more sensitive assay for adverse effects used to trigger regulatory requirements, and real-time monitoring of ex-posed populations and ecosystems are some of the potential applications discussed in the chapter. These promising applications raise important policy issues relating to data and methods validation, appropriate levels of regulatory stringency, avoidance of false positives, and reporting requirements.

In the second chapter by Kerry Dearfield, William Benson, Kathryn Gallagher, and Jeremy Johnson, these and other potential regulatory applications highlighted by Marchant are discussed from the perspective of policy makers at the U.S. Environmental Protection Agency. The chapter covers several EPA-supported activities and policy initiatives, including the Agency's Interim Policy on Genomics and its technical framework for developing methods and standardizing approaches for assessing genomic information submitted to EPA.

Several other stakeholder interests and perspectives inform environmental policy and will shape how genomics is incorporated into ongoing regulatory practices. In chapter 3, Richard Phillips explores the application of genomics to environmental policy and regulation from the perspective of regulated industries, with special attention to the use of genomic data to assess chemical safety. In chapter 4, John Balbus provides a contrasting public interest perspective on the use of toxicogenomic data in environmental policy. Like Phillips, Balbus highlights potential regulatory impediments that could delay or misdirect beneficial uses of toxicogenomics, such as unduly burdensome validation requirements or lack of public access to toxicogenomic databases. He concludes by calling for active involvement of public interest organizations in the development and application of toxicogenomic data.

The second part of the book examines specific legal issues raised by new genomic data. In chapter 5, Lynn Bergeson discusses the importance and legal relevance of technology standardization, data modeling, and protocol validation. She argues that resolving these critical scientific issues is essential to the successful application of genomic data to regulatory standard-setting. Using the example of adverse effects reporting under the Toxic Substances Control Act to anchor her discussion, Bergeson frames several key challenges facing attorneys, regulators, and the regulated community in the genomic era.

Chapter 6 covers the implications of toxicogenetics and toxicogenomics for the law of toxic torts. There, Andrew Askland and Marchant explore several legal considerations introduced by Bergeson and consider how gene expression data may play a role in establishing causation and documenting exposure to toxic substances. Data on genetic susceptibility may also affect assessments of causation and could introduce important questions about a defendant's duty to warn various parties about known hazards, plaintiff's assumption of risk, and the treatment of "idiosyncratic" responses to toxic agents. In addition to discussing the far-reaching implications of genomics for tort law, the authors discuss limitations of the emerging science that must be addressed before it can be used effectively in the legal arena.

In chapter 7, Marchant and Jamie Grodsky adopt a broader perspective and evaluate the implications of genetic susceptibility for the law and normative goals of environmental justice. The authors grapple with the question of whether environmental justice should focus on disproportionate exposure to toxic substances (as in the traditional environmental justice model), on disproportionate risk, or on some combination thereof. They conclude that environmental justice must continue to focus on disparate exposures borne by politically disadvantaged groups. However, where susceptibilities exacerbate risk in these disparately burdened groups, such data arguably may be relevant to proving disparate impacts in legal settings or for designing effective remedial policies. This raises the crucial question of whether susceptibility data gathered on the basis of race or ethnicity can be used to help remedy the effects of discrimination without reifying outmoded social categories or reinforcing unfounded notions of biological difference among human populations.

In chapter 8, Gary Marchant examines what is likely to be one of the first major regulatory contexts in which genetic susceptibility data will be used, namely, in the setting of national ambient air quality standards. Marchant reviews the legal and scientific status of using genetic data in setting air quality standards and then discusses the evidentiary and normative issues that will need to be addressed in applying genomic data in this context. Focusing on this specific regulatory context, Marchant illustrates how many of the larger legal issues discussed in the preceding chapters may arise in practice.

The third part of the book examines the manner in which genomic technologies may affect the workplace. In chapter 9, Paul Schulte discusses the workplace use of genetic information (both inherited genetic factors and acquired genetic effects) focusing on the following categories: research, practice, regulation, and litigation. Schulte suggests that occupational safety and health researchers, practitioners, and policy makers should be particularly cautious in applying genetic susceptibility data to the workplace and that worker confidentiality and decision-making rights need to be protected.

Chapter 10, by Marc Weinstein, covers the first of the areas examined by Schulte in more detail, focusing on the growing importance of human genome–related epidemiological research to public health and occupational medicine. Weinstein argues that such research will significantly expand the number of human subpopulations in which risk can be well characterized. In broad-based public health initiatives, that prospect may be of lesser value, but in the occupational realm this possibility may be much more significant. Building on this idea, the chapter details the legal and regulatory atmosphere surrounding genetic screening in the workplace from both the employer's and the worker's perspectives.

In chapter 11, Mark Rothstein expands upon Schulte's discussion of regulatory considerations in the workplace and explores how technological advances will affect overarching legal themes, including regulating in the face of scientific uncertainty, the benefits and burdens of alternative regulatory interventions, conflicts between autonomy and paternalism, and the respective rights of employees and employers. The chapter focuses on the implications of genomics for the Occupational Safety and Health Act, the Americans with Disabilities Act, and state and federal laws addressing genetic discrimination.

This part of the book concludes with an in-depth case analysis of issues posed by genetic susceptibility to ionizing radiation. Ionizing radiation presents an important case study as it is probably the best-characterized human carcinogen. Researchers have identified a subpopulation of individuals who are particularly sensitive due to genetic and other factors. In chapter 12, Kenneth Mossman discusses policy approaches for protecting these sensitive individuals in the workplace. He proposes a targeted strategy whereby individual workers who declare a sensitivity to radiation can avail themselves of additional protections.

The last part of the book examines a number of broad philosophical questions raised by the application of genomic technologies to environmental regulation. The first chapter presents perhaps the most contrarian analysis developed in the book. Andrea Smith and Jason Robert challenge several widely accepted views about genomics, human exposure to toxic substances, and gene-environment interactions. They argue that if toxicogenomics is to make good on its promise to transform environmental regulation, it must be situated within the larger contexts of developmental and evolutionary biology, social ecology, politics, and economics. The importance of framing genomics within a broader range of contextual considerations is defended as critical to successfully integrating genomics into environmental regulation in a manner that is not only scientifically robust, but socially responsible.

In chapter 14, David Resnik begins with a different set of philosophical concerns and considers the role of the precautionary principle in applying genomics to environmental protection. This principle is often viewed as a useful guide for making regulatory policy decisions in the absence of conclusive scientific evidence and frequently underlies debates about environmental regulation, food and drug safety, uses of biotechnology, and public safety. Although the precautionary principle has its roots in a common-sense view of risk management, critics object that it is too vague to serve as a basis for environmental regulation. Resnik examines competing views on the role of the precautionary principle in science policy and defends its utility as a guide to new regulatory applications of genomics.

James Nickel, in chapter 15, offers a political philosophy perspective, examining how the application of genomics to environmental protection will affect rights-based claims to a safe environment. Competing philosophical views on the right to a safe environment are discussed, with an emphasis on debates about the potential scope and interpretation of this right. Nickel maintains that the potentially enormous economic costs of protecting exceptionally vulnerable persons require a reassessment of any claimed universal right to a safe environment. The chapter develops a novel conception of the right to a safe environment that takes into account the feasibility and cost of recognizing such a right.

In chapter 16, Carl Cranor examines moral and political philosophies influencing deliberations about environmental law and regulatory policy. The chapter discusses how these underlying moral positions not only inform particular views on the need to protect individuals from toxic harm but also shape our moral imaginations regarding available policy options and alternatives. In contrast to Nickel, Cranor defends the need to protect everyone, even the most susceptible, from harms caused by environmental toxicants. The chapter concludes by exploring how this protectionist position might be best represented in various legal and regulatory structures.

In the concluding chapter of the book, Adam Finkel proposes what he considers a "middle-ground position" that would accommodate many of the stakeholder interests and philosophical positions articulated in the preceding chapters. To avoid many of the potential discriminatory, psychological, and policy problems that would result from more widespread use of genetic susceptibility information, he proposes new kinds of confidentiality measures.

To assist readers who are new to genomics and its application to environmental regulation, we have included as an appendix the executive summary of a recent National Research Council report, *Applications of Toxicogenomic Technologies to Predictive Toxicology and Risk Assessment.* In addition to presenting a concise overview of the current state of the science, this material considers the types of genomic discoveries that are likely to be made in the near future and some of the uncertainties that exist regarding the pace of genomic research and its application to predictive toxicology and environmental regulation. Our hope is that this material will allow readers to engage the text more critically and better appreciate aspects of genomics of particular relevance to environmental regulators.

In a rapidly changing field like contemporary genomics, it is impossible to predict all emergent policy challenges. Nevertheless, our aim in this book is to clarify several critical issues and to develop new lenses through which to peer into an uncertain future. Responsible technology development demands nothing less.

As part of this project, the editors initially identified critical topics and convened a conference that brought together leading scientists, policy makers, environmental advocates, lawyers, and ethicists concerned about the implications of genomics for the future of environmental policy. The conference was held at Arizona State University on January 13–14, 2005, and was supported by the National Human Genome Research Institute and National Institute of Environmental Health Sciences of the National Institutes of Health. In addition to those who have contributed to this volume, we would like to thank others who attended the conference and participated in our discussions, including Anthony DeCaprio, David Eaton, Kelly Fryer-Edwards, Robert Kavlock, Steven Kleeberger, Mary Lyndon, Susan Poulter, William Rodgers, Raymond Tennant, and Brenda Weis. We would also like to thank Ernie Hood, David Landy, Wendy Harris, and Michele Callaghan for their help in preparing the book for publication.

CONTRIBUTORS

About the Editors

Richard R. Sharp is director of bioethics research at the Cleveland Clinic. Dr. Sharp received his training in philosophy and medical ethics at Michigan State University. Before joining the Cleveland Clinic in 2007, Sharp taught bioethics at Baylor College of Medicine and the National Institute of Environmental Health Sciences, one of the National Institutes of Health, where he directed the Program in Environmental Health Policy and Ethics. His professional interests center on the promotion of informed patient decision making in clinical research, particularly research that involves genetic analyses. He regularly lectures on advanced topics in research ethics and has served on advisory committees for the American Thoracic Society, the European Respiratory Society, the Alpha One Foundation, the Woodrow Wilson Center, and the National Institutes of Health. At the Cleveland Clinic, Sharp participates in the teaching of clinical ethics to medical students, residents, and fellows.

Gary E. Marchant is Lincoln Professor of Emerging Technologies, Law, and Ethics at Arizona State University College of Law and executive director of the ASU Center for the Study of Law, Science and Technology. He has a Ph.D. in genetics from the University of British Columbia, an M.P.P. from the Kennedy School of Government, and a law degree from Harvard. Before joining the ASU faculty in 1999, he was a partner in a Washington, D.C., law firm, where his practice focused on environmental and administrative law. Marchant teaches and researches in the subject areas of environmental law, risk assessment and risk management, genetics and the law, and law, science, and technology. He has published several articles in legal and scientific journals on the role of genomics in environmental regulation and toxic torts. He was the principal investigator on a research grant examining the role of genetic susceptibility in environmental regulation supported by the National Human Genome Research Institute and National Institute of Environmental Health Sciences.

Jamie A. Grodsky is an associate professor of law at the George Washington University Law School, where she specializes in environmental law, natural resources law, science and technology law, and genetics. She joined the George Washington law faculty in 2006 after serving on the faculty of the University of Minnesota Law School. Prior to entering academia, Professor Grodsky served as a counsel to the U.S. House Committee on Natural Resources, counsel to the U.S. Senate Judiciary Committee, and the senior advisor to the general counsel at the U.S. Environmental Protection Agency. Previously, she was an analyst at the congressional Office of Technology Assessment. Her scholarship focuses on implications of emerging technologies for environmental law, including award-winning legal journal articles on the role of genomics in toxic tort and regulatory law. Her work has appeared in the *Stanford Law Review, the California Law Review,* the *Minnesota Law Review,* and the *Yale Journal on Regulation,* among others. Professor Grodsky holds a B.A. from Stanford University, an M.A. from the University of California, Berkeley, and a J.D. from Stanford Law School.

About the Contributors

Andrew Askland is the director of the Center for the Study of Law, Science, and Technology at the College of Law at Arizona State University, where he teaches privacy, economics and the law, and advanced research topics in law, science, and technology. He earned an M.A. and a Ph.D. in philosophy at the University of Colorado at Boulder and a J.D. at the University of Maryland, Baltimore. He received a B.A. in philosophy from Holy Cross College and a B.S. in economics from the University of Maryland.

John M. Balbus, M.D., M.P.H., is senior scientist and director of the Health Program for Environmental Defense. Before joining Environmental Defense, he spent seven years at the George Washington University, where he was founding director of the Center for Risk Science and Public Health and served as acting chair of the Department of Environmental and Occupational Health. Balbus received a B.A. in biochemistry from Harvard University, an M.D. from the University of Pennsylvania, and an M.P.H. from the Johns Hopkins University.

William H. Benson, Ph.D., is director of the National Health and Environmental Effects Research Laboratory's Gulf Ecology Division within the U.S. Environmental Protection Agency's Office of Research and Development. Benson obtained a B.S. in biology from Florida Institute of Technology and an M.S. and a Ph.D. in toxicology from the University of Kentucky. Benson is a past president of the Society of Environmental Toxicology and Chemistry and a fellow of the American Association for the Advancement of Science.

Lynn L. Bergeson is a founder and shareholder of Bergeson & Campbell, P.C., a Washington, D.C., law firm concentrating on chemical product approval, regulation, litigation, and associated chemical product business issues. Bergeson is a graduate of Michigan State University (B.A.), and the Columbus School of Law, the Catholic University of America. Bergeson is a member of the Bar Association of the District of Columbia; American Bar Association (Section of Environment, Energy, and Resources); Women's Bar Association of the District of Columbia; and the Women's Council on Energy and the Environment.

Carl Cranor, Ph.D., professor of philosophy at the University of California, Riverside, did his undergraduate work in mathematics and physics at the University of Colorado and his graduate work in philosophy at the University of California, Los Angeles. He received a Master of Studies in Law from Yale Law School. He is the author of several books, including *Regulating Toxic Substances: A Philosophy of Science and the Law* (Oxford University Press, 1993) and *Are Genes Us? The Social Consequences of the New Genetics* (Rutgers University Press, 1994). In 1998 he was elected a fellow of the American Association for the Advancement of Science.

Kerry L. Dearfield, Ph.D., was a senior scientist for science policy in EPA's Office of the Science Advisor, in Washington, D.C. He received a Ph.D. in pharmacology from the George Washington University School of Medicine. He cochaired the U.S. Environmental Protection Agency Genomics Task Force Workgroup while at EPA. He is currently the scientific advisor for risk assessment in the U.S. Department of Agriculture's Food and Safety Inspection Service.

Adam M. Finkel is currently a professor of environmental and occupational health at the University of Medicine and Dentistry of New Jersey (UMDNJ) School of Public Health and is also a fellow and executive director of the Penn Program on Regulation at the University of Pennsyl-

vania Law School. At the time of the conference, he was a visiting professor at the Woodrow Wilson school of Public and International Affairs
at Princeton University. He has an Sc.D. in environmental health sciences, an M.P.P., and an undergraduate degree in biology, all from Harvard University, and is a certified industrial hygienist. Finkel was director
of regulatory programs at the U.S. Occupational Safety and Health Administration from 1995 to 2000 and regional administrator for the Rocky
Mountain states from 2000 to 2003.

Kathryn Gallagher received her Ph.D. in Marine Science in 1995
through the Department of Environmental Chemistry at the College of
William and Mary's Virginia Institute of Marine Science and conducted
her postdoctoral research in comparative toxicology using transgenic
species at the National Institute of Environmental Health Sciences. Her
work at EPA has included developing the Office of Pesticide Program's
approach to probabilistic risk assessment for aquatic systems and coordinating research on toxicants for the Chesapeake Bay Program. She has
co-authored numerous peer-reveiwed scientific papers and technical reports, primarily focusing on the impacts of anthropogenic chemicals on
ecosystems. She currently works in EPA's Office of the Science Advisor
on cross-agency initiatives including genomics, nanotechnology, expert
elicitation, and probabilistic risk assessment.

Jeremy D. Johnson is a toxicologist and human health risk assessor for
the Environmental Services Division in the Environmental Protection
Agency's (EPA) Kansas City regional office. He received a B.S. in environmental science from the University of Arizona and an M.S. in Toxicology from the University of Kansas Medical Center. In 2004 and 2005,
Mr. Johnson assisted with the implementation of EPA's genomics
initiatives.

Kenneth L. Mossman, Ph.D., is professor of health physics in the
School of Life Sciences and affiliate member of the Center for the Study
of Law, Science, and Technology at Arizona State University in Tempe.
He is also an administrative judge on the Atomic Safety and Licensing
Board of the United States Nuclear Regulatory Commission. From 1990
to 1992, he served as assistant vice president for research at Arizona State,
and from 1997 to 2004 served as director, University Office of Radiation
Safety. From 1973 to 1990, he was on the faculty at Georgetown University and was professor and founding chair of the Department of Radia-

tion Science in Georgetown's Graduate School. In 2001, Mossman was elected a fellow of the American Association for the Advancement of Science. His research interests include radiological health and safety and radiation risk assessment and management.

James W. Nickel is professor of law and affiliate professor of philosophy at Arizona State University. He was professor of philosophy at the University of Colorado, Boulder, from 1982 to 2002, where he served as director of the Center for Values and Social Policy from 1982 to 1986 and as chair of the Philosophy Department from 1992 to 1996. Nickel has held visiting positions at the University of California, Berkeley, School of Law and the University of Utah. His recent work addresses questions about human rights, personal autonomy, and political liberty.

Richard D. Phillips, Ph.D., DABT, has more than twenty-five years of experience in toxicology. He is a senior scientific advisor in toxicology at ExxonMobil Biomedical Sciences, Inc., where he provides expertise in the mechanistic toxicology and risk assessment and chair's ExxonMobil's Occupational Exposure Limit Committee. Phillips is a diplomate of the American Board of Toxicology and vice president of administration for the Toxicology Forum.

David B. Resnik, Ph.D., is a bioethicist at the National Institute of Environmental Health Sciences at the National Institutes of Health. He has a Ph.D. in philosophy from the University of North Carolina and a J.D. from Concord School of Law. He also is an adjunct professor of philosophy at North Carolina State University and associate editor of the journal *Accountability in Research.* Resnik has published four books and more than a hundred articles on various topics in the philosophy of science and medicine, bioethics, and research ethics.

Jason Scott Robert, Ph.D., is with the Bioethics Program at the School of Life Sciences, Arizona State University. Robert is a member of the Stem Cell Network in Canada and serves on the Institute Advisory Board for the Institute of Population and Public Health, part of the Canadian Institutes of Health Research. He also serves on the Advisory Committee on Ethical, Legal, and Social Issues of the Canadian Lifelong Health Initiative. In addition, Robert is one of the coeditors for Philosophy of Biology of the *Stanford Encyclopedia of Philosophy.*

Mark A. Rothstein, J.D., holds the Herbert F. Boehl Chair of Law and Medicine and is director of the Institute for Bioethics, Health Policy and

Law at the University of Louisville School of Medicine. He has served as an advisor to the National Institutes of Health, Centers for Disease Control and Prevention, U.S. Department of Energy, U.S. Congress, the Institute of Medicine, National Conference of State Legislatures, and numerous other public and professional entities. He is the author or editor of nineteen books.

Paul A. Schulte, Ph.D., director of the Education and Information Division of the National Institute of Occupational Safety and Health, is an epidemiologist with interests in quantitative risk assessment, health communication, use of biological markers in epidemiologic research, intervention research, and genetics. He is the editor of a widely used textbook in epidemiology, *Molecular Epidemiology: Principles and Practices.*

Andrea O. Smith is a graduate student in the Department of Community Health and Epidemiology at Dalhousie University. She received her B.A. from St. Thomas University. With Jason Scott Robert, she currently is examining the impact of genomics on population health. Her Ph.D. thesis is analyzing ethical, philosophical, and social dimensions of epidemiological studies of environmental risk.

Marc Weinstein, Ph.D., is at the Charles H. Lundquist School of Business of the University of Oregon. He received a Ph.D. from the Massachusetts Institute of Techonology. At the University of Oregon he teaches courses in compensation, negotiations, and conflict resolution. He is involved in a number of research projects studying the role of international and national institutions in the economic transition in Central Europe and has just begun a project examining conflict resolution in private sector health and safety committees.

GENOMICS AND ENVIRONMENTAL REGULATION

Introduction

Environmental Policy in the Age of Genomics

RICHARD R. SHARP, GARY E. MARCHANT,
AND JAMIE A. GRODSKY

For decades, scientists have recognized that individuals can differ significantly in their susceptibility to environmental toxicants. Using information and tools produced by recent genomic initiatives such as the Human Genome Project, risk assessors may soon be able to conduct far more systematic investigations of individual susceptibilities to toxic substances, potentially transforming environmental risk assessment. Whereas in the past risk assessment was limited to characterizing risks for large, biologically heterogeneous groups, applications of genomics hold the promise of understanding biological features of discrete subpopulations and perhaps even of opening the door to a new era of personalized risk assessment.

Although genomics has the potential to make environmental regulation more accurate and precise, its application in regulatory contexts requires that a number of daunting technical and scientific challenges first be overcome. Regulatory applications of genomics will also raise difficult ethical, legal, and policy issues. This book aims to elucidate some of these challenges and to foster ongoing analysis of the scientific, ethical,

legal, social, and policy issues raised by the application of genomic technologies to environmental regulation (which we view broadly to include
hazard identification, risk assessment, risk management, risk communication, and rule making). Emphasis is placed on the emerging field of
toxicogenomics, defined as the application of genomic technologies to
the identification and understanding of human and environmental toxicants (Marchant, 2003a). If genomic technologies are to be integrated successfully into ongoing risk-assessment and risk-management efforts, the
broader social impact of these applications must be carefully examined
and thoughtfully addressed.

Genomics and Environmental Regulation

By reducing some of the many uncertainties that currently impede risk
assessment, genomic data have the potential to greatly improve the precision and effectiveness of environmental regulation (Henry et al., 2002).
At the same time, the application of genomic data within the existing
matrix of environmental statutes and regulations will raise fundamental
issues regarding the validity, reliability, and biological significance of
these new data (Bergeson, Campbell, and Bozof, 2002; Marchant, 2003b;
Grodsky, 2005).

To encourage discussion of these issues, the U.S. Environmental Protection Agency (EPA) has developed an Interim Policy on Genomics (U.S.
Environmental Protection Agency [EPA], 2002). This policy conveys the
agency's enthusiasm for the potential use of genomic data for risk assessment and regulatory decisions. For example, the interim policy states that
genomic data can be helpful in exploring "the possible link between exposure, mechanism(s) of action, and adverse effects" of potentially toxic
substances and "in setting priorities, in ranking of chemicals for further
testing, and in supporting possible regulatory actions." At the same time,
the interim policy adopts a cautionary approach with respect to regulatory applications of genomic data, given the many uncertainties that
currently exist. The agency notes that at present, such data alone are insufficient for regulatory decision making and that the agency "will consider genomics information on a case-by-case basis" (EPA, 2002).

One of the most important regulatory applications of genomics, particularly gene expression data, will be in providing more sensitive
measurements of adverse effects of exposure to pollutants and other haz-

ardous substances. Many existing regulatory requirements are triggered by the lowest detectable "adverse effect." For example, the Clean Air Act allows national ambient air quality standards to be set at a level that will avoid adverse effects in sensitive populations. Regulatory standards to be set for many noncarcinogens are based on their reference concentrations or reference doses, which are derived by applying a series of uncertainty factors to what is known as the "no observed adverse effect level" or lowest observed adverse effect level. Similar reporting requirements under statutes such as the Toxic Substances Control Act and the Federal Insecticide, Fungicide and Rodenticide Act also require product manufacturers to report to EPA new findings on adverse effects.

A critical question to be resolved is when, if ever, systemic changes in gene expression should be considered an adverse effect under these and other regulatory programs (Grodsky, 2005; Kramer, Cullen, and Faustman, 2006). There are existing regulatory precedents in which subclinical molecular changes have been viewed as adverse effects. For example, molecular changes in erythrocytein levels in response to lead exposure were classified as an adverse effect under the Clean Air Act (*Lead Industries Association,* 1980). To the extent that certain changes in gene expression qualify as an adverse effect, calls for more stringent regulatory standards may result. This is because, on the one hand, gene expression changes are expected at lower dose levels than the morphological or functional adverse effects on which current standards generally are based. On the other hand, some gene expression changes reflect adaptive changes or normal human variation and thus should not qualify as an adverse effect for regulatory purposes. Differentiating gene expression changes that are toxicologically significant from those that represent innocuous cellular responses will therefore be central to regulatory applications of gene expression data.

Toxicogenomic data also have the potential to help fill in many gaps and uncertainties in current regulatory risk assessments. Examples include species-to-species extrapolations, low-dose-to-high-dose extrapolations, and risk assessment of chemical mixtures. Genomic tools may also be useful in evaluating the toxicity of chemicals that have not been tested using standardized tests, such as the rodent chronic bioassay, or in making regulatory decisions based on limited toxicological data. Finally, toxicogenomic methods could be useful for prioritizing contaminated sites, listing chemicals under various statutory programs, and in providing "early warning" or potential toxicological impacts in exposed human populations or ecological communities (Frederickson et al., 2001).

In all these applications, a critical issue, examined in detail in this book, is whether and when toxicogenomic data are adequately informative and validated to be used for making high-stakes regulatory decisions. As reflected in EPA's Interim Policy on Genomics, regulatory agencies are unlikely to base hazard identification classifications and other regulatory decisions exclusively on toxicogenomic data at this time (Dix et al., 2006). A remaining question is under what circumstances genomic data could alter regulatory decisions or criteria that would ordinarily be based on other available evidence.

Other types of genomic information beyond gene expression data will have applications for environmental regulation. Most significantly, the findings of widespread variation in genetic susceptibility to toxic substances will present major challenges to setting regulatory standards under those statutes that require protection of the most susceptible groups within the population (Marchant, 2003a; Grodsky, 2005). Examples of statutory programs that require consideration or protection of the most sensitive subgroups include national ambient air quality standards under the Clean Air Act, pesticide regulations under the Food Quality Protection Act, and drinking water standards established under the Safe Drinking Water Act. As genetic polymorphisms are associated with significant risks of disease at pollutant levels far below levels than are considered safe for the general population, regulatory agencies will face difficult choices. Although economic and other practical considerations may make it infeasible to protect the most genetically vulnerable among us, knowingly adopting regulatory standards that place identifiable subpopulations at risk may be unacceptable to many members of the public.

Moreover, some will suggest that information on susceptible groups should also have implications for environmental justice programs, particularly in select cases in which disease-related polymorphisms occur disproportionately in groups sharing a common geographic heritage. And it is indisputable that genomic data will be increasingly used by both plaintiffs and defendants in toxic tort cases involving exposure to environmental toxicants.

These considerations suggest that the potential applications of toxicogenomic data for environmental regulation are numerous and diverse. Regulatory agencies such as EPA will need to proceed deliberatively to ensure that genomic data are adequately confirmed, validated, and reliable before these data are used in regulatory decision making. At the same time, regulators will need to avoid undue caution that would stifle the development of this promising technology, as has occurred in the past for other types of new risk-assessment data and methodologies (National Research Council, 1994).

Ethical and Social Considerations

The current system of environmental protection, and the implicit ethical, political, economic, legal, and social principles that support it, were developed long before the recent emergence of genomics. Our present system of environmental laws was designed to protect the citizenry as a whole and not to address the unique needs of individuals and small groups (though under certain circumstances laws may authorize protection of broadly defined sensitive subgroups within the general population, such as children or asthmatics). As our knowledge of individual and group sensitivities to environmental exposures expands, such information may lead to rising expectations of levels of environmental protection that cannot be delivered under existing laws and regulations. Such expectations may fuel new demands for limiting concentrations of environmental chemicals, remediating environmental damage, monitoring occupational exposures, and compensating for toxic injuries (Grodsky, 2007).

Requests for enhanced environmental protection may come from individuals or specific populations with genetic sensitivities to identifiable environmental agents. It remains unclear, however, who should bear the social and economic costs of maintaining higher levels of environmental quality, particularly where the risks fall disproportionately on those with rare genetic sensitivities to hazardous environments. The availability of toxicogenomic information will force regulators to reexamine the social costs of protecting the most vulnerable among us, raising pressing issues with respect to social justice and the equitable distribution of public resources.

A related issue is whether specially targeted environmental regulations can successfully protect susceptible individuals (or narrowly defined subpopulations) without changing regulatory requirements designed to protect the population as a whole. In cases where residual risks are concentrated largely in susceptible subpopulations, one could argue that it would be more efficient and cost-effective to focus on interventions for those subgroups. Yet where this is not the case, such a shift in regulatory focus would not only depart from current practices but would also introduce several larger questions. One such question is the extent to which susceptible individuals should be expected to rely on self-help measures such as avoiding certain products in lieu of (or as a supplement to) regulatory requirements imposed on manufacturers. Given the current paradigm that it is the responsibility of industry and governmental regulators to protect all citizens from environmental risks, any shift to toward greater reliance on self-help measures is certain to be controversial even when such an approach is economically attractive. An additional question concerns the nature of the duty of manufacturers to test their products for potential effects on genetically susceptible subgroups or to issue warnings directed at susceptible consumers.

Employers, risk managers, and environmental regulators will face difficult decisions regarding the appropriate balance to strike between segregating genetically sensitive individuals from adverse environments and working to improve environmental conditions. In some cases, targeted efforts to protect individuals and subpopulations with heightened genetic sensitivities to environmental agents could divert risk-management resources away from the improvement of unhealthy environmental conditions in favor of individual exclusion or self-help approaches. For example, rather than trying to make chemical products safer for all users, manufacturers may increasingly rely on labels to warn genetically susceptible consumers to avoid using particular products.

One set of overarching considerations relates to the relative merits of emphasizing genetic over environmental contributions to disease. This trend, which has been described as an aspect of genetic reductionism or the "geneticization" of disease (Lippman, 1991), could foster mistaken beliefs that environmentally associated diseases result primarily from genetic causes. This reduction of complex social problems to a narrow universe of biological problems could change how people think about social priorities. For example, if certain diseases are viewed as attributable to inherent genetic predispositions, employers may be held less accountable for improving workplace conditions. Similarly, a singular emphasis on genetic causes of disease could shift the focus of disease prevention from reducing hazards in the workplace to reliance on the choices and actions of individual workers (Draper, 1991). Following this logic, research funding could be diverted from preventive strategies for improving public health (Edlin, 1987).

Reflecting another aspect of the question of the relative responsibility for environmental risk, environmental protection efforts often focus on categories of risks deemed "involuntary" or beyond individual control (e.g., clean air and water), as opposed to risks that individuals "voluntarily" impose on themselves (e.g., health risks associated with cigarette smoking). As tests for genetic sensitivities to environmental agents become more widely available, individual choices to remain in high-risk environments may increasingly be perceived as voluntary, raising new questions about personal and governmental responsibilities in the genomic age.

Finally, the genomic revolution may affect historically disadvantaged communities in disproportionately burdensome ways. Of particular concern are potential associations between genetic susceptibilities and social categories such as race or ethnicity. Such associations could result in stigmatization and threaten employment and insurance opportunities for members of such groups (Rothstein, 1997). On the one hand, genomic information could strengthen environmental justice claims and reveal new opportunities to improve health through hazard avoidance. On the other hand, this information could perpetuate discredited conceptions of biological difference and undermine the egalitarian goals that environmental justice seeks to achieve. Moreover, if it becomes possible to identify genetic susceptibilities to environmental exposures but only those with significant financial resources could afford preventive steps, toxicogenomics could be viewed as contributing to the existing social disadvantage of underserved individuals and communities.

REFERENCES

Bergeson, L.L., L.M. Campbell, and R.P. Bozof. 2002. Toxicogenomics. *Environmental Forum* 19(6):28–29.

Dix, D.J., K. Gallagher, W.H. Benson, B.L. Groskinsky, J.T. McClintock, K.L. Dearfield, and W.H. Farland. 2006. A framework for the use of genomics data at the EPA. *Nature Biotechnology* 24:1108–11.

Draper, E. 1991. *Risky business: Genetic testing and exclusionary practices in the hazardous workplace.* New York: Cambridge University Press.

Edlin, G. 1987. Inappropriate use of genetic terminology in medical research: A public health issue. *Perspectives in Biology and Medicine* 31:47–56.

Frederickson, H.L., et al. 2001. Towards environmental toxicogenomics: Development of a flow-through, high-density DNA hybridization array and its application to ecotoxicity assessment. *The Science of the Total Environment* 274:137–49.

Grodsky, J.A. 2005. Genetics and environmental law: Redefining public health. *California Law Review* 93:171–270.

Grodsky, J.A. 2007. Genomics and toxic torts: Dismantling the risk-injury divide. *Stanford Law Review* 59:1671–1734.

Henry, C.J., R. Phillips, F. Carpanini, et al. 2002. Use of genomics in toxicology and epidemiology: Findings and recommendations of a workshop. *Environmental Health Perspectives* 110:1047–50.

Kramer, C.B., A.C. Cullen, and E.M. Faustman. 2006. Policy implications of genetic information on regulation under the clean air act: The case of particulate matter and asthmatics. *Environmental Health Perspectives* 114:313–19.

Lead Industries Association v. EPA 1980. 647 F.2d 1130 (D.C. Cir.), *cert. denied,* 449 U.S. 1042.

Lippman, A. 1991. Prenatal genetic testing and screening: Constructing needs and reinforcing inequities. *American Journal of Law and Medicine* 17:15–50.

Marchant, G.E. 2003a. Genomics and toxic substances: Part I—Toxicogenomics. *Environmental Law Reporter* 33:10071–93.

Marchant, G.E. 2003b. Genomics and toxic substances: Part II—Toxicogenetics. *Environmental Law Reporter* 33:10641–67.

National Research Council. 1994. *Science and judgment in risk assessment.* Washington, DC: National Academies Press.

Rothstein, M.A. 1996. Preventing the discovery of plaintiff genetic profiles by defendants seeking to limit damages in personal injury litigation. *Indiana Law Journal* 71:877–910.

U.S. Environmental Protection Agency. 2002. Interim Policy on Genomics. Available at http://epa.gov/osp/spc/genomics.pdf.

PART I

ENVIRONMENTAL POLICY PERSPECTIVES

CHAPTER 1

Toxicogenomics and Environmental Regulation

GARY E. MARCHANT

Toxicogenomics seeks to better understand toxic substances and their effects on living systems, with the ultimate objective of improving human health and environmental protection. This objective will in large part be accomplished through environmental regulation, and thus environmental regulation is an important context for the application of toxicogenomics. This chapter explores potential applications of toxicogenomic data in environmental regulation. For the purpose of this analysis, the primary focus will be on gene expression data, but many of the issues could also apply to other types of toxicogenomic data, such as proteomics and metabonomics. Toxicogenomic data have the potential to make environmental regulation more effective, efficient, and fair, but at the same time present many new evidentiary, policy, and ethical challenges.

Regulatory Applications of Toxicogenomics
Enhancing Regulatory Risk Assessment

Major uncertainties and data gaps limit the utility and credibility of risk assessment for informing regulatory decisions (Latin, 1988; Hornstein, 1992). These uncertainties include extrapolating results from animals to humans and from high-dose to more typical low-dose human exposures, understanding the mechanism of action of a toxicant and its implications for risk assessment, determining the shape of the dose-response curve, and estimating the exposure levels for actual human populations (National Research Council, 1983). Gene expression data have the potential to help address many of these unknowns.

Toxicogenomic data can improve risk assessment in several ways. First, gene expression data, by providing a characteristic "fingerprint" of different toxicological mechanisms, can be used to characterize the mechanism or mode of action of a toxicant (Aardema and MacGregor, 2002). Regulatory agencies such as the U.S. Environmental Protection Agency (EPA) have recently focused on mode of action as a key factor in risk assessment, because this information is critical for addressing the issues raised above and for deciding whether an agent is likely to exhibit a threshold below which there is no significant toxicity (Gallagher et al., 2006). As noted in EPA's 2002 Interim Policy on Genomics, toxicogenomics will "likely provide a better understanding of the mechanism or mode of action of a stressor and thus assist in predictive toxicology, in the screening of stressors, and in the design of monitoring activities and exposure studies" (U.S. Environmental Protection Agency, 2002, p. 3).

Second, gene expression data will be useful in extrapolating results obtained in animal and epidemiology studies that typically involve higher dose levels than those more relevant for the general human population. Until now, low-dose effects have generally been refractory to empirical analysis, and risk assessors have had to rely on models to extrapolate results from high to low dose levels. A finding that gene expression changes characteristic of the carcinogenic response of a particular agent at high doses are also observed in low-dose groups, even though those low-dose animals may not develop tumors, may indicate that low-dose exposures present a carcinogenic risk in large populations. Alternatively, the absence of any characteristic gene expression response in low-dose animals may suggest that the carcinogenic response occurs only at high doses (Farr and Dunn, 1999).

Third, gene expression patterns may help to assess the relevance of animal studies for humans (Aardema and MacGregor, 2002). Most toxicology data comes from animal studies, which are often but not always relevant to humans. By providing a quick and inexpensive test of whether a chemical is causing a similar response in rodents and humans, gene expression assays can help prevent false positives for chemicals that cause toxicity in rodents but not humans and false negatives for chemicals that cause toxicity in humans but not rodents.

Fourth, gene expression data may also be beneficial for exposure assessment. Many types of environmental exposures lack adequate exposure data, which severely limits the ability to accurately determine the relationship between dose and response that underlies risk-assessment estimates. By characterizing gene expression patterns in exposed persons, microarrays have the potential to provide more precise quantitative estimates of exposure to specific toxic substances in contemporaneous and prospective human studies (Nuwaysir et al., 1999).

Fifth, gene expression profiling may be particularly useful for evaluating the toxicity of chemical mixtures, which is difficult to do with traditional chemical-by-chemical toxicological methods. DNA microarrays permit the simultaneous monitoring of all gene expression changes within a cell in a single experiment, thus they are "particularly suitable to evaluate any kind of combinational effect resulting from combined exposure to toxicants" (Feron and Groten, 2002, p. 834).

These potential applications of gene expression data may help reduce many of the most important uncertainties in risk assessment, although by no means eliminating such uncertainties altogether. The effect may be to give risk regulation greater credibility and certainty, which will allow environmental regulation to more directly target the most serious risks to human health and the environment.

High-Throughput Toxicity Screening of Chemicals

The majority of chemicals in commercial use in the United States have not been comprehensively tested for human toxicity and carcinogenicity potential (Environmental Defense Fund, 1997). EPA and the chemical industry have begun to address this data gap for chemical risk assessment with the high-production volume (HPV) chemical testing initiative. However, given that there are now some 80,000 chemicals in commerce, it is not feasible to conduct full toxicological testing for all or even most of these chemicals using existing methods (Olden, 2004). As the then–director of the National Institute of Environmental Health Sciences testified to Congress in 2002, many commercial products require additional testing, but "we can never satisfy this testing requirement using traditional technologies" (Olden, 2002, p. 6).

Gene expression assays have the potential to provide a rapid, inexpensive, and high-throughput screening of chemicals for a wide range of genotoxic and nongenotoxic responses (Aardema and McGregor, 2002; Freeman, 2004; Gallagher et al., 2006). Microarrays can be used to interrogate the gene expression of cells either in tissue culture or in living laboratory animals that have been treated with putative toxic agents. The resulting gene expression profiles can be used to classify those chemicals in specific toxicological categories to characterize likely risks (Hamadeh et al., 2002; Yang et al., 2006). In addition to their relatively low cost and rapid results, microarrays offer possible advantages as a screening assay. Microarrays can monitor changes in the expression of all genes within a cell, potentially permitting simultaneous evaluation of all toxicological endpoints in a single assay, something that is not possible with traditional toxicological technologies. In addition, microarrays allow a more sensitive assay of potential toxicity, because they test for the initial molecular events in a toxic response. This is more sensitive than other assay methods that tend to monitor clinical effects that do not occur until much later in the disease process.

Initially, gene expression assays will need to be conducted in association with traditional toxicity testing until a sufficiently robust and validated data set has been accumulated to reliably correlate specific gene expression profiles with particular toxicological mechanisms and endpoints (Henry et al., 2002). Used in conjunction with traditional toxicology tests, gene expression data have the potential to improve the sensitivity and interpretability of the standard tests (Nuwaysir et al., 1999). After an adequate relational database has been established, gene expression assays might replace some or all of the current toxicological screening and testing assays or at least select the specific assays indicated by the observed gene expression pattern.

One possible initial regulatory application of this gene expression technology—which would help build the necessary database to validate gene expression data—would be to require companies submitting premanufacturing notices for new chemical substances under section 5 of the Toxic Substances Control Act (TSCA) to include the results of a gene expression assay in their submission (Marchant, 2003). Currently, companies are not required to generate any new data to support premanufacturing notices; they are only required to submit relevant data already in their possession. Requiring a manufacturer of a new substance to conduct and submit a gene expression assay would not be unduly burdensome and would begin to build an experiential database of chemical-specific gene expression data that would then be available to EPA. Such a database would be most useful if the submitted data were roughly consistent and comparable, so some form of standardization of microarray platforms and methods would be desirable.

Screening of chemicals using DNA microarrays has a number of other potential regulatory applications. For example, those chemicals to be included on the Toxic Release Inventory list of reportable substances might be based at least in part on the results of DNA microarray analyses. Similarly, wastes considered hazardous based on the characteristic of toxicity could be identified by a quick and inexpensive microarray assay that evaluates whether the waste induces a gene expression profile that is characteristic of a known toxicity mechanism. Under the Food Quality Protection Act, EPA must combine all pesticides that share the same mechanism of toxicity in a single cumulative risk assessment. Toxicogenomic data may indicate which pesticides should be grouped together for such assessments.

Gene expression data may also aid in prioritizing contaminated sites. Indeed, in the foreseeable future EPA could consider adding gene expression assays to its hazard ranking scheme for establishing the National Priorities List under Superfund. Gene expression data may also be useful in assessing risks and selecting appropriate cleanup options at individual waste sites. Many abandoned waste disposal sites contain large quantities of soils and sediments with moderate or low levels of contamination that present uncertain risks but very large cleanup costs. Microarray evaluations of changes in expression of stress response genes in model systems exposed to samples from the contaminated soils or sediments could be used for ranking and prioritizing cleanup sites (Frederickson et al., 2001).

Finally, in addition to these potential regulatory screening applications of microarrays, industry will be able to use the technology to screen potential future products for toxicity. Pharmaceutical companies are already using toxicogenomic technologies to screen candidate substances based on their toxic potential (Freeman, 2004). Companies producing new chemicals and products with the potential for environmental release or human exposure could similarly use toxicogenomics to identify potential hazards early in the development cycle before any harm is done (Pennie et al., 2001).

Calculation of Reference Dose

EPA traditionally uses Reference Doses (RfDs) or Reference Concentrations (RfCs) as regulatory targets for noncarcinogenic chemicals. An RfD or RfC is defined as the level of human exposure that "is likely to be without an appreciable risk of deleterious effects during a lifetime" (U.S. Environmental Protection Agency, 2005). RfDs and RfCs are calculated by applying a series of uncertainty factors to the "no observed adverse effect level," or in the absence of such a level, the "lowest observed adverse effect level." In other words, regulatory levels are based on the concentration at which a pollutant creates an "adverse" health effect. A key issue in the implementation of toxicogenomics will be determining whether a gene expression change that occurs at levels below more traditional toxicity endpoints is to be considered an adverse effect.

In some cases, gene expression changes may represent simply an adaptive response of the cell or organism to a chemical exposure that is reversible and is not indicative of a true toxicological response (Dybing et al., 2002). In other cases, gene expression changes may be a valid and early biomarker of toxicity. Distinguishing between these two possibilities will often be difficult and controversial, with no bright line available to demarcate adverse and adaptive responses. The situation is further complicated by the likelihood that the same exposure may produce different responses in different people due to factors that affect susceptibility, such as genetics, health, weight, other toxic exposures, age, gender, or nutritional status (Dybing et al., 2002). The determination of whether a particular gene expression change is adverse will likely require expert judgment on a case-by-case basis (Lewis et al., 2002).

If EPA does determine that a change in gene expression is an "adverse effect" in a particular case, the next question is whether EPA should adjust the uncertainty factors it typically uses to calculate the RfC or RfD based on this new, lower level adverse effect (Marchant, 2003). EPA traditionally has not taken into consideration the severity of an adverse effect when calculating an RfD or an RfC, although the agency has occasionally reduced the overall uncertainty factor in a given instance for adverse effects of low severity (Alexeeff et al., 2002). It could be argued that the validation of gene expression changes as an adverse effect should not change estimates of a chemical's toxic potential but rather just provide a more sensitive and early marker of the toxicity that was already detected by subsequent changes. Under this view, EPA should compensate for the more sensitive test by reducing the otherwise applicable uncertainty factors to compensate for the low severity of the critical adverse effect. Conversely, it could be argued that a gene expression change that is "adverse" demonstrates that the chemical adversely affects the body at a concentration lower than previously appreciated, and thus the RfD or RfC and regulations based on those values should be tightened accordingly (Gallagher et al., 2006).

Real-Time Surveillance

In many cases, environmental risks are not discovered until long after the damage is done and exposed individuals have become sick or have died. Microarray assays may provide an early warning of potentially dangerous exposures before adverse health effects occur by providing "a rapid means of assessing the bioavailability and potential toxicity of complex mixtures of chemicals released into the air and into groundwater" (Bartosiewicz, Penn, and Buckpitt, 2001). Early detection of potentially hazardous exposures would facilitate more timely and effective interventions to monitor and treat affected persons as well as to minimize further exposures. This type of surveillance program using microarray assays could be applied to individuals living near a polluting facility or hazardous waste site, workers employed in a hazardous workplace, consumers exposed to a potentially hazardous product, or citizens who may have been exposed to toxics released by an industrial accident (Marchant, 2003; Travis, Bishop, and Clarke, 2003).

Microarray technology may also be used to monitor pollutant effects on nonhuman organisms, such as aquatic species (Travis et al., 2003). For example, one study demonstrated that an estrogenic compound produced a characteristic pattern of changes in the expression of estrogen-responsive genes in sheepshead minnows, allowing the species to be used as a sentinel for the presence of endocrine-disruptive chemicals in coastal habitats (P. Larkin et al., 2002). Another study showed that characteristic changes in gene expression in tadpoles can be detected from laboratory exposure to the herbicide acetochlor before the development of overt morphological changes brought about by the endocrine disruption effect of the herbicide (Crump et al., 2002).

Gene expression assays have several advantages over traditional toxicological endpoints for real-time surveillance of potentially at-risk populations (Gallagher et al., 2006). Microarrays have the potential to provide immediate, on-site estimates of both exposure and risk. In particular, it may be possible, using high-throughput gene expression screening, to quantify the potential exposures of a large number of people in a quick and minimally intrusive manner. Another important advantage of microarrays for real-time surveillance is that microarrays provide a more sensitive and earlier indication of a potential risk than do traditional methods. Of course, one of the inevitable consequences of using a more sensitive assay is that the results will require careful interpretation and judgment by both regulators and companies to avoid false alarms while recognizing truly significant early toxicological responses.

The potential for real-time surveillance provided by microarrays may trigger questions about some existing regulatory requirements for product safety surveillance by manufacturers. For example, section 8(e) of the TSCA requires the manufacturer of a substance or mixture to report to EPA information received that "reasonably supports the conclusion that such substance or mixture presents a substantial risk of injury to human health or the environment." Similarly, section 6(a)(2) of the Federal Insecticide, Fungicide and Rodenticide Act (FIFRA) requires pesticide registrants to report "factual information regarding unreasonable adverse effects" associated with their products. It is unclear whether a gene expression change, standing alone, could ever trigger a duty to report the findings under TSCA or FIFRA (Marchant, 2003). EPA has indicated that such reporting may not be required until the gene expression change has been clearly tied to a traditional toxicological endpoint. However, the agency has not yet provided industry with a definitive and clear statement on its policy with respect to such reporting requirements.

Setting Environmental Standards

Several environmental statutes require risk-based standards that protect the public health against adverse effects. For example, section 109 of the Clean Air Act requires EPA to establish national ambient air quality standards that protect the public health with an adequate margin of safety, which has been defined by legislative history, agency action, and judicial decisions to mean protection against adverse effects resulting from exposure to air pollutants (U.S. Congress, 1970). Regulatory and judicial precedent holds that an adverse effect under the Clean Air Act need not involve clinical symptoms. When EPA first promulgated its ambient air quality standard for lead in 1978, the D.C. Circuit Court of Appeals upheld the agency's finding the subclinical elevation of erythrocytein protoporphyrin levels in the blood qualified as an adverse effect, holding that EPA need not show that an effect caused by exposure to an air pollutant was "clearly harmful" to health (*Lead Industries Association v. EPA,* 1980). Instead, it was sufficient, according to the court, that the chemical changes relied on by EPA indicated that "lead has begun to affect one of the basic biological functions of the body" (*Lead Industries Association v. EPA,* p. 1139).

The precedent established in the *Lead Industries* case suggests that an effect need not be clinically detectable or clearly harmful to be considered adverse, and that an effect can be adverse if it occurs solely at the molecular level. It therefore appears that at least some gene expression changes may be considered adverse. It remains to be seen, however, how this new category of data will affect regulatory standard-setting given that the existing criteria and precedents for such standards were established in the pregenomic era.

Toxicogenomics: Caveats and Limitations

Gene expression profiling using DNA microarrays and other toxicogenomic methods has much potential and many applications for environmental risk assessment and regulation. Some of these applications will be available in the very near future, and in some cases are available now, at least in "proof of concept" form, while other applications are farther into the future. Nevertheless, many obstacles and uncertainties remain to be addressed before toxicogenomic data can be given widespread practical and legal effect in the regulatory world. Foremost among these challenges is the need for the toxicological significance of gene expression changes to be validated (Corvi et al., 2006), which is not an easy undertaking given the rapid pace at which microarray technology is still evolving. As one commentator has noted: "New chips can be developed faster than chips can be validated. Validation is a significant underpinning of the quality of toxicology data today. If microarray technology moves faster than the validation technology, how will we use these data for the development of new products and the development of data to assess safety and efficacy?" (Schwetz, 2001, p. 6). Validation will involve evaluating the robustness and reproducibility of toxicogenomic assays between or across different laboratories, species, individuals, tissues, development stages, exposure levels, and exposure durations, all of which could potentially affect gene expression patterns (Fielden and Zacharewski, 2001; King and Sinha, 2001).

Microarray analyses need not only distinguish "real" changes in gene expression from background fluctuations but also need to discriminate reversible and adaptive gene expression changes from true toxic responses (Marchant, 2003; Freeman, 2004). One important factor to be considered is the extent to which gene expression changes have been correlated or "anchored" with traditional observed effects of toxicity (Henry et al., 2001; Waters and Fostel, 2004).

There will ultimately be a need to standardize DNA microarrays and other toxicogenomic platforms (Gallagher et al., 2006), although premature standardization may carry its own risks by freezing a rapidly developing technology before it matures. Many different microarray platforms, methodologies, and content have been developed and used by commercial companies and individual laboratories, making interlaboratory comparison and reconciliation of results difficult. For example, different microarray platforms have been shown to produce inconsistent results, although recent attempts to harmonize approaches have shown significant improvement in obtaining consistent results between laboratories and platforms (Bammler et al., 2005; Irizarry et al., 2005; J.E. Larkin et al., 2005).

Another limitation in the development of toxicogenomics is industry concerns about potential premature regulatory use of the resulting data and also the potential for retrospective liability (Freeman, 2004). Companies may fear generating toxicogenomic data if EPA, state agencies, environmental organizations, and the media will construe any change in gene expression as evidence of toxicity. Moreover, companies may have legitimate fears that any toxicogenomic data they generate today of unknown or uncertain toxicological significance could be used against them in future litigation, when hindsight might suggest that the data were an early warning of a problem. These concerns are likely to significantly diminish the incentives of companies to generate and make public toxicogenomic data.

EPA's (2002) Interim Policy on Genomics provides some reassurance to companies by stating that the agency will not rely on genomic data alone to make regulatory decisions at this time. EPA might be able to provide more guidance to regulated parties, without unduly tying its hands with rigid regulatory requirements, by producing more detailed "points to consider" or "best practices" guidelines that provide specific guidance on how microarray data should be developed and used for regulatory purposes (Henry et al., 2002). An alternative approach for the time being might be for EPA to expressly provide a "safe harbor" for toxicogenomic data, in which the agency encourages the development and submission of such data but commits not to take enforcement action for the failure to submit gene expression data or otherwise use the data for enforcement purposes until the methodology has been adequately validated (Rajeski, 2002).

Conclusion

Toxicogenomics offers a tool of unprecedented power to look within the black box of the cell and directly observe the earliest stages of the toxicological response with information that is both highly specific and sensitive. While the potential applications and benefits of toxicogenomics for environmental regulation are enormous, the use of this technology in such contexts is not without limitations and without the need for caution. In particular, toxicogenomics has the potential to produce too much information—in that it has the potential to identify too many chemicals and products that are interacting with biological systems and too many people who are experiencing gene expression changes as a result of exposures to environmental agents—to permit practical decisions and priority-setting based on gene expression changes alone. Careful judgment and rigorous validation will be needed to discriminate those gene expression changes that warrant public health concern from those with no public health significance that merely reflect innocuous adaptive responses and normal fluctuations within dynamic cells.

ACKNOWLEDGMENTS

Preparation of this chapter was supported by Grant number 1 R01 ES12577-01 from the National Institute of Environmental Health Sciences (NIEHS) and the National Human Genome Research Institute (NHGRI) of the National Institutes of Health (NIH). The contents of this chapter are the responsibility of the author and do not necessarily represent the official views of NIEHS or NIH.

REFERENCES

Aardema, M.J., and J.T. MacGregor. 2002. Toxicology and genetic toxicology in the new era of "toxicogenomics": Impact of "-omics" technologies. *Mutation Research* 499:13–25.

Alexeeff, G.V., R. Broadwin, J. Liaw, and S.V. Dawson. 2002. Characterization of the LOAEL-to-NOAEL uncertainty factor for mild adverse effects from acute inhalation exposures. *Regulatory Toxicology and Pharmacology* 36:96–105.

Bammler, T., R.P. Beyer, S. Bhattacharya, et al. 2005. Standardizing global gene expression analysis between laboratories and across platforms. *Nature Methods* 2:351–56.

Bartosiewicz, M., S. Penn, and A. Buckpitt. 2001. Applications of gene arrays in environmental toxicology: Fingerprints of gene regulation associated with calcium chloride, benzo(a)pyrene, and trichloroethylene. *Environmental Health Perspectives* 109:71–74.

Corvi, R., H.J. Ahr, S. Albertini, et al. 2006. Validation of toxicogenomics-based test systems: ECVAM-ICCVAM/NICEATM considerations for regulatory use. *Environmental Health Perspectives* 114:420–29.

Crump, D., K. Werry, N. Veldhoen, G. Van Aggelen, and C.C. Helbing. 2002. Exposure to the herbicide acetochlor alters thyroid hormone-dependent gene expression and metamorphosis in Xenopus laevis. *Environmental Health Perspectives* 110:1199–1205.

Dybing, E., J. Doe, J. Groten, et al. 2002. Hazard characterisation of chemicals in food and diet: dose response, mechanisms and extrapolation issues. *Food and Chemical Toxicology* 40:237–82.

Environmental Defense Fund. 1997. "Toxic ignorance." At www. environmentaldefense.org/documents/243_toxicignorance.pdf.

Farr, S., and R.T. Dunn. 1999. Gene expression applied to toxicology. *Toxicological Science* 50:1–9.

Feron, V.J., and J.P. Groten. 2002. Toxicological evaluation of chemical mixtures. *Food and Chemical Toxicology* 40:825–39.

Fielden, M.R., and T.R. Zacharewski. 2001. Challenges and limitations of gene expression profiling in mechanistic and predictive toxicology. *Toxicological Science* 60:6–10.

Fredrickson, H.L., E.J. Perkins, T.S. Bridges, et al. 2001. Toward environmental toxicogenomics: Development of a flow-through, high-density DNA hybridization array and its application to ecotoxicity assessment. *Science of the Total Environment* 274:137–49.

Freeman, K. 2004. Toxicogenomics data: The road to acceptance. *Environmental Health Perspectives* 112:A678–85.

Gallagher, K., W.H. Benson, M. Brody, et al. 2006. Genomics: Applications, challenges, and opportunities for the U.S. Environmental Protection Agency. *Human and Ecological Risk Assessment* 12:572–90.

Hamadeh, H.K., P.R. Bushel, S. Jayadev, et al. 2002. Gene expression analysis reveals chemical-specific profiles. *Toxicological Science* 67:219–31.

Henry, C.J., R. Phillips, F. Carpanini, et al. 2002. Use of genomics in toxicology and epidemiology: Findings and recommendations of a workshop. *Environmental Health Perspectives* 110:1047–50.

Hornstein, D.T. 1992. Reclaiming environmental law: A normative critique of comparative risk analysis. *Columbia Law Review* 92:562–633.

Irizarry, R.A., D. Warren, F. Spencer, et al. 2005. Multiple-laboratory comparison of microarray platforms. *Nature Methods* 2:345–50.

King, H.C., and A.A. Sinha. 2001. Gene expression profile analysis by DNA microarrays; promise and pitfalls. *Journal of the American Medical Association* 286:2280–88.

Larkin, J.E., B.C. Frank, H. Gavras, R. Sultana, and John Quakenbush. 2005. Independence and reproducibility across microarray platforms. *Nature Methods* 2:337–44.

Larkin, P., L.C. Folmar, M.J. Hemmer, A.J. Poston, H.S. Lee, and N.D. Denslow. 2002. Array technology as a tool to monitor exposure of fish to xenoestrogens. *Marine Environmental Research* 54:395–99.

Latin, H. 1988. Good science, bad regulation, and toxic risk assessment. *Yale Journal of Regulation* 5:89–148.

Lead Industries Association v. EPA. 1980. 647 F.2d 1130 (D.C. Cir.), *cert. denied,* 449 U.S. 1042.

Lewis, R.W., R. Billington, E. Debryune, A. Gamer, B. Lang, and F. Carpanani. 2002. Recognition of adverse and nonadverse effects in toxicity studies. *Toxicologic Pathology* 30:66–74.

Marchant, G.E. 2003. Genomics and toxic substances: Part I—Toxicogenomics, *Environmental Law Reporter* 33:10071–93.

National Research Council. 1983. *Risk Assessment in the Federal Government: Managing the Process.* Washington, DC: National Academies Press.

Nuwaysir, E.F., M. Bittner, J. Trent, J.C. Barrett, and C.A. Afshari. 1999. Microarrays and toxicology: The advent of toxicogenetics. *Molecular Carcinogenesis* 24:153–59.

Olden, K. 2002. *NIH Environmental Health Prevention Research,* Prepared Testimony before the Subcommittee on Public Health, U.S. Senate Committee on Health, Education, Labor, and Pensions, March 6, 2002.

Olden, K. 2004. Genomics in environmental health research: opportunities and challenges. *Toxicology* 198:19–24.

Pennie, W.D., N.J. Woodyatt, T.C. Aldridge, and G. Orphanides. 2001. Application of genomics to the definition of the molecular basis for toxicity. *Toxicology Letters* 120:353–58.

Rejeski, D. 2002. Exploring the genomics frontier. *Risk Policy Report* (Aug. 20): 24–26.

Schwetz, B. 2001. Toxicology at the Food and Drug Administration: New century, new challenges. *International Journal of Toxicology* 20:3–8.

Travis, C.C., W.E. Bishop, and D.P. Clarke. 2003. The genomic revolution: What does it mean for human and ecological risk assessment? *Ecotoxicology* 12:489–95.

U.S. Congress. 1970. S. Rep. 1196 1970. 91st Cong., 2d Sess.

U.S. Environmental Protection Agency. 2002. Interim Policy on Genomics. At http://epa.gov/osa/spc/pdfs.genomics.pdf.

U.S. Environmental Protection Agency. 2005. Integrated Risk Information System, Glossary of IRIS Terms. At www.epa.gov/iris/gloss8.htm.

Waters, M.D., and J.M. Fostel. 2004. Toxicogenomics and systems toxicology: Aims and prospects. *Nature Reviews Genetics* 5:936–48.

Yang, Y., S.J. Abel, R. Ciurlionis, and J.F. Waring. 2006. Development of a toxicogenomics *in vitro* assay for the efficient characterization of compounds. *Pharmacogenomics* 7:177–86.

CHAPTER 2

Addressing Genomic Needs at the U.S. Environmental Protection Agency

KERRY L. DEARFIELD, WILLIAM H. BENSON,
KATHRYN GALLAGHER, AND JEREMY D. JOHNSON

The data and information emanating from the various genomic technologies (speaking generally here as encompassing all aspects of genomics, proteomics, metabolomics, and systems biology) present many exciting opportunities as well as challenges for the U.S. Environmental Protection Agency (EPA). To deal efficiently and fairly with the information generated by genomic technologies, EPA has initiated many activities. The agency has taken measures to address policy positions; to identify effects on regulatory, research, and risk-assessment activities; and to create working groups to explore many of the needs for EPA to address this information.

EPA Interim Policy on Genomics

A major consideration EPA had to address was what to do with information being generated by genomic technologies. A large amount of this information is already available, with an increasing amount on the horizon. However, it is not readily usable for EPA purposes, including use in regulations that require the identification of adverse human health or ecological risks. As it stands, much of the genomic information is not correlated with effects the regulatory community historically considers "adverse" (e.g., for human health: cancer, reproductive effects; for ecological health: growth, reproductive effects). This challenge to correlate responses seen in genomic data with adverse effects recognized by the agency must be met for EPA to base regulatory decisions on genomic information alone.

Therefore, in June 2002 EPA issued a policy position, called the *Interim Policy on Genomics,* to help address what to do with available genomic-related information (U.S. Environmental Protection Agency, 2002). This interim policy states that EPA encourages and supports continued genomic research as a powerful tool for understanding the molecular basis of toxicity and for developing biomarkers of exposure, effects, and susceptibility. However (and this is the major statement of the interim policy), genomic data alone are currently insufficient as a basis for risk-assessment and management decisions. The document further states that genomic data may be useful in a weight-of-evidence approach for human health and ecological health risk assessments. Consequently, genomic information will be used in concert with all of the other information EPA considers for a particular assessment or decision. The interim policy will be revisited when EPA can evaluate what genomic data mean relative to adverse effects of concern to EPA. It should be kept in mind, though, that there may be other areas, particularly environmental monitoring, where genomic data can be useful.

EPA Actions Associated with the Interim Policy

EPA initiated several actions immediately after it issued the interim policy. For example, EPA began to address the ethical aspects, such as privacy and fairness concerns, that are associated with emerging genomic data (Marchant, 2003a, 2003b; Orphanides and Kimber, 2003; Robert and Smith, 2004).

One such action was to reorganize agency programs that dealt with genomic issues. EPA has many research activities associated with genomic technologies, in both the human health and ecological arenas. It was clear that these research activities could be better coordinated across the agency and aligned with EPA regulatory responsibilities. EPA analyzed this situation and through a major reorganization initiative created the Computational Toxicology Program (U.S. Environmental Protection Agency, 2003). This program serves to facilitate the introduction of genomics and computational tools into the practical issues facing the agency and to provide leadership in the application of these tools to regulatory decisions at the agency.

In response to a charge by EPA senior managers, a Genomics Task Force was formed within the agency to develop a white paper (U.S. Environmental Protection Agency, 2004) on regulatory implications and to highlight additional actions needed. The rest of this chapter will highlight findings from the white paper and subsequent activities.

The Genomics Task Force and the White Paper

Anticipated regulatory and risk-assessment applications and the implications of genomics for EPA are identified in the white paper. It also includes an overview of current agency science activities that may support these applications (which are not discussed here). The white paper then identifies the science and research needed to advance genomics to support agency activities.

Identified Regulatory Applications

Three major general regulatory applications identified in the EPA white paper will likely benefit from genomic information. The first relates to prioritization applications used by many agency programs. These applications are important to EPA, helping to focus agency efforts on the greater risks of concern and to properly allocate resources to address those greater risks. Genomic data can be used as part of the body of information considered in EPA prioritization efforts, including screening for potential risks, testing to more fully investigate a risk, and making one particular decision versus another. For example, one prioritization effort that could make use of genomic data is EPA's voluntary high-production volume program, in which chemicals manufactured in large amounts are identified and are candidates for examination of risk. Here, genomics (primarily microarray technologies) may be part of a suite of tools to help validate category groupings of HPV chemicals and to identify which chemicals (or groups of chemicals) may present greater risks within future high-volume screening processes. As another example, genomic data may play a role in prioritizing pathogens for EPA's Contaminant Candidate List, based on the presence of virulent genes and their corresponding gene products.

A second identified regulatory application relates to EPA's monitoring activities. EPA obtains, requests, and receives many types of environmental data for both assessment and compliance purposes. Monitoring activities may be among the nearer-term applications that use genomic data. Many types of environmental monitoring data could be generated using genomics-based techniques, and some applications are already being tested. For example, microarrays could be used to screen for host-specific markers that can be used in microbial source tracking (MST). Recently, a research consortium including state of California regulatory agencies, public utilities, and EPA participated in a study comparing the performance of various genomics-based methods designed to identify the source of fecal material in ambient waters using an MST approach (Griffith et al., 2003). MST work will help address the issue of beach closures; current microbial methods require several days to complete and do not distinguish between bacteria from humans and those from other sources, such as seagulls or seals. Another example of a monitoring application of genomics is in the area of development of multigene arrays of model animals. Future toxicity testing for compliance with discharge requirements could involve using gene chips for species such as fathead minnow to determine whether a water sample resulted in a toxic pattern of response in exposed fish.

A third regulatory application is concerned with reporting provisions under EPA statutes (e.g., Toxic Substances Control Act section 8(e) and Federal Insecticide, Fungicide, and Rodenticide Act section 6(a)(2)). Before the interim policy was released, it was unclear whether data generated from genomic technologies would trigger EPA provisions that require reporting any data to EPA indicating that a substance may present an unreasonable risk to human health or the environment. Consistent with the interim policy, because genomic data are not currently well correlated with adverse effects, these data alone do not trigger these reporting provisions at this time. However, as the predictability and validity of genomic methods increase, EPA will reevaluate this stance on reporting provisions.

Identified Risk-Assessment Applications

Genomic data may be able to aid several risk-assessment activities of interest to EPA, such as helping identify modes of action (MOA) of chemicals and stressors, identifying and helping assess effects on susceptible populations and life stages, and improving mixtures assessments. Gene, protein, or metabolite profiles may be developed that can advance the screening of individual chemicals and allow faster, more accurate categorization into defined classes according to their MOA. For example, genomic data may help elucidate the many possible modes of carcinogenic action, such as mutagenicity, mitogenesis, inhibition of cell death, cytotoxicity with regenerative cell proliferation, and immune suppression. Genomic data may also be useful in improving extrapolations between high- and low-dose exposures by helping to refine pharmacokinetic or pharmacodynamic models and in enhancing interspecies comparisons that characterize the relevance of animal data to humans and the relevance of data on one wildlife species compared with another. For these reasons, genomic data are very attractive for use in MOA-derived analyses.

Genomic information presents a tremendous opportunity to identify individuals who may have increased susceptibility to any number of environmental stressors. Among individuals, there are likely to be small differences in gene sequence in the same gene, variations known as single nucleotide polymorphisms (SNPs). These differences can have a range of effects, from inconsequential to dramatic, on whether one person or organism may be more vulnerable to an adverse effect than another person or organism. Susceptibility may or may not be defined based upon the presence of a single SNP in a single gene. Many multifactorial conditions involve multiple SNPs. Nonetheless, genomic technologies have the potential to yield information about the distribution of SNPs within the human population and how they affect responses of genes to various environmental contaminants. The interaction of genetic variants with environmental conditions can affect an individual's susceptibility to a variety of diseases such as cancer, diabetes, and heart disease and can promote sensitivity to disease from exposure (Bishop et al., 2001). Further, exposure during an individual's susceptible life stage (e.g., early development) could result in higher risk during that portion of the individual's life or could influence an outcome at a later life stage. For wildlife species, genomic technologies may allow the examination of toxicological responses across species for prediction of susceptibilities in untested organisms.

It is recognized that, with humans and wildlife, exposures are usually cumulative involving many stressors, particularly mixtures of stressors, rather than exposure to single chemicals. Genomic technologies hold the promise of improving risk assessment of mixtures. For example, the toxicity of a test mixture could be evaluated through genomic biomarkers that have been linked to known adverse effects from individual chemicals. Constructed test mixtures can also be examined with genomic technologies to assay how chemicals in the mixture may interact in terms of their additivity, synergism, or antagonism. Further, genomic indicators may be useful for identifying unidentified components of chemical mixtures through the use of a genomic fingerprint database. Differences in gene expression elicited between a mixture of known chemicals and a test mixture containing unknown chemicals could point to specific known chemicals with known adverse effects or to unknowns that may need further examination.

EPA Technical Framework Workgroups

The white paper not only identifies regulatory and risk assessment applications of genomic data but also highlights some of the challenges and needs EPA should address. Research needs include linkage of genomic responses to adverse effects, proper interpretation of genomic data, examination of acceptance criteria for genomic data submissions to EPA, management and storage of the huge amount of genomic information EPA is projected to handle, and training of EPA risk assessors and managers in how to interpret and understand genomic data. Technical framework workgroups are now established at EPA under the auspices of the Genomics Task Force to address these challenges and needs. An overarching Coordinating Committee for the Task Force coordinates and provides oversight to these technical workgroups. Also, all of these workgroup efforts coordinate with the Computational Toxicology Program, as well as with efforts on these issues in other federal agencies and elsewhere.

Performance-Based Quality Assurance Workgroup

The Performance-Based Quality Assurance Workgroup is charged with developing a universal set or sets of data quality and performance-based considerations for genomics-based technologies. Genomic data will be generated by multiple laboratories and procedures, and the agency realizes there is a need for these data to be reviewed consistently and without bias. Therefore, performance and data quality considerations are critical in ensuring the generation of high quality data and consistent evaluation of the data. This workgroup is scanning and reviewing existing technologies and procedures to glean common quality assurance and performance considerations, so that generation of genomic data is not unnecessarily tied to a specific technique or platform. Because genomic technologies are rapidly progressing, it is realized that this will be a continual effort over the coming few years and that a set of performance standards will not be immediately forthcoming. However, in the near term, general data quality and performance objectives will be considered. For example, draft interim guidance for microarray-based assays relating to data submission, quality, analysis, management, and training considerations is being assembled.

Data Submission Workgroup

The Data Submission Workgroup has been tasked with defining the format for data submission to EPA for its consideration in risk-assessment activities. The goal is to develop a consistent format for data submission, so that risk assessors in EPA can concentrate on the content of the submission, without needing to wonder where the salient points in a submission are located or whether sufficient information has been submitted to permit a complete evaluation. This will also make it easier for submitters to organize their data for submission to EPA. The details necessary for a complete data submission are being defined. Elements of a complete data submission may include experimental and array design, treatment and manipulation of biological materials, quality assurance and quality control measures, and data measurement and analysis. The U.S. Food and Drug Administration (FDA) issued a guidance for industry pharmacogenomic data submissions (U.S. Food and Drug Adminstration, 2005). The EPA workgroup has been working with FDA for understanding and lessons learned in their experience with this issue.

Data Analysis Workgroup

Once data are submitted to EPA in a consistent format, the data will need to be analyzed. The Data Analysis Workgroup has been tasked with facilitating and guiding the development of the tools (e.g., guidance, computational) necessary for risk assessors and other scientists to analyze, process, and integrate the large quantity and various types of genomic information submitted to EPA. The goal is to point risk assessors toward a consistent, transparent approach to genomic data analyses. To do this, the workgroup will be striving toward developing guidance and tools from the risk assessor's point of view and will focus on methods that will be used to analyze and interpret the data to be used in risk assessments.

Data Management Workgroup

EPA expects a great volume of genomics-related data will be submitted. The Data Management Workgroup has been tasked with addressing the need to coordinate the storage of and access to submitted data, particularly the need to consider a cross-agency databank or repository for storage and retrieval of information. To address data storage and access needs, this group is developing a set of guidelines and recommendations for genomic data management. For example, EPA could maintain its own storage of data and identify its information technology needs for such storage and retrieval. Another option would be to partner with other organizations and agencies for data storage, management, and mining, such as with the Chemical Effects in Biological Systems knowledge base being developed by the National Institute of Environmental Health Sciences (Waters et al., 2003). Issues affecting confidentiality and public availability are also important considerations. Currently, this group is beginning to address the data mining aspects of bioinformatics, including examining promising bioinformatics mining utilities, such as those associated with FDA's ArrayTrack (Tong et al., 2003).

Training Workgroup

The charge to the training workgroup is straightforward: to lead the development of materials and appropriate delivery mechanisms for training agency risk assessors and managers to understand and interpret genomic data in the context of a risk assessment. The workgroup is developing a library of training materials, presentations, and modules to be used as a resource by EPA personnel. These training resources will range from the basics in molecular biology and genetics to advanced training in data analysis and more advanced genomic techniques. Given the potential impact of genomic information, training is being geared toward target audiences ranging from nonscientists and managers to research scientists and risk assessors. Additional target audiences may include state and tribal risk assessors and managers. Because a wealth of training and educational materials is already available, the workgroup will glean relevant information that will be most useful for EPA assessors and managers from the literature and outside sources. EPA is working particularly with partners in FDA to create similar, harmonized training materials and presentations.

Conclusion

The advent of the genomic revolution and the burgeoning amount of genomics-related data present opportunities and challenges to EPA regulatory and risk assessment responsibilities. Because of this, EPA initiated many activities to properly address genomic information in its everyday activities. The agency reorganized its research activities into a coordinated Computational Toxicology Program. Its Interim Policy on Genomics provided guidance on how currently available genomic information will be considered at EPA for the present time. The genomics white paper outlined potential implications of genomics for regulatory and risk-assessment applications at EPA. Finally, a technical framework has started that will develop formats, methodologies, and consistent approaches for dealing with genomic information that will be submitted to EPA.

REFERENCES

Bishop, W.E., D.P. Clarke, and C.C. Travis. 2001. The genomic revolution: What does it mean for risk assessment? *Risk Analysis* 21:985–87.
Griffith, J.F., S.B. Weisberg, and C.D. McGee. 2003. Evaluation of microbial source tracking methods using mixed fecal sources in aqueous test samples. *Journal of Water and Health* 1:141–52.
Marchant, G.E. 2003a. Genomics and toxic substances: Part I—Toxicogenomics. *Environmental Law Reporter* 33:10071–93.

Marchant, G.E. 2003b. Genomics and toxic substances: Part II—Toxicogenetics. *Environmental Law Reporter* 33:10641–67.

Orphanides, G., and I. Kimber. 2003. Toxicogenetics: Applications and opportunities. *Toxicological Sciences* 75:1–6.

Robert, J.S., and A. Smith. 2004. Toxic ethics: Environmental genomics and the health of populations. *Bioethics* 18:493–514.

Tong, W., X. Cao, S. Harris, et al. 2003. ArrayTrack: Supporting toxicogenomic research at the FDA's National Center for Toxicological Research (NCTR). *EHP Toxicogenomics* 111:1819–26.

U.S. Environmental Protection Agency. 2002. Interim Policy on Genomics. At www.epa.gov/osa/spc/htm/genomics.htm.

U.S. Environmental Protection Agency. 2003. A Framework for a Computational Toxicology Research Program in ORD. At www.epa.gov/comptox/comptox_framework.html.

U.S. Environmental Protection Agency. 2004. Potential Implications of Genomics for Regulatory and Risk Assessment Applications. At www.epa.gov/osa/genomics.htm.

U.S. Food and Drug Administration. 2005. Guidance for Industry, Pharmacogenomic Data Submissions. At www.fda.gov/cder/guidance/index.htm.

Waters, M.D., G. Boorman, P. Bushel, et al. 2003. Systems toxicology and chemical effects in biological systems knowledge base. *Environmental Health Perspectives* 111:811–24.

CHAPTER 3

Application of Genomics for Health and Environmental Safety of Chemicals

An Industry Perspective

RICHARD D. PHILLIPS

The advent of genomic technologies has facilitated major advances in our understanding of the molecular details of normal biology and holds the promise of providing new insights into molecular mechanisms of a variety of toxicities. These "-omics" technologies provide many potential benefits for assessment of chemical safety. Among the more promising areas are opportunities for more effective screening and priority setting for chemicals. In addition, it is possible to identify biomarkers of chemical exposure at the molecular level and potential interactions of chemicals and effects at low doses. Genomics will likely lead to an improved understanding of mechanisms of action, thereby reducing uncertainty and improving chemical risk assessments, and of the use and limitations of toxicological models. This will enable the application of computational toxicology models in risk assessment. Finally, it will be possible to identify and quantify susceptible populations for protection in unique instances as appropriate.

Although we anticipate the many important applications listed above, much is still to be done in developing and applying of these technologies before we realize their full benefit. As the technologies develop, we'll need to proceed with caution to avoid overinterpretation and inefficiency, which could delay progress. A rigorous and disciplined scientific approach will be needed to realize the benefits as quickly as possible.

Henry et al. (2002) reported the outcome of a multiple-stakeholder workshop that considered the issues regarding the application of genomic technologies to toxicology and epidemiology. The workshop identified challenges, opportunities, and possible areas for high value research. Among the global challenges was the enormous volume of information generated and how that information should be managed and assimilated in a productive manner. In addition, the need for standardized methods and platforms was seen as critical. Cunningham and colleagues (2003) observed that the barriers to the broad application of "-omics" include the lack of publicly available databases, the paucity of validated technologies, and the lack of comparative data on experimental platforms, experimental approaches, and study design. Other challenges include the immaturity of robust tools for data analysis and uncertainty about the direct relationship between transcripts and toxicity and about regulatory applications. Yet another major challenge that needs to be addressed is the method of analyzing complex data sets that require sophisticated bioinformatics to unravel how small changes in gene expression relate to disease development. This level of analysis then needs to be linked, both qualitatively and quantitatively, to the association between gene and protein changes following exposure to chemicals and the ultimate outcome of disease.

Other potential obstacles include the high cost of replicate measures and collection of the data as dichotomous variables (e.g., the gene expression level exceeds a predefined threshold or it does not). Also, there is the difficult task of integrating the vast amount of data into meaningful patterns overlaid on top of background fluctuations in cell cycle, diurnal cycles, developmental maturation, and aging.

Understanding complex diseases has challenges as well. Large population case control studies may well detect some individual genetic determinants associated with moderate relative risks of specific diseases. However, these genetic determinants may not act independently. Understanding the combined quantitative contributions of alleles at many specific loci to polygenic traits, and interactions among loci, will require overcoming substantial multiple comparison problems in studies in which effects at thousands of loci are investigated.

Notwithstanding these challenges, several key opportunities presented by genomic technologies were identified by Henry et al. (2002), among them, improved understanding of mechanism or mode of action of chemical interaction with biological systems. This will ultimately lead to improved risk assessments by reducing key uncertainties such as dose-response relationships leading to adverse or toxic effects, threshold responses, and the relationship of responses in surrogate species to target species. This type of information will improve our understanding of mode of action and the biologic plausibility of exposure-effect relationships.

Identification of biomarkers of chemical exposure and effects is another important need for improving risk assessment. "-Omics" tools should inform the search for useful biomarkers of effect and exposure and better characterize their relationship.

Information gleaned from "-omics" may also improve our ability to predict toxicity. There is the opportunity for development of toxicity screens, the characterization of chemical-related toxicity, the selection of candidate molecules with lower toxicity in chemical discovery or product formulation (thereby reducing cycle time), and the elucidation of mechanisms of toxicity. This information may be useful for prioritizing chemicals for further evaluation. Improvements in study design and dose-response assessments, and increased sensitivity in detecting adverse effects, are also possible.

It will also likely be possible to identify and quantify susceptible populations. This could occur by identifying metabolic differences or genetic polymorphisms between individuals within a population. Also, -omics will help to identify differences in the way individuals respond to a chemical exposure. However, knowledge of the functional impact of genetic differences on a toxicologic response will be necessary prior to using such information in the context of risk assessment.

Predictive Toxicology, Screening, Signatures

One of the most promising applications of genomic technologies is the potential to generate chemical-specific or mechanism-specific molecular signatures of toxicity. To this end, the National Center for Toxicogenomics is developing genomic technologies in collaboration with other research institutes such as the International Life Sciences Institute/Health and Environmental Sciences Institute, and through cooperative agreements with industry (Tennant, 2002). The National Center for Toxicogenomics is focusing on a proof of principle program to determine whether gene expression profiles can be used to generate chemical-specific profiles that can distinguish across and within compound classes or groups. Initially, NCT examined whether gene expression profiles could distinguish peroxisome proliferator- and barbiturate-treated animals. The peroxisome proliferators included Wyeth-14643, clofibrate, and gemfibrozil, and the barbiturates included phenobarbital and hexobarbital. The investigators' approach included multiple dose levels and time course information. Multiple bioinformatics tools were used to classify compounds using previously derived data. Samples were analyzed in a blinded fashion. Of twenty-three blinded samples, twelve were correctly classified as being similar to another compound of the same class. Ten were correctly classified as not being similar to a "toxic profile" in the database (Hamadeh et al., 2002a, 2002b). These "proof of principle" experiments suggest that it may be possible to identify the toxicological potential and mechanism of an otherwise unknown chemical based on its toxicogenomic signature.

Mechanisms and Modes of Action

In recent years, regulatory risk-assessment procedures have given increased weight to the mechanism or mode of action of a toxic substance for purposes such as hazard identification and dose-response modeling. Genetic technologies may be useful in identifying the mechanism and mode of action of a chemical. Heinloth and colleagues (2004) examined the possible use of gene expression profiling for identifying doses at which "subtoxic" changes could be detected. Such changes would typically not be detected by classical means such as abnormal clinical chemistry and histopathology. The investigators used acetaminophen as a model hepatotoxicant. Patterns of gene expression were found that indicated cellular energy loss as a consequence of acetaminophen treatment. Elements of these patterns were apparent even after treatment to "subtoxic" doses. With increasing dosage, the magnitude of changes increased, and additional components of the same biological pathway were differentially expressed.

The ideal biomarker should provide an indication of potential toxicity at times or doses preceding adverse effects such as overt tissue damage, toxicity, or disease initiation. Such changes in gene expression patterns could be predictive of toxicity if they reflect perturbations of vital cellular pathways, such as was the case in the "subtoxic" dosing of acetaminophen discussed above. With increasing severity of the insult, the degree of disturbance of these pathways would be expected to increase, ultimately resulting in overt tissue damage as detected by traditional measurements of toxicity. The threshold between subtoxic adverse effects and toxic tissue injury would be marked by additional gene expression alterations leading to events in pathways such as apoptosis, necrosis, or inflammation.

Sawada, Takami, and Asahi (2005) demonstrated important advancement in the application of toxicogenomics in two ways. First, they provided new mechanistic insight into an important phenomenon, drug-induced phospholipidosis, and second, they used the validated genomic results to develop an in vitro rapid screening system to evaluate the potential for compounds to elicit this effect. The group performed large-scale gene expression analyses in human hepatoma *Hep*G2 cells to understand more completely the pathogenesis of drug-induced phospholipidosis, a condition in which excess phospholipids accumulate in cells. The study established four important pathways that were altered and thereby contributed to the development of phospholipidosis. Interpretation of these results suggests that phospholipidosis occurs from the combination of events involving both increased synthesis and decreased degradation of phospholipids.

Although the genomic data identified important mechanistic events, the authors extended this work to the practical application of developing an in vitro screening test. They identified a set of twelve marker genes for predicting phospholipidosis. The approach differs from other recent attempts at establishing biomarkers and phospholipidosis in that they used genomics technology in place of analytical chemistry techniques (Mortuza et al., 2003) or metabonomic applications (Nicholls et al., 2000). These marker genes included functions for degradation of phospholipids, cholesterol biosynthesis, fatty acid transport, proteolysis, and endopeptidase inhibition. More important, these marker genes provided an accurate predictor of drug-induced phospholipidosis, and the in vitro assay requires a smaller quantity of the substance being evaluated than do standard in vivo tests. This work of Sawada et al. (2005) thus demonstrates the utility of toxicogenomic approaches for understanding mechanistic aspects in toxicology and provides a valuable approach for the development of markers of toxicity.

Another example involves dibutyl phthalate (DBP), a male reproductive toxicant in the rat that primarily targets the developing testis (Mylchreest et al., 1998, 1999, 2000). Shultz and colleagues hypothesized that DBP induces its antiandrogenic effects by altering both androgen-dependent and -independent signaling pathways during male reproductive development (Shultz et al., 2001). Alterations in gene expression induced by DBP in the developing fetal testes were examined and compared with alterations elicited by flutamide, a known nonsteroidal antiandrogen.

Shultz et al. demonstrated that DBP exposure in utero resulted in altered expression of a number of genes in fetal testes development. The role of these genes in DBP toxicity remains to be determined. Additional studies are needed to examine the dose-response of gene expression alterations and its relation to DBP toxicity. The investigators confirmed the expression of a select group of genes known to play a significant role in testicular development. Alterations in expression of these genes can be linked to the actions of DBP in the developing male reproductive tract, including reduced testicular testosterone, Leydig cell hyperplasia, and gonocyte degeneration. However, the diverse cell populations within the fetal testes as well as the dramatic changes in gene expression and cell function that occur normally during fetal testicular development complicates efforts to understand the mechanism of DBP-induced male reproductive toxicity. This will likely be an issue for other toxicities and tissues as well.

These examples demonstrate that genetic technologies can provide important insights and markers of toxicological mechanisms and modes of action. Such information can be useful in the assessment and management of chemical risks. At the same time, these initial studies also further demonstrate the complexity of biological systems and the challenges that will be involved in elucidating toxicological responses in such systems.

Risk Assessment Challenges

Risk assessment is evolving from a process dependent on traditional toxicologic testing paradigms into one that incorporates more scientific understanding of mechanistic data and biologically based computational models. In this regard, greater emphasis is being placed on early markers—

that is, indicators that signal preclinical events in biological systems. There are at least two approaches being used to incorporate genomic data in toxicology and identify such biomarkers. The first is a targeted approach in which one assesses the expression levels of key biochemical pathways identified a priori. The second is a "shotgun" approach in which gene expression profiling is coupled with bioinformatics techniques to identify these key pathways based on the identification of genes that are up- or down-regulated in response to a particular exposure. It is the latter approach for which the incorporation of genomic data into quantitative risk assessments is uncertain but is expected to be significant.

These -omics technologies will be useful for assessing tissue status in response to toxicants at the gene expression level, in order to establish and validate hypothesized modes of action and dose-time response dependencies. They will also provide information for assessing across-species comparisons. In contrast to the current paradigms for assessing risk of noncancer toxic endpoints (i.e., the use of safety or uncertainty factors), information on genetic variability has the potential to improve quantification of individual and population-based interindividual variability in susceptibility to different diseases or toxicants.

Approaches to risk-benefit analysis being taken by regulatory agencies are evolving, and the science of genomics is stimulating the development and formation of improved strategies for safety assessment. For regulatory purposes, it will be necessary to establish the relationships between the new genomics-based endpoints and known health outcomes, develop more established methodologies, and characterize the biologic relationships of the endpoints in laboratory animal models to use with humans. For full integration of genomic information into risk and safety assessment, regulatory bodies also will need to gain confidence in the accuracy, sensitivity, and robustness of these new methods. To gain regulatory acceptance it will be necessary for consensus to emerge from the larger scientific community and then form within the responsible centers within the various agencies. Guidance, guidelines, and regulations will then result from such consensus.

Genetic Variability and Susceptibility

Genetic polymorphisms are variations in DNA sequences (e.g., substitutions, insertions, and deletions) that are present at a frequency greater than 1 percent in a population. These variations are common in all genes, though in many cases the variation will not have a functional significance. From a risk-assessment perspective, what is important are the functional variations that affect the internal dose of a chemical, target organ damage, or other responses to exposure, and eventually, an adverse health outcome. Identification of susceptible groups that may be at much greater increased risk from exposure than the general population is especially important. Knowledge of mechanism and characterization of genetic susceptibility will be useful in risk assessment.

Gentry and colleagues recently focused on chemical metabolism and genetic polymorphisms (Gentry et al., 2002). The default uncertainty factor for human variability used in noncarcinogen risk assessment includes a subfactor that addresses difference in either metabolizing the chemical to a more toxic form or metabolizing it to a safer or less active form. The purpose of the project was to develop a more accurate approach that incorporates information on how genetic differences affect metabolism. To do this, the researchers first conducted literature searches to identify genes that are known to code for metabolizing enzymes that exist in more than one genetic form in the general population. The researchers then identified substances that are known to be metabolized by these enzymes.

They further evaluated four chemicals for which the metabolic pathways were well-characterized (e.g., the key metabolizing enzymes were known), the effect of genetic differences on metabolism were understood, and physiologically based pharmacokinetic models were available. They conducted detailed case studies with two of these chemicals, parathion and warfarin. Using pharmacokinetic models, the researchers estimated the concentrations of these chemicals and their metabolites, in blood following a single oral dose of the compounds. The team used statistical techniques (probabilistic Monte Carlo methods) to evaluate the extent that both common genetic differences and physiological differences (e.g., body weight, blood flow rate) contributed to the overall variation in internal dose among individuals in the population. The models provided estimates of the distributions of levels of the active form of the chemical, supporting efforts to predict how many people would exhibit higher, lower, or average sensitivity to the chemicals due to genetic differences.

This approach is significant for chemical risk assessment, because many chemicals regulated by various agencies are metabolized through pathways that are influenced by genetic differences. Data on the incidence of these genetic differences in human populations and their effects on metabolic pathways are becoming more readily available. This research demonstrates that data on polymorphisms can be combined with other information to improve the accuracy of the human variability uncertainty factor applied by EPA and other regulatory agencies in their chemical risk assessments for noncancer health effects.

Evaluations of human variability in response to specific toxic chemical exposures remain complex and controversial. The project described here identifies data needs and demonstrates a successful, systematic method for analyzing how human genetic differences may affect susceptibility to a particular chemical. This approach can lead to a decision framework for incorporating information on genetic differences, which will help in prioritizing resources for data collection and analysis. The research also will improve cancer risk assessments, because the approach enables risk assessors to use data on genetic differences to more accurately predict tissue doses for populations.

In addition, any human work should be done under widely accepted human research subject protections such as the Common Rule, which are the regulations for human subject protection that apply to federally funded research. While that rule is not legally binding on all research, it may be considered unethical to proceed without equivalent protection for human participants. At a future point, when some of the tests become "validated" for use as screening or diagnostic tools, a different set of bioethical codes apply. Those codes are based on the same fundamental bioethical principles. Paul Schulte addresses these and some of the workplace dilemmas in his chapter in this volume, "Genetics and Workplace Issues." Harrison's book is another excellent resource (Harrison, 1998).

Conclusion

The emergence of genomic technologies has the potential to lead to major advances in human understanding of normal biology and holds the promise of providing new insights into mechanisms of a variety of toxicities. The potential benefits of "-omics" include more scientifically precise and robust assessment of risk. However, much is still to be done in the development and application of these technologies before their full benefit is realized. As the technology develops, caution will be needed to avoid overinterpretation and inefficiency, which could delay progress by deterring development and reliance on the technology. A rigorous scientific approach will be needed to realize the benefits from -omics as quickly as possible.

REFERENCES

Cunningham, M.L., M.S. Bogdanffy, T.R. Zacharewski, and R. N. Hines. 2003. Workshop overview: Use of genomic data in risk assessment. *Toxicological Sciences* 73:209–15.

Gentry, P.R., C. E. Hack, L. Haber, A. Maier, and H.J. Clewell III. 2002. An approach for the quantitative consideration of genetic polymorphism data in chemical risk assessment: Examples with warfarin and parathion. *Toxicological Sciences* 70:120–39.

Hamadeh, H.K., P.R. Bushel, S. Jayadev, et al. 2002a. Gene expression analysis reveals chemical-specific profiles. *Toxicological Sciences* 67:219–31.

Hamadeh, H.K., P.R. Bushel, S. Jayadev, et al. 2002b. Prediction of compound signature using high density gene expression profiling. *Toxicological Sciences* 67:232–40.

Harrison, M.C. 1998. *Implications of genetic testing for medical examinations in the workplace.* Washington, DC: Joseph Henry Press.

Heinloth, A.N., R.D. Irwin, G.A. Boorman, et al. 2004. Gene expression profiling of rat livers reveals indicators of potential adverse effects. *Toxicological Sciences* 80:193–202.

Henry, C.J., R. Phillips, F. Carpanini, et al. 2002. Use of genomics in toxicology and epidemiology: Findings and recommendations of a workshop. *Environmental Health Perspectives* 110:1047–50.

Mortuza, G.B., W.A. Neville, J.W. Delany, C.J. Waterfield, and P. Camilleri. 2003. Characterization of a potential biomarker of phospholipidosis from amiodarone-treated rats. *Biochimica et Biophysica Acta* 1631:136–46.

Mylchreest, E, R.C. Cattley, and P.M.D. Foster. 1998. Male reproductive tract malformations in rats following gestational and lactational exposure to di(n-butyl) phthalate: An antiandrogenic mechanism? *Toxicological Sciences* 43:47–60.

Mylchreest, E., M. Sar, R.C. Cattley, and P.M.D. Foster. 1999. Disruption of androgen-regulated male reproductive development by di(n-butyl) phthalate during late gestation in rats is different from flutamide. *Toxicology and Applied Pharmacology* 156:81–95.

Mylchreest, E., D.G. Wallace, R.C. Cattley, and P.M.D. Foster. 2000. Dose-dependent alternations in androgen-regulated male reproductive development in rats exposed to di(n-butyl) phthalate during late gestation. *Toxicological Sciences* 55:143–51.

Nicholls, A.W., J.K. Nicholson, J.N. Haselden, and C.J. Waterfield. 2000. A metabonomic approach to the investigation of drug-induced phospholipidosis: An NMR spectroscopy and pattern recognition study. *Biomarkers* 5:410–23.

Sawada, S., K. Takami, and S. Asahi. 2005. A toxicogenomic approach to drug-induced phospholipidosis: Analysis of its induction mechanism and establishment of a novel in vitro screening system. *Toxicological Sciences* 83:282–92.

Shultz, V.D., S. Phillips, M. Sar, P.M.D. Foster, and K.W. Gaido. 2001. Altered gene profiles in fetal rat testes after in utero exposure to di(n-butyl) phthalate. *Toxicological Sciences* 64:233–42.

Tennant, R.W. 2002. The national center for toxicogenomics: Using new technologies to inform mechanistic toxicology. *Environmental Health Perspectives* 110:A8–10.

CHAPTER 4

Toxicogenomics and the Public Interest

Technical and Sociopolitical Challenges

JOHN M. BALBUS

New scientific tools spawned by the genomics revolution promise to improve our ability to identify causative factors in human diseases. Transcriptomics (the analysis of messenger RNA transcripts), proteomics (the global analysis of cellular or biofluid proteins), and metabolomics (the global analysis of tissue, cellular, or biofluid metabolites) all share the potential to examine early processes in the pathways to toxicity in a comprehensive fashion. These tools are expected to allow more rapid screening of chemicals for toxic effects and to provide insight into toxicological mechanisms for a greater range and earlier stage of adverse outcomes associated with chemical exposures. But the reliance on computational methods may make it harder for scientists trained in traditional toxicology to integrate this new knowledge into existing paradigms. In addition to barriers within the scientific community, the emergence of these new technologies is taking place in a political context that involves a variety of stakeholders with separate agendas. Despite major advances in the science and technology of these new toxicogenomic tools, these scientific and political complexities threaten to delay the use of toxicogenomics to further the public interest or, worse, to advance its use initially to weaken the regulation and safety of widely used chemicals.

Why We Need Toxicogenomics? What Are the Problems in Need of Solution?
Lack of Cheap, Effective Tests

Current toxicological testing batteries fall short of meeting public needs because they are expensive and take too long. The testing battery that pesticides must undergo costs as much as ten million dollars and requires a minimum of three years to complete (Culleen, 1994). With tens of thousands of chemicals in commerce, most of which unlike pesticides are not legally required to be tested before marketing, these cost and time constraints have been an important factor in the persistence of ignorance regarding the toxicity of chemical products. Given the time and expense required to evaluate and understand the properties of individual chemicals, it is not surprising that limited resources have been available to study the complex mixtures to which humans are actually exposed.

Traditional toxicological tests provide useful information on which to base risk-management decisions, but they are far from perfect. Because readily observable pathological changes must develop before toxic effects can be detected, the test protocols maximize the likelihood of creating such advanced toxic effects while minimizing the number of animals used in each study. This leads to dosing that is generally well above the anticipated level of environmental, or even occupational, exposures. Questions about the applicability of effects observed at high doses to low-dose exposure scenarios generate controversy about the level of uncertainty and risk. This leads to unproductive legal and scientific battles between regulators and the regulated industries.

Reliance on rodent models in traditional toxicological tests leads to similar controversy and opportunities for action-inhibiting debates. On the one hand, our current level of toxicological sophistication requires us to study whole animals, because we are otherwise unable to simulate the complex interplay between toxic exposures and defense mechanisms that operate in living creatures. On the other hand, limitations in our ability to apply observations in rodent responses to predictions of human responses inject uncertainty into the risk-assessment process and again provide grist for debates between government and industry scientists and cause subsequent stalling of measures to reduce risk. In addition, the emergence of groups whose goal is to eliminate the use of animals in chemical testing and assessment has heightened the controversy over the best ways to identify and manage the risks from harmful chemicals.

How Could Toxicogenomics Serve the Public Interest?

The three data-generating fields of toxicogenomics—transcriptomics, proteomics, and metabonomics—all share the potential to address the shortcomings of traditional toxicological testing. In theory, cellular- and organ-level responses to toxic exposures can be described at the earliest stages by changes in expression of genes that are up- or down-regulated. Transcriptomics, by detecting these changes in a comprehensive fashion, should be highly sensitive to early stages in the pathological processes arising from toxic exposures. Those changes in gene expression should also be reflected by changes in levels of proteins. Proteomic analysis also has the theoretic advantage of capturing changes in biological function that may not be easily detected by analyzing gene expression, because substantial modification of biological function is brought about by posttranslational changes in proteins, such as the addition of small molecules like methyl groups or sugars. And metabonomics has the theoretical advantage of incorporating factors that are not fully mediated through genes and proteins, such as nutritional status. This massive increase in the amount and types of data able to be generated about responses to toxic exposures offers several potential advantages over traditional methods:

- By detecting earlier changes in pathological processes, toxicogenomics should shorten test durations.
- By increasing the sensitivity of testing systems, thereby enhancing the ability to detect small changes earlier in pathological processes, toxicogenomics should allow the use of lower, more relevant doses and avoid the debates around interpreting changes observed in high-dose studies.
- By analyzing states of the exposed organism in a global manner, toxicogenomics should prove to be more comprehensive than traditional, histology-based toxicology that tends to focus on a relatively limited set of endpoints.

- By providing large amounts of data on mechanisms, toxicogenomics methods should enhance scientists' ability to extrapolate changes observed in experimental systems (either using a wider range of animals or laboratory-derived cell lines) to effects in humans or other species of interest.
- By being shorter or less expensive than traditional tests (to the extent that this turns out to be true) or providing unique signatures of toxicity for specific chemicals, toxicogenomic tests will make it easier to study chemical mixtures, a longtime shortcoming of traditional regulatory toxicology.
- By combining with the parallel growth of knowledge and technical ability in analyzing genetic variability, toxicogenomics should enhance scientists' ability both to describe the range of responses within humans at various life stages and of varying genetic makeup and to identify those within the population who are most at risk from specific exposure scenarios.

The downside of having the ability to detect early changes in biological responses on a global scale is that an enormous quantity of data is generated, and our limited understanding of mechanisms in their full complexity renders it difficult to interpret. The heightened sensitivity of the testing systems makes their results more variable due to small differences in testing equipment and techniques, as well as to background "noise"—changes in measurements due to random variation. For these reasons, the ability to apply these techniques to the most complex problems of predictive toxicology will require years of data generation, greater experience with the technologies, and consensus building regarding the interpretation of data.

This does not mean, however, that there aren't uses for these technologies in the short term. Applications that don't require full mechanistic understanding or dose-response characterization are less complex and more realistic for the near term. For example, hazard screening, which is currently performed using high doses and whole animals, may be initially augmented and ultimately partially replaced by toxicogenomic methods. Hazard screening using toxicogenomics is already used in the drug development process by the pharmaceutical industry, as toxicogenomic techniques are sufficiently reliable and less expensive to provide a screening indication of specific types of toxicity in this setting. Examples of proof of concept studies using toxicogenomic techniques to assess hazard categories of environmental toxins include studies of periox-isome proliferators and hepatotoxins (Hamadeh et al., 2002; Huang et al., 2004).

Another application that could be pursued at the present time is valida-tion of the grouping of chemicals into categories for the purposes of large-scale chemical screening programs like the High Production Volume Chemical Challenge, an EPA program to "challenge" companies to produce health and environmental data on chemical produced in the United States in quantities of one million pounds or more per year. As now practiced, industry consortia group together chemicals for data gathering based on structural and, in some cases, physicochemical considerations. Original data generated for members of a chemical category presumed to represent ex-tremes are then interpolated to other members of the class that are pre-sumed to have properties that are intermediate between the extremes. But it is clear that even subtle differences in structure can lead to huge differ-ences in toxicity. Sensitive screening methods could provide a means of recognizing outliers in chemical categories, placing these categories on a more rigorous scientific footing and enhancing their acceptability.

With simpler applications feasible now, and with more complex ap-plications not likely to be feasible for some years, it makes sense to im-plement toxicogenomic technologies as a sequence of applications that steps up in complexity over time. Initial steps could include those that do not require characterization of dose-response or full description of ei-ther toxicity or susceptibility. Intermediate steps will include the initial development of mechanistic dose-response models based on toxicoge-nomic data and the partial characterization of individual susceptibility. Ultimately, the acquisition of experience and extensive data may enable more complex exposure and risk modeling. It is critical that the current inability to use toxicogenomics to assess dose-response relationships not preclude simpler applications. The data generated and experience gained through applying toxicogenomics to these simpler questions will help promote the development of more complex applications and models.

Transferring Technology from Drug Development to Regulatory Chemical Screening

Among other factors, different regulatory requirements have led to dif-ferent levels of interest in developing toxicogenomic methods in the pharmaceutical and chemical industries. Knowing that toxicity made evident by extensive and mandatory premarket testing will prevent commercialization of novel compounds, pharmaceutical companies have a strong financial incentive to prescreen compounds early in the drug development process and eliminate those likely to cause toxicity before significant resources have been expended in their development. It is not essential in this scenario to detect all possible toxicity, nor is it essential to be near perfect in either detecting toxicity or exonerating compounds. If a testing method fails to detect toxicity in the screening process, subsequent extensive animal and human testing would provide a more reliable backstop. Conversely, if it inappropriately labels a relatively safe compound as toxic, this is allowable for business purposes so long as other effective compounds that are relatively safe are correctly identified for further marketing. The cost savings that arise from avoiding more costly toxicity testing through the use of toxicogenomic prescreening is largely what has driven the development of these methods in the pharmaceutical industry.

In the course of developing methods for screening new therapeutic compounds, the pharmaceutical companies and the biotechnology companies that support them have acquired technical expertise, as well as databases that have considerable utility for the application of toxicogenomics to the assessment of nontherapeutic chemical compounds. But this transfer of methods and databases will be impeded by a number of barriers and limitations. First, as mentioned above, the toxicity screening of candidate compounds for potential therapeutics can be effective even with a limited number of endpoints. The majority of databases developed for this purpose have focused on hepatotoxicity; limited work has been done to predict other organ toxicity. Accurate prediction of chemical toxicity will likely require assays for a broader spectrum of toxicological endpoints.

In addition, pharmaceutical companies need to detect toxicity in a relatively limited dose range around the therapeutic dose. Chemical companies must assess toxicity over a broader range of exposures, from the high doses of workplace accidents to the lower doses occurring when chemicals are gradually released into the ambient environment. Thus, toxicogenomic assessment of chemicals will have to either directly assess lower-level exposures or facilitate extrapolation to lower-level exposures to be useful.

Last, business interests may interfere with the transfer of capability from the pharmaceutical industry to the control of chemical toxicity. For many of the biotechnology companies, the databases and the analytic algorithms they have developed constitute their main business product. As such, they regard much of the data and software as proprietary and avoid sharing the complete data sets they have developed. Furthermore, while the cost savings in the drug discovery and development process produced by earlier toxicity screens are simple to demonstrate, the financial incentives for screening chemicals, especially existing chemicals already enjoying commercialization, are less clear. Chemical companies may look to more thorough toxicity evaluations as a means of lowering potential liability, but the lack of a required and extensive set of animal and human tests that must be passed before commercialization of chemicals (other than pesticides) removes a substantial part of the financial incentive to prescreen.

What Are the Barriers to Application of Toxicogenomics?

In the short term, the first barrier is cost. While many look to toxicogenomics as providing data that are "too cheap to meter," that is not the present situation. Gene chips can still cost as much as a thousand dollars apiece, and the equipment required to create individual gene microarrays or perform proteomic or metabolomic analyses can require multimillion-dollar investments. In the current phase of standardization, validation, and transition from traditional animal testing, the need to conduct traditional animal tests in parallel further escalates the required investment. To fulfill its promises, toxicogenomic techniques must prove to be reliable, reproducible, and ultimately inexpensive enough to make them attractive as a means of lowering liability risk for industry.

The next major hurdle is validation. While it is clear that any set of test methods intended for regulatory use must be validated, it would be a mistake to consider validation to be a yes/no process. On the way to formal validation, toxicogenomic techniques will go through a series of stages, including demonstrations of reproducibility and biological relevance, that should allow their use in increasingly complex applications. Initially, toxicogenomic data might be combined with data from traditional sources to provide additional weight-of-evidence support for applications such as hazard identification and prioritization. Intermediate steps could include use of toxicogenomic data for screening unknown chemicals for indications for further testing. Full replacement of animal testing data for the purposes of regulatory risk assessment or product registration will clearly require greater familiarity with the techniques and more formal validation procedures that guarantee superior performance compared with existing methods. Most traditional toxicological tests did not have to go through formal validation procedures but entered regulatory use through extensive experience and comfort with their methods and results (National Institute of Environmental Health Sciences, 2005). Rigorous assessments of their biological relevance have come retrospectively, and it has been difficult to get an accurate estimation of their sensitivity and specificity for human health endpoints. It is critical that the potential power of toxicogenomic analysis not be held captive by a prolonged and formal validation process.

One initial hurdle toxicogenomic methods must vault on the path to validation is demonstration that the techniques are reproducible and reliable. It must be shown that the same equipment gives the same results each time the same experiment is run and that different laboratories and different platforms or ways of generating data also produce comparable results. Some initial papers suggesting shortcomings in reproducibility of gene expression arrays have attracted attention and have been cited by some as reasons to hold back on promoting development of microarrays for chemical testing (Petricoin et al., 2002; Shi et al., 2004). A more recent series of papers, however, suggests that much of the lack of reproducibility can be explained either by different analysis methods or by the use of less well-standardized dotted microarrays (Bammler et al., 2005; Irizarry et al., 2005; Larkin et al., 2005; Sherlock, 2005). The authors of these papers suggest that the assays return consistent interpretations of data from a biological relevance standpoint when standardized procedures are followed.

Two principles should inform public interest stances on reproducibility. First, to the extent that there are inconsistencies, they represent problems to be solved aggressively, not reasons for delaying development of the techniques. Second, as with all dynamic and developing technologies, it is nearly certain that manufacturing methods will improve and equipment variability will be ironed out in a relatively short period of time. Such improvements can be anticipated as work to address other aspects of validation progresses.

The U.S. Interagency Coordinating Committee on the Validation of Alternative Methods (ICCVAM) and the European Centre for the Validation of Alternative Methods (ECVAM) addressed the question of validation at a joint workshop (European Centre for the Validation of Alternative Methods et al., 2005). Their approach separates the validation process into technical validation of the equipment, techniques, and protocols of data generation and biological validation of the interpretation of toxicogenomic data. They recommend a step-wise validation process, starting with single or small sets of gene or protein expression based biomarkers. These biomarkers can then be compared with and validated in comparison to standard clinical biomarkers, thereby working within a system more familiar to regulatory bodies. With time, refinement of equipment and techniques and additional generation of data will "facilitate development and validation of more complex expression Asignatures" as indicators of toxicity.

The ICCVAM/ECVAM workshop report emphasizes the need to embark on the validation process now, while the development of toxicogenomic techniques is ongoing, so that early problems can be identified and data necessary for validation can be generated. Recognizing that the technologies are dynamic and constantly improving, workshop participants recommended a series of studies aimed at transcending questions of interlaboratory and interplatform performance. In particular, they recommended the parallel running of toxicogenomic assays in conjunction with standard regulatory testing, so that a database relevant to assessing biological relevance can be accumulated.

Are the Needed Data Being Generated?

Interviews with a multisectoral group of experts (Balbus, 2005) revealed widely held beliefs that successful incorporation of toxicogenomic data into risk assessment and chemical safety would require a huge initial investment in generating massive data sets that tied toxicogenomic data to presently accepted measures of pathology, whether from traditional toxicological tests or from clinical epidemiological settings. Such data sets need to have significant redundancy to address concerns about reproducibility and reliability. The need for these databases leads to two questions: Who

will do the laboratory work to create them? And are those parties investing enough resources to complete the task in a timely fashion?

As discussed above, some pharmaceutical and related biotechnology companies are investing large amounts of money to develop the laboratory capability to perform toxicogenomic analyses of candidate drug compounds.
Companies like GeneLogic and Iconix have developed large databases that
they market to the pharmaceutical industry for use in compound screening.
These databases, developed mainly by running both known toxins and novel
candidate compounds through gene expression assays, should be relevant
to the screening and assessment of environmental chemicals, although there
are important differences. For the most part, these databases have been designed to detect a limited array of toxic effects. Companies are working on
multiple organ toxicity screens, but the best-developed and most widely
published screens are thus far limited to hepatotoxicity. Because there is
more concern about environmental chemicals causing cancer or neurological, immune, and reproductive toxicity than about hepatotoxicity, these databases will need to be expanded to include these other outcomes to be most
useful. Similarly, the ability of short-term assays to predict more chronic effects from environmental exposures needs to be demonstrated.

More important, the development of these databases by for-profit entities raises serious concerns about their commercialization and about
proprietary restrictions on them. For many companies, the database itself is their primary intellectual capital—the likelihood that these companies will make their databases fully available is therefore quite low. In
addition, many of the large pharmaceutical companies closely guard data
on candidate compounds, as competitors could theoretically use the data
to gain intelligence on the types of compound being explored. Thus far,
some companies have made some data from assays of common chemicals available. The disincentives for openly sharing most of their data,
however, are likely to greatly limit the contribution of pharmaceutical
and biotechnology companies to the creation of the large databases necessary for the development and validation of toxicogenomic techniques
for environmental chemical screening and assessment.

Governmental Efforts

The federal government, through both regulatory and research agencies,
is playing several critical roles in the development of toxicogenomics for

the public interest. The first is encouraging the incorporation of toxicogenomics data into the regulatory review of new drugs and chemicals. Both
FDA and EPA have published guidance on the submission of toxicogenomic
data in the process of new product review (U.S. Environmental Protection
Agency, 2002; U.S. Food and Drug Administration, 2005b). Because toxicogenomic methods are still in the process of validation, a delicate balance
must be achieved. Companies must be given incentives to go to the extra
trouble and expense to generate toxicogenomic data, assuring them that the
data will not be interpreted haphazardly. But at the same time, a framework must be set up that will take advantage of any superior features of
toxicogenomic studies as they are validated. Drug companies are already
using toxicogenomics to screen compounds, indicating that they believe
there is an economic advantage to generating these data. For FDA, the challenge is to encourage submission of any toxicogenomic data that have been
generated during the research and development process. This has led to
FDA's "safe harbor" approach described below.

Chemical companies, on the other hand, have no predetermined testing requirements for new products other than pesticides, giving them little incentive to invest in toxicogenomic screening methods. Chemical
industry representatives have indicated that their perceived benefit from
the application of toxicogenomic techniques to assessment of environmental chemicals is the "reduction of uncertainty" surrounding already
regulated chemicals. Research that emphasizes elucidation of mechanisms conducted by the Hammer Institutes for Health Science may reflect this different focus. The challenge for EPA, and for the public interest
community, is therefore to ensure that toxicogenomic techniques are used
to strengthen protections that are currently too weak, as well as to identify standards or other protective measures that are overly conservative.
At this stage, given the difficulties assessing dose-response through toxicogenomic methods, EPA guidance is necessarily nonprescriptive.

FDA Regulations and Toxicogenomics

FDA's current policies describe in some detail when toxicogenomic
data must be submitted. According to FDA's Guidance for Industry Pharmacogenomic Data Submissions (FDA, 2005b), submission of pharmacogenomic data in an investigational new drug application is required if

(1) the results arise from a specific clinical or animal trial that is being used to support safety decisions (such as dosing, subject selection, etc.), (2) the results are being used to support scientific arguments pertaining to mechanism of action or other safety or efficacy arguments, or (3) test results constitute a known valid biomarker for human or animal studies (Food and Drug Administration, 2005a). Conversely, submission of toxicogenomic data is not required if the data are not supporting a regulatory decision or argument or if the test results use biomarkers whose validity is not clearly established.

Because pharmaceutical companies are primarily using toxicogenomics for preliminary toxicity screening, most pharmacogenomic data are considered exploratory and are not significant in determining the safety or effectiveness of a particular drug. Under current guidance, such data are unlikely to be required for submission to FDA. The only way FDA has access to such data is if industry scientists submit Voluntary Genomic Data Submissions (VGDSs). The primary review body for VGDSs is the Interdisciplinary Pharmacogenomic Review Group, whose mission is to establish a scientific and regulatory framework for reviewing genomic data. VGDSs received by FDA are processed and sent directly to the IPRG, with the general policy that submitted information will not be used for regulatory decision making on investigational and marketing and licensing applications, providing a de facto safe harbor for such data submissions.

In theory, VGDSs should be mutually beneficial to FDA and industry scientists alike. By submitting information now, industry scientists could help ensure that regulatory bodies are prepared to evaluate future, more critical genomic data as the understanding and application of toxicogenomics increases. FDA has received several submissions of genomic data. It is not entirely clear, however, whether these data were being used to support regulatory decisions or whether they were "model" data sets voluntarily submitted for the benefit of the agency scientists (U.S. Food and Drug Administration, 2005a). Pharmaceutical companies may be concerned that submitting genomic data might slow down approval of drug applications. There is also concern that FDA will overreact to single gene changes. For example, a large number of drugs are known to elevate the expression of the oncogene ras, although none have been shown to cause cancer at therapeutic levels (Freeman, 2004).

EPA Toxicogenomic Guidance

EPA's position on the submission of toxicogenomic data for regulatory purposes is set forth in its 2002 Interim Policy on Genomics (U.S. Environmental Protection Agency [EPA], 2002). This four-page document expresses many of the anticipated applications of toxicogenomic data to hazard and risk assessment for chemicals, but it offers little in the way of specific guidance for chemical companies to use in deciding whether to incorporate toxicogenomic assays into any laboratory testing of products they may decide to do. The interim policy expresses the view that "the relationships between changes in gene expression and adverse effects are unclear at this time and may likely be difficult to elucidate" (EPA, 2002, p. 2). For this reason, EPA states that it may consider toxicogenomic data as part of a weight-of-evidence decision, but that "[toxicogenomic] data alone are insufficient as a basis for decisions" (p. 2). This stated uncertainty regarding interpretation of toxicogenomic data is most likely to have a chilling effect on the submission of toxicogenomic data by chemical companies. With concerns that retrospective interpretation of data may indicate toxicity of a product at some point in the future, with subsequent consequences for legal liability, it is unlikely that companies will risk submitting data in the absence of some kind of safe harbor arrangement.

Governmental Research Initiatives

While it appears that current federal regulatory policies are presently doing little to encourage the use of toxicogenomic techniques to evaluate drugs and chemicals for clearance procedures, the research laboratories within EPA and National Institutes of Health have begun to increase investment in and sophistication of efforts to do the types of research and to create the types of databases needed to transition toxicogenomics into chemical regulatory use.

The EPA Office of Research and Development established the National Center for Computational Toxicology (NCCT), an entity designed to coordinate and implement research being funded and conducted by EPA in its Computational Toxicology Research Program. The mission of the NCCT is (1) to provide scientific expertise and leadership related to the application of mathematical and computational tools and models; (2) to improve the predictive capabilities of the methods, models, and measurements that constitute the input materials to the computational models; (3) to conduct or sponsor research to provide models for fate and transport of chemicals, environmental exposures to humans and wildlife, delivery of the chemical to the target site of toxicity, molecular and cellular pathways of toxicity, and ultimately systems level understanding of biological processes and their perturbation; and (4) to maintain a strong emphasis on the development of partnerships with other government and private organizations (Kavlock, 2005). The NCCT operates through transfer of funds to other EPA and government labs, as well as through external contracts and grants.

An example of a partnership between the Computational Toxicology Research Program and a private organization was announced in January 2005, shortly after the creation of NCCT. Iconix Pharmaceuticals was awarded a contract by EPA to use its chemogenomics platform, originally designed for drug development, to predict toxicity to the liver, and potentially to the heart and kidneys, of five chemicals. With gene expression, biological pathway, toxicology and pharmacology information on over 650 compounds, Iconix has developed a reference database that it uses to compare compounds and predict the toxicity of chemicals and the pathologies they might induce (Iconix, 2005). The terms of the contract, with Iconix receiving $250,000 to analyze the five chemicals of interest, indicate that the cost of using toxicogenomics might be prohibitively high at this early stage. However, the only way to break through existing financial and technical hurdles to using toxicogenomics is to continue its development and application.

In its new road map documents, the National Toxicology Program of the National Institutes of Environmental Health Sciences envisions making toxicogenomic assays a central part of its ongoing chemical studies (National Toxicology Program, 2004). Specifically, the National Toxicology Program intends to begin incorporating genomic analyses into its current studies, targeting endpoints being addressed using more traditional methods to further develop knowledge of mechanisms of toxicity. New research activities will focus on creating high-throughput screening methods to evaluate chemicals quickly using in vitro biological systems. This type of screening will focus on screening alterations to mechanistic targets through toxicogenomic assays.

Analyzing the Individual: Toxicogenetics and Pharmacogenetics

During interviews with experts, many respondents voiced concerns that societal forces would hinder the implementation and use of toxicogenomic advances. Most frequently mentioned was the concern that the development of societal mechanisms for addressing the ethical, legal, and social aspects of toxicogenomics (and toxicogenetics) was lagging behind the technological advances. Many respondents also worried that privacy concerns and mistrust among the general public would impede the development of methods to determine and understand susceptibility.

These concerns are especially great when individual genetic data are being collected, as in the field of toxicogenetics, the study of individual and population differences in susceptibility to toxic insults. Just as pharmaceutical companies are at the forefront of toxicogenomics, they are also leading in the closely related fields of toxicogenetics and pharmacogenetics. Pharmacogenetics promises individualized medicine based on each patient's ability to respond to specific pharmaceutical therapies, as determined by genetic and biochemical biomarkers. Currently, pharmacogenetic testing is being used routinely in a few specialized applications, such as genotyping for specific polymorphisms of the enzyme thiopurine S-methyltransferase, which is important in metabolizing drugs used to fight acute lymphocytic leukemia (Ensom et al., 2001). However, as the body of knowledge grows, there will be more widespread application of pharmacogenetic information in diverse areas such as hypertension treatment, estrogen therapy, and psychiatry (Melzer et al., 2005). In addition to wider use by physicians, pharmacogenetic testing is being marketing directly to consumers as a tool to diagnose and screen for adverse drug reactions.

Because the same enzymes that metabolize pharmaceuticals also metabolize toxins, as information becomes available for pharmacogenetic purposes, it will also inform decision making on potential effects of exposure to environmental contaminants. One potential application of this information at the population level is the opportunity for better characterization of variability in metabolism of toxins, allowing for stronger estimations of uncertainty factors for chemical risk assessments (Dorne et al., 2005). However, this information will almost certainly be used at an

individual level as well. For example, "normal" functioning of the cy-
tochrome P450 2C9 (*CYP*2C9) enzyme has been found to be associated
with increased risk of colon cancer, possibly because the carcinogenic
polycyclic aromatic hydrocarbons and heterocyclic aromatic amines are
*CYP*2C9 substrates (Martinez et al., 2001). Polymorphisms in the gene
coding for *CYP*2C9 also affect a patient's response to warfarin, the most
widely used oral anticoagulant, and there is widespread interest in pharmacogenetic testing for this purpose (Hall and Wilkins, 2005). Genetic
testing for the polymorphisms in the gene coding for *CYP*2C9 is already
being marketed directly to consumers in the United States, despite the
lack of consensus on appropriate counseling and follow-up. As pharmacogenetic testing becomes more prevalent and the body of literature on
toxicogenetics grows, individual-level information on susceptibility to
environmental threats will grow, raising a host of issues on how individuals and society should best address this information.

Some of the potential applications and implications of widespread genetic testing are beginning to be addressed. Health insurance plans are
interested in incorporating genetic information into their predictive modeling to manage costs (Sipkoff, 2005). In a response to concerns about
misuse of genetic information, legislation is pending in the U.S. Congress
that would ban employers and health insurance providers from discriminating on the basis of that information (Sipkoff, 2005). The potential effects of the availability of toxicogenetic data on environmental law,
however, have remained largely unaddressed. The Environmental
Genome Project identified a number of ethical, legal, and social issues
related to its work identifying genes conferring susceptibility to environmental toxins, including the broad categories of informed consent, privacy and confidentiality, disclosure of results, application of findings,
and shifting the burden of prevention from those producing environmental hazards to those susceptible to those hazards (Robert and Smith, 2004).

Robert and Smith criticized the makers of this list for failing to
address a number of other questions. One of the consequences of identifying and tailoring interventions toward genetically susceptible populations is that overall exposures to toxins among those not deemed
susceptible may rise. This could lead to overall decreases in the health
of the public, especially through increased exposure to toxins that cause
harm through multiple pathways, but where only a subpopulation susceptible to one pathway is fully protected. Robert and Smith also point

out that widespread applications of toxicogenetics could create newly identified vulnerable populations (Robert and Smith, 2004). The responsibility of regulatory agencies to protect these newly identifiable subpopulations under current environmental law and the public's willingness to protect them are unclear (Grodsky, 2005). The potential effects of widespread data on individual genetic susceptibility on protecting the public from environmental toxins are profound. One of the great potential barriers to successful incorporation of toxicogenomic data into chemical regulatory practice is the possibility of backlash against this information due to misuses and misinterpretations of the data. All sectors involved—private, public, academic, and nonprofit—have barely begun to address these critical societal issues, but the need for greater focus is clear.

Conclusion

Toxicogenomic tools promise to increase our understanding of the mechanisms of toxicity, especially at the early stages, and to allow faster, more comprehensive, and more accurate screening of chemicals than do traditional toxicology testing methods. However, there are a number of obstacles to implementing toxicogenomic testing for evaluation of environmental toxins. Technical barriers include high cost, uncertainty about reproducibility, and the need for development and sharing of databases that go well beyond the limited and propriety databases developed specifically for screening by pharmaceutical companies. Sociopolitical barriers include ensuring that use of toxicogenomic testing is not bogged down in an overdrawn validation process and that regulatory agencies are equipped to interpret the results. In addition, ethical concerns need to be addressed. As variations of susceptibility among humans become an important part of assessing toxicity, individualized genetic information will become more easily available, and potential abuse of this information by insurance companies, employers, or others could lead to a backlash by the public to any use of genomic data in this context. To ensure that new advances in toxicogenomics are exploited to the fullest extent, the public interest community needs to actively advocate a research agenda and funding that serve public policy needs, act as a watchdog in the discussions between government agencies and industry, and help to keep the public fully informed about the potential benefits and limitations of the technology.

ACKNOWLEDGMENTS

I would like to acknowledge the assistance of Stephanie Mickelson, M.P.H., and Yewlin Chee in the preparation of this chapter.

REFERENCES

Balbus, J. 2005. Toxicogenomics: Harnessing the power of new technology. At www.environmentaldefense.org/pdf.cfm?ContentID=4549&FileName=toxico genomics.pdf.

Bammler, T., R.P. Beyer, S. Bhattacharya, et al. 2005. Standardizing global gene expression analysis between laboratories and across platforms. *Nature Methods* 2:351–56.

Culleen, L.E. 1994. Pesticide registration in the United States: Overview and new directions. *Quality Assurance* 3:291–99.

Dorne, J.L., K. Walton, and A.G. Renwick. 2005. Human variability in xenobiotic metabolism and pathway-related uncertainty factors for chemical risk assessment: A review. *Food and Chemical Toxicology* 43:203–16.

Ensom, M.H., T.K. Chang, and P. Patel. 2001. Pharmacogenetics: The therapeutic drug monitoring of the future? *Clinical Pharmacokinetics* 40:783–802.

European Centre for the Validation of Alternative Methods, U.S. Interagency Coordinating Committee on the Validation of Alternative Methods, and National Toxicology Program Interagency Center for the Evaluation of Alternative Toxicological Methods. 2005. Workshop on the validation principles for toxicogenomics-based test systems: An overview. At http://ecvam.jrc.it/index.htm.

Freeman, K. 2004. Toxicogenomics data: The road to acceptance. *Environmental Health Perspectives* 112:A678–85.

Grodsky, J.A. 2005. Genetics and environmental law: Redefining public health. *California Law Review* 93:171–270.

Hall, A.M., and M.R. Wilkins. 2005. Warfarin: A case history in pharmacogenetics. *Heart* 91:563–64.

Hamadeh, H.K., P.R. Bushel, S. Jayadev, et al. 2002. Gene expression analysis reveals chemical-specific profiles. *Toxicological Sciences* 67:219–31.

Huang, Q., X. Jin, E.T. Gaillard, B.L. Knight, F.D. Pack, J.H. Stoltz, S. Jayadev, and K.F. Blanchard. 2004. Gene expression profiling reveals multiple toxicity endpoints induced by hepatotoxicants. *Mutation Research* 549:147–67.

Iconix. 2005. Iconix awarded EPA contract for novel toxicology screening platform. At www.iconixpharm.com/newscenter/news_release.php?newsID=37.

Irizarry, R.A., D. Warren, F. Spencer, et al. 2005. Multiple-laboratory comparison of microarray platforms. *Nature Methods* 2:345–50.

Kavlock, R. 2005. Computational toxicology overview. At www.epa.gov/comptox/bosc_review/2005/files/2_overview_kavlock.pdf.

Larkin, J.E., B.C. Frank, H. Gavras, R. Sultana, and J. Quackenbush. 2005. Independence and reproducibility across microarray platforms. *Nature Methods* 2:337–44.

Martinez, C., E. Garcia-Martin, J. M. Ladero, J. Sastre, F. Garcia-Gamito, M. Diaz-Rubio, and J.A.G. Agúndez. 2001. Association of CYP2C9 genotypes leading to high enzyme activity and colorectal cancer risk. *Carcinogenesis* 22:1323–26.

Melzer, D., A. Raven, T. Ling, D. Detmer, and R.L. Zimmern. 2005. Pharmacogenetics: Policy needs for personal prescribing. *Journal of Health Services Research and Policy* 10:40–44.

National Institute of Environmental Health Sciences. 2005. Validation and regulatory acceptance of toxicological test methods: A report of the ad hoc Interagency Coordinating Committee on the Validation of Alternative Methods. At http://iccvam.niehs.nih.gov/docs/guidelines/validate.pdf.

National Toxicology Program. 2004. A national toxicology program for the 21st century: A roadmap for the future. At http://ntp.niehs.nih.gov/index.cfm?objectid=B4DA3C38-F1F6-975E-7168BAC6475F1E5B.

Petricoin, E.F., J.L. Hackett, L.J. Lesko, et al. 2002. Medical applications of microarray technologies: A regulatory science perspective. *Nature Genetics* 32 Suppl.:474–79.

Robert, J.S., and A. Smith. 2004. Toxic ethics: Environmental genomics and the health of populations. *Bioethics* 18:493–514.

Sherlock, G. 2005. Of fish and chips. *Nature Methods* 2:329–30.

Shi, L., W. Tong, F. Goodsaid, F.W. Frueh, H. Fang, T. Han, J.C. Fuscoe, and D.A.Casciano. 2004. QA/QC: Challenges and pitfalls facing the microarray community and regulatory agencies. *Expert Review of Molecular Diagnostics* 4:761–77.

Sipkoff, M. 2005. Predictive modeling and genomics: Marriage of promise and risk. *Managed Care* 14:63–64, 66.

U.S. Environmental Protection Agency, Science Policy Council. 2002. Interim Policy on Genomics. At http://epa.gov/osa/spc/htm/genomics.htm.

U.S. Food and Drug Administration. 2005a. FDA works to speed the advent of new, more effective personalized medicines. At www.fda.gov/bbs/topics/news/2005/NEW01167.html.

U.S. Food and Drug Administration Center for Drug Evaluation and Research, Center for Biologics Evaluation and Research, and Center for Devices and Radiological Health. 2005b. Guidance for industry: Pharmacogenetic data submissions. Rockville, MD: Center for Drug Evaluation and Research, Food and Drug Administration.

PART II

LEGAL PERSPECTIVES

CHAPTER 5

Challenges in Applying Toxicogenomic Data in Federal Regulatory Settings

LYNN L. BERGESON

Both the legal and the scientific literatures are replete with assessments of the implications of toxicogenomics for many aspects of human and ecological health. Based on a review of the research and writings in this area, there is consensus that toxicogenomic data will find their greatest application in at least three areas: susceptibility—identifying subpopulations and life stages uniquely susceptible to environmental factors; predictive toxicology—facilitating high-throughput chemical screening for potential adverse impacts and hence assisting in prioritizing chemicals believed to be most potentially toxic; and understanding disease mechanisms—helping to elucidate a substance's mode of action to define better its dose-response continuum.[1]

Similarly, the application of high-throughput genomic data to toxicology is progressing, and the generation of large quantities of toxicogenomic data seems to be well along. The good news is that some of the important technical issues associated with collecting toxicogenomic data, such as how to manufacture microarrays, have been addressed. Database construction and maintenance are mature for genetic and genomic data, and microarray databases are developing.

Many challenges remain, however. For example, these databases do not consistently incorporate data relevant to toxicology, including exposure, dose, or time parameters. Similarly, statistical models applicable to large data sets are only now developing and do not yet include in all cases dose and time effects at toxic and nontoxic exposures. The next scientific frontier in genomics and bioinformatics will be conquering key challenges such as standardizing methods, nomenclature, and database construction; automating data collection; integrating toxicological with gene expression data; developing statistical models applicable to gene expression data that consider dose and time; and, perhaps most important, validating all of the above. In short, additional scientific, policy, ethical, and legal concerns remain to be addressed. This brief summary of some of these issues is not intended to suggest that these challenges are readily amenable to solution, quite the contrary.

Until these challenges are addressed, the true utility and promise of toxicogenomic data will remain unfulfilled in four areas the U.S. Environmental Protection Agency (EPA) identified as the most likely to be influenced by the generation of genomic information: prioritization of contaminants and contaminated sites, monitoring, reporting requirements, and risk assessment. EPA acknowledged this in its 2004 report *Potential Implications of Genomics for Regulatory and Risk Assessment Applications at EPA,* prepared by the Genomics Task Force Workgroup of EPA's Science Policy Council (SPC; U.S. Environmental Protection Agency, 2004c). As EPA notes, "understanding genomic responses with respect to adverse ecological and/or human health outcomes is far from established."[2]

Accordingly, the application of genomic data any time soon for any regulatory standard-setting purpose, and the use of gene expression data to classify toxic and nontoxic effects, would seem unwise, if not entirely premature. Nonetheless, despite their nascent stage of development, the temptation to use these data early will be hard to resist, and undoubtedly some will succumb. To benefit from the full potential of genomic data, many scientific challenges need to be overcome.

Outlined below are selected illustrations of the types of challenges that agencies and stakeholders in human and ecological health areas can expect to confront when using genomic data in regulatory settings. No attempt is made here to put too fine a point on whether these challenges are fundamentally "legal," "regulatory," or "attitudinal" in nature.

Information Quality and Peer Review

A threshold issue for all federal agencies is the weight toxicogenomic data and related information should be given in regulatory and federal decision-making contexts. The EPA SPC's Genomics Task Force was formed expressly to explore the broader implications genomics is expected to have for EPA programs and policies and to attempt to gain "further understanding of the appropriate usage of these data and the potential consequences of their use, as well as to identify possible infrastructure needs."[3]

EPA's consideration of the use of genomic information generally must be guided by and consistent with a broader federal mandate required under the Information Quality Act (IQA), a federal law directing all federal agencies to ensure and maximize the quality, objectivity, utility, and integrity of the information they disseminate.[4]

How exactly EPA and other agencies will evaluate the quality, objectivity, utility, and integrity of genomic data and information against the emerging body of legal precedent developed under the IQA is a matter of considerable significance and uncertainty. Set forth below are a few thoughts as to why this is.

As a one-sentence rider to an appropriations bill, the IQA is unlike other federal laws. It has no legislative history, and its scant language has been the subject of a great deal of commentary and speculation to the point that tea leaf reading skills are in high demand. The IQA directs the Office of Management and Budget (OMB), and ultimately the Office of Information and Regulatory Affairs (OIRA) at OMB, to provide guidance on exactly what Congress meant by the one-sentence law.[5]

OMB issued government-wide guidelines regarding how to implement the IQA in interim form in 2001[6] and in final form in 2002.[7] In general, the guidelines provide a "basic standard of quality . . . as a performance goal" and require agencies to develop predissemination review procedures, to report certain information annually to OMB, and to establish a petition process enabling aggrieved parties to correct information that they believe does not comply with OMB or agency guidelines implementing the IQA.

More recently, OMB issued its *Final Information Quality Bulletin for Peer Review* on December 15, 2004 (U.S. Office of Management and Budget, 2004). The final bulletin sets forth minimum requirements for peer reviewing scientific information and stricter minimum requirements for the peer review of "highly influential scientific assessments" disseminated by the federal government. As a rule, each agency must conduct a peer review of all influential scientific information that it intends to disseminate. In assessing the adequacy of a peer review, each agency must give due consideration to "the novelty and complexity of the science to be reviewed, the importance of the information to decision making, the extent of prior peer reviews, and the expected benefits and costs of additional review."[8] The bulletin's forty-one pages provide much more explicit guidance on specific issues, including peer review mechanisms; selection of peer reviewers; and how to assess and ensure balance, independence, and transparency.

Of particular relevance is the bulletin's insistence on additional peer review requirements for "highly influential scientific assessments." These are assessments that "could have a potential impact of more than $500 million in any year" or are "novel, controversial, or precedent-setting or [have] significant interagency interest."[9] The bulletin defines a "scientific assessment" as an "evaluation of a body of scientific or technical knowledge, which typically synthesizes multiple factual inputs, data, models, assumptions, and/or applies best professional judgment to bridge uncertainties in the available information."[10] Peer reviews of highly influential scientific assessments are considered by OMB to be most rigorous and leave less consideration regarding the form of peer review to the agency's discretion. Other, more rigorous, conditions also apply to highly influential scientific assessments regarding the composition of the peer review panels and opportunity for public comment.[11]

Genomic Data and Peer Review

EPA's initial and ongoing forays into initiatives that rely on gene expression data for regulatory purposes would seem almost certain to trigger the most stringent level of peer review. At face value, this seems like an entirely logical and appropriate result. Application of these standards in practice, however, raises challenging questions. For example, it is not clear whether EPA program offices are applying guidelines found in the bulletin or how each office is actually interpreting and applying the standards set out under the bulletin for "influential scientific information" and "highly influential" scientific assessments with the context of their respective federal enabling statutes and the regulatory frameworks that have evolved under each. Nor is it clear whether the decision-making process used to make these selections is applied uniformly among program offices, and if not, why not.

One recent EPA action illustrates the challenges the agency faces in this regard. EPA's Office of Pesticide Programs (OPP), the program office charged with implementing the Federal Insecticide, Rodenticide, and Fungicide Act (FIFRA), reportedly relied on several published articles involving genomic information in response to a data package submitted to OPP by a FIFRA registrant to support a pesticide product registration. The data were submitted "to propose an alternative mode of action that would affect human health assessment conclusions."[12]

This event is significant for several reasons and illustrates the difficulty of applying the bulletin's peer review framework to scientific decisions routinely made by EPA program offices. First, that EPA's OPP may have accepted and relied on genomic information in confirming an alternative mode of action (MOA) for a pesticide is noteworthy in itself. It is not clear from the reference in the Genomics Task Force white paper what the alternative MOA involved, or on what genomics data EPA may have relied in making its decision. That such data were used in a regulatory decision-making context involving a pesticide is significant given the nature of the data and that the data were used to support an alternative MOA theory.

Second, it is not clear what standard of peer review OPP applied. OPP may have considered the information "influential scientific information," a standard most deferential to the agency intending to disseminate the information. It may have considered the information "highly influential," in which case a more rigorous peer review standard would apply. Nor is it clear how OPP went about deciding which category of scientific information the MOA data fell within for purposes of peer review, or even whether, as a threshold matter, the bulletin applies to information that is disseminated as part of a FIFRA registration. Under the bulletin, agencies need not peer review information that is "disseminated in the course of an individual agency adjudication or permit proceeding (including a registration . . .), unless the agency determines that peer review is practical and appropriate and that the influential dissemination is scientifically or technically novel or likely to have precedent-setting influence on future adjudications and/or permit proceedings."[13]

Assuming either EPA determined that the bulletin applied, or EPA determined that dissemination of the information was likely to have precedent-setting influence and waived the exemption, it is unclear whether EPA's apparent reliance on the registrant-supplied genomic data conferred on them the status of "influential scientific information," thus subjecting them to more rigorous peer review. Presumably, because the genomic data were included in published articles, they were peer reviewed in some fashion. It is not clear, however, whether the peer review given them for publication purposes would be considered sufficiently robust and at a level of scrutiny commensurate with the level contemplated under the OMB bulletin.

Similarly, it is not clear whether OPP's scientific assessment of the registrant-submitted genomic data constituted a "highly influential scientific assessment" triggering the highest level of peer review. Given the limited information available, it is not possible to assess whether the registration decision, whether favorable or not from the registrant's perspective, had a potential impact of 500 million dollars in any year or was deemed sufficiently "novel, controversial, or precedent-setting" to trigger the standard of peer review reserved for highly influential scientific assessments. Again, the application of these criteria to any fact pattern raises many questions at each step of the analysis, but absent more specific information, we can only speculate as to the thought process that was used ultimately to enable OPP comfortably to rely on these data for regulatory purposes.

Of interest is the lack of transparency regarding the process for making this one, discrete OPP decision, which is not especially isolated or uncharacteristic of EPA's implementation of the spirit, if not the letter, of OIRA's many missives implementing the IQA. Indeed, it is not clear in most cases whether and, if so, how EPA's various program offices have taken to heart the dictates of OMB's various bulletins and guidelines issued under the IQA. This is disconcerting, particularly given OMB's many efforts incentivizing federal agency transparency through requests for correction petitions, Web postings, reporting obligations, and other avenues of information correction made available under the IQA. As noted, the registration process is more in the spirit of an individual permit proceeding and thus less amenable to traditional disclosure mechanisms. Nonetheless, to the extent the registration and reregistration of chemicals regulated under FIFRA invite some of the most challenging and controversial intersections of science policy and law, it is interesting that the disciplined application of IQA policies and procedures is as fluid as it is seven years after IQA's enactment.

Resolution of these issues, and related others, is an open question under the bulletin. As federal agencies begin to use and rely on genomic data for regulatory purposes, as they are expected to do in the years to come, questions almost certainly will arise regarding whether the high standards of the bulletin have been met. Similarly, private parties need to think carefully about the implications of submitting genomic data to federal agencies for regulatory purposes and of IQA policies when designing and implementing research initiatives to support product registrations and approvals and about the impact of these policies on other scientific data generated in connection with regulatory outcomes. How these questions will be answered, and in what forum, is anyone's guess.

Genomic Data and Adverse Effects Reporting

Another vexing question of particular concern to chemical producers relates to the lack of adequate EPA guidance on the relevance of genomic data for reporting purposes under the Toxic Substances Control Act (TSCA) section 8(e) and its counterpart under FIFRA section 6(a)(2). This lack of guidance has been noted repeatedly in articles over the past several years, but is now perhaps even more compelling in light of EPA's enforcement actions filed in 2004 against E.I. DuPont de Nemours and Company (DuPont) under TSCA section 8(e)[14] and more recent claims asserted against 3M Company for violations of TSCA section 8(e) and related TSCA provisions.[15] The enforcement actions filed against DuPont in particular, and DuPont's subsequent settlement of them, broke new ground on several fronts.[16] Among the concerns raised by EPA's allegations are how an adverse effect is defined for purposes of section 8(e) reporting obligations and the potential liability a company might face for establishing a voluntary internal standard.

Under TSCA section 8(e), any person who manufactures, imports, processes, or distributes a chemical substance or mixture, and who obtains information that reasonably supports the conclusion that the chemical substance or mixture poses a substantial risk of injury to human beings or the environment, must provide the information to EPA immediately.[17] EPA's policy on section 8(e) reporting addresses two types of reportable information—human health effects information and environmental contamination. EPA's policy identifies the human health effects that warrant reporting as follows:

> The Agency considers effects for which substantial-risk information should be reported to include the following.
>
> (a) *Human health effects.* (1) Any instance of cancer, birth defects, mutagenicity, death, or serious or prolonged incapacitation, including the loss of or inability to use a normal bodily function with a consequent relatively serious impairment of normal activities, if one (or a few) chemical(s) is strongly implicated.
>
> (2) Any pattern of effects or evidence which reasonably supports the conclusion that the chemical substance or mixture can produce cancer, mutation, birth defects or toxic effects resulting in death, or serious or prolonged incapacitation.[18]

EPA identifies in its policy the nonemergency situations involving environmental contamination that warrant reporting:[19]

> The agency considers effects for which substantial-risk information should be reported to include the following. . . .
>
> (b) Non-emergency situations involving environmental contamination; environmental effects—(1) Non-emergency situations of chemical contamination involving humans and/or the environment. Information that pertains to widespread and previously unsuspected distribution in environmental media of a chemical substance or mixture known to cause serious adverse effects, when coupled with information that widespread or significant exposure to humans or non-human organisms has occurred or that there is a substantial likelihood that such exposure will occur, is subject to reporting. The mere presence of a chemical in an environmental media, absent the additional information noted above, would not trigger reporting under section 8(e). Information concerning the detection of chemical substances contained within appropriate disposal facilities such as treatment, storage and disposal facilities permitted under RCRA should not be reported under this part.[20]

To fall within the type of environmental effect information that is reportable under TSCA, the information must pertain to "widespread" and
"previously unsuspected distribution in environmental media." As anyone familiar with TSCA will attest, there has been an abundance of con-
fusion regarding the application of section 8(e) reporting obligations to
contaminated media. EPA has sought to clarify its position through various Q & A documents and in other contexts, but on the whole, the area
is not a paradigm of regulatory clarity.

The DuPont Case and Adverse Effects Reporting: Hints of the Future?

Enter the DuPont case, which dealt with DuPont's use of the chemical perfluorooctanoic acid (PFOA). All of the alleged TSCA violations
pertain to data relating to this especially controversial molecule, which
has been the subject of significant EPA regulatory attention since data
were first released showing a general background level of five parts per
billion (ppb) in the blood of the U.S. population. Because PFOA has been
associated with certain adverse effects, including cancer and reproductive toxicity, knowledge that just about everyone's bodily fluids contain
detectable levels of PFOA was not great news.

The nature of the government's allegations against DuPont sent shock
waves throughout chemical producers because these allegations represented the first time EPA took the position that a company's exceedance
of a voluntarily set company exposure guideline can be TSCA section
8(e) reportable, even if the information does not show an exceedance of
a government-set exposure standard and even when small or minor ex-
ceedances of government-set standards may generally not be reportable.
EPA also alleged that DuPont's failure to report the placental transfer of
PFOA, information known to EPA long before the DuPont case, was ac-
tionable under TSCA section 8(e). This allegation raised questions concerning the circumstances under which the mere presence of a chemical
in bodily fluids might be considered a reportable event under TSCA section 8(e), even when no effect other than the presence has been asserted.
In the DuPont case, EPA alleged facts that tied the presence of PFOA in
blood to the defined dose determined in the contaminated drinking water of those whose blood samples were at issue and made broader state-

ments that could signal a future new approach to determining the re-
portability of biomonitoring data.

Many have expressed concern that EPA's position as inferred from the
allegations in the DuPont cases could discourage the development and
adoption of internal health and safety standards that are more restrictive
than government-established standards. Similarly, the allegation of placental transfer of PFOA raises new issues regarding traditional interpretations
of what constitutes a "significant adverse effect" for purposes of TSCA section 8(e) reporting and precisely when information is already known to
EPA. Because EPA and DuPont settled their differences, the appropriateness and legality of EPA's interpretation of TSCA section 8(e) under the circumstances presented in the DuPont cases will not be further litigated.

Nonetheless, the case is useful in that it illustrates the pressing need
for greater clarity regarding the application of TSCA section 8(e) to genomic information, as well as the growing body of information deriva-
tive of a wide range of emerging technologies including, for example,
genomics and nanotechnologies. In its *Interim Policy on Genomics,* EPA
encouraged and supported continued genomic research, clarified that genomic data alone are "insufficient as a basis for decisions," and stated
that changes in gene expression "can be informative when a weight-of-
evidence approach for human and ecological health assessments is performed" (U.S. Environmental Protection Agency, 2002, p. 2). It remains
unclear, however, how EPA will interpret genomic information, under
what specific circumstances might these data be reportable, and whether
new interpretations and guidance are necessary to fulfill the congressional goals that inspired these statutory reporting obligations. It is also
unclear whether EPA will communicate these new interpretations in the
context of enforcement actions or other, less contentious and perhaps
more interactive and productive venues. The *Interim Policy on Genomics*
is correctly termed "interim," properly telegraphing EPA's desire for flex-
ibility and timeliness, as EPA and other stakeholders continue to assess
the biological relevance of genomics and the utility of genomic information in regulatory contexts. Nonetheless, the interim policy is short on
detail with respect to the relevance of genomic data and the circumstances under which such data may be deemed reportable, particularly
when read against the backdrop of the DuPont cases.

Better guidance would help address growing concerns with the lack
of clarity of EPA's evolving legal position in this area and provide much-

needed clarity. In the Genomics Task Force white paper, EPA wisely observes that "there is a need to interpret how these TSCA and FIFRA provisions apply to genomics data. . . . As the predictability and validity of genomics methods increase, EPA may need to re-evaluate its stance on these reporting provisions."[21] EPA might pick up the Food and Drug Administration's (FDA) lead. FDA issued guidance in November 2003 entitled *Guidance for Industry Pharmacogenomic Data Submissions.* The guidance is "intended to facilitate scientific progress in the field of pharmacogenomics and to facilitate the use of pharmacogenomic data in informing regulatory decisions" (U.S. Food and Drug Administration, 2003, p. 1). The guidance notes that study sponsors are subject to FDA requirements that were developed before the advent of genetic or gene expression testing and thus "do not specifically address when such data should be submitted."[22] The guidance is offered to bridge the gap and assist "in advancing the field in a manner that will benefit both drug development programs and public health."[23] EPA may wish to consider developing such guidance with interested stakeholders.

The Need for Collaboration

EPA's Science Advisory Board (SAB) convened a workshop on December 1–2, 2004, entitled *Nanotechnology, Biotechnology, and Information Technology: Implications for Future Science at EPA.*[24] The workshop was convened to enable SAB members to "learn more about recent developments in nanotechnology, biotechnology and information technology [and] to educate and inform the SAB, so that it may better understand the potential applications and implications of these technologies for science and research programs at EPA."[25] It is good that the SAB is focusing on these matters, and the workshop yielded many constructive suggestions regarding how best to proceed in these challenging areas (Science Advisory Board, 2005).

The Need for New Paradigms to Assess Risks and Benefits of Emerging Technologies

Among the many useful comments repeated over the course of the two-day meeting were statements expressing the importance of and the need to disseminate scientific information. Also, the need for EPA and others to consider "new paradigms" was discussed, not only how to develop consensus on what is an adverse effect based on genomic data but also how to ensure that legal and regulatory conventions keep pace with scientific and technological advances. There is legitimate concern that the legal, regulatory, and administrative process, and the ethical considerations that must inform how genomic data will be used and interpreted in legal and regulatory contexts, are simply not proceeding at a pace that will fulfill the promise of these data.

EPA's Genomics Task Force suggested that EPA's reevaluation of adverse effects reporting may be "best approached in a multi-stakeholder process to ensure scientific consensus around the understanding of adverse effects based on genomics data."[26] This suggestion would seem to be equally relevant to many other areas in which consensus would appear to be both necessary and desirable. For example, *standardization* and *validation* are terms and concepts that mean different things to different people. The need for scientific consensus, however, is critical to paving the way for use of genomic data in regulatory contexts.

The urgent need for better consensus-building mechanisms is similarly apparent in other areas, particularly in assessing the human health and environmental consequences of other transformative technologies, including nanotechnology, biotechnology, and cognitive sciences that are related to this technology. The lightning speed of technological developments in these areas stands in sharp contrast to the glacial pace at which conventional government premarket review of new products proceeds. How these emerging technologies converge and the consequences of this convergence on our legal and regulatory infrastructure invite the very real concern that our infrastructure is ill prepared to accommodate what is coming down the road.

To unlock the true potential of genomic data, many scientific challenges need to be resolved. Equally important, however, are the challenges confronting the legal, regulatory, ethical, and policy communities to develop consensus-driven frameworks within which genomic data can be interpreted and applied in legal settings. These same frameworks, or at the least the process used to develop them, hold promise to help ensure that our legal and regulatory infrastructure will be able to address the many issues posed by other emerging transformative technologies, such as nanotechnology, in a timely fashion, and not represent a delay to the many benefits these scientific advances offer society.

NOTES

1. Marchant, 2003a, 10071; Marchant, 2003b, 10641; Science Advisory Board, 2005, Grodsky, 2005, 171.

2. U.S. Environmental Protection Agency (EPA), 2004c, vii.

3. Ibid., 1.

4. Pub. L. No. 106-554; § 515(a), 114 Stat. 2763, 2763A, 153-154 (2000).

5. Ibid.

6. 66 *Fed. Reg.* 49718 (Sept. 28, 2001).

7. 67 *Fed. Reg.* 8452 (Feb. 22, 2002).

8. U.S. Office of Management and Budget (OMB), 2004, 35.

9. Ibid., 36.

10. Ibid., 35.

11. Ibid., 36–38.

12. EPA, 2004c, 4.

13. OMB, 2004, 40.

14. EPA, 2004a, 2004b.

15. *In Re 3M Company,* Docket Number TSCA-HQ-2006-5004, available at www.epa.gov/compliance/resources/cases/civil/tsca/3m.html. In this case, EPA claimed, among the 244 counts against 3M, that 3M failed to provide timely information required under TSCA section 8(e).

16. The first complaint includes two violations of TSCA section 8(e) and one violation of the Resource Conservation and Recovery Act (RCRA). EPA alleges that DuPont's failure to submit toxicological information it obtained regarding perfluorooctanoic acid (PFOA) used in the manufacturing process for fluropolymers at its Washington Works facility in West Virginia violates provisions in the Company's RCRA Corrective Action Permit. See *In Re E.I. du Pont de Nemours and Company,* TSCA-HQ-2004-0016, RCRA-HQ-2004-0016 (July 8, 2004) (First Complaint), available at www.epa.gov/compliance/ resources/complaints/civil/ mm/dupont-pfoa-complaint.pdf. The second complaint alleges an additional TSCA section 8(e) violation for failing to report the results of a blood serum analysis. *In Re E.I. du Pont de Nemours and Company,* TSCA-HQ-2005-5001 (December 6, 2004), Complaint and Notice of Opportunity for Hearing, available at www.epa.gov/compliance/resources/complaints/civil/mm/dupont2-pfoa-complaint.pdf (Second Complaint).

17. TSCA § 8(e), 15 U.S.C. § 2607(e).

18. 68 *Fed. Reg.* 33129, 33138 (June 3, 2003).

19. EPA requirements governing emergency incidents of environmental contamination are not addressed here.

20. 68 *Fed. Reg.,* 33138. Four other types of "environmental effects" also are identified by EPA as effects for which substantial-risk information should be reported, including measurements and indicators of pronounced bioaccumulation, ecologically significant changes in species' interrelationships, and facile transfor-

mation or degradation to a chemical having an unacceptable risk (68 *Fed. Reg.*, 33138). Effects related to the environment do not appear applicable to measurements of worker blood or to workplace air concentrations, nor are we aware based on our review of any instance in which EPA has asserted a different conclusion.

21. EPA, 2004c, 15.

22. Ibid., 2.

23. U.S. Food and Drug Administration (FDA), 2003, 2.

24. 69 *Fed. Reg.* 65428 (Nov. 12, 2004).

25. Ibid.

26. EPA, 2004c, 15.

REFERENCES

Grodsky, J.A. 2005. Genetics and environmental law: Redefining public health, *California Law Review* 93:171.

Marchant, G.E. 2003a. Genomics and toxic substances: Part I—Toxicogenomics. *Environmental Law Review* 33:10071.

Marchant, G.E. 2003b. Genomics and toxic substances: Part II—Toxicogenetics. *Environmental Law Review* 33:10641.

Science Advisory Board. 2005. *Nanotechnology, biotechnology, and information technology: Implications for future science at EPA.* Washington, DC: U.S. Environmental Protection Agency.

U.S. Environmental Protection Agency. 2002. *Interim policy on genomics.* At www.epa.gov/osa/spc/pdfs/genomics.pdf.

U.S. Environmental Protection Agency. 2004a. "EPA press advisory: EPA files new claim alleging DuPont withheld PFOA information" (Dec. 6, 2004).

U.S. Environmental Protection Agency. 2004b. "EPA press advisory: EPA takes enforcement action against DuPont for toxic substances reporting violations" (July 8, 2004).

U.S. Environmental Protection Agency. 2004c. *Potential implications of genomics for regulatory and risk assessment applications at EPA* (Genomics Task Force White Paper). At www.epa.gov/OSA/genomics.htm.

U.S. Food and Drug Administration. 2003. *Guidance for industry pharmacogenomic data submissions.* At www.fda.gov/cder/guidance/5900dft.pdf.

U.S. Office of Management and Budget. 2004. *Final information quality bulletin for peer veview* (Final Bulletin). At www.whitehouse.gov/omb/inforeg/peer 2004/peer_ bulletin.pdf.

CHAPTER 6

Genetic Data and Toxic Torts

Intimations of Statistical Reductionism

ANDREW ASKLAND AND GARY E. MARCHANT

Rapid advances in our knowledge about genomics are affecting many areas of legal policy and practice. This knowledge encompasses the structure and function of genes and their products and also the impacts of genes on conditions and behavior. The condition component includes both etiological accounts for how conditions arise and predictions about avoiding harmful outcomes and promoting beneficial outcomes.

The etiological studies are important for tort law because they affect its ability to causally link conduct that may be tortious to detrimental effects on individuals who were exposed to apparently dangerous substances. The matters considered controversial include what level of exposure occurred, what level of exposure can cause harm generally or caused harm to a particular plaintiff, and also what role genetic susceptibility plays in assessing arguably wrongful conduct and apparently harmful consequences. In short, can we prove that this substance causes harm in general, that it caused harm to this plaintiff, and that the harm it caused is better explained by the defendant's actions than by the plaintiff's special genetic vulnerabilities?

The focus is the interaction of substances that the defendant controls with the genes of the plaintiff, which may demonstrate the level of her exposure, the impact of that exposure on her health, and her special susceptibilities to the substance to which she was exposed. As to the susceptibility question, many substances are dangerous for all who are exposed if the level of exposure is sufficiently high but are dangerous to only a smaller number of genetically vulnerable people at lower exposures. We are concerned with the combination of a polymorphism (or particular genetic variation) and an occupational or environmental exposure that together increase the risk of illness. These combinations are the focus of much current toxicological research, both with regard to the expression of genes in response to exposure to a toxic substance (toxicogenomics) and the identification of genetic variations affecting susceptibility to these toxic substances (toxicogenetics).

Potential Uses of Genomic Data

One major application of genomic data for toxic torts is gene expression data and other types of biomarkers, including proteomics and metabolomics. DNA microarrays increasingly will be used to monitor the expression of genes in response to toxic agents. Gene expression patterns may provide signature profiles of specific toxicants or mechanisms of effects. Another major application concerns susceptibility genes. Genetic polymorphisms affect susceptibility to exposure to toxic substances via variations in processes such as xenobiotic metabolism and detoxification, DNA repair, and receptors. This chapter considers various uses of these two types of data in toxic tort cases in which one or more individuals (the plaintiffs) seek compensation for injuries allegedly resulting from toxic exposures created by a business or governmental entity (the defendant). Gene expression data are relevant to issues in general causation, specific causation, quantifying exposure, demonstrating absence of exposure, medical monitoring, and duty to test. Susceptibility gene data are relevant to issues of specific causation, duty to warn, idiosyncratic defenses, assumption of risk, alternative causation, multiple causation, damages, and class certification. We shall consider these issues seriatim.

Gene Expression Data and Toxic Torts

A recurring problem for plaintiffs in toxic tort suits is proving causation, that is, that the substance to which the plaintiff has been exposed does in fact cause harm (general causation) and did in fact cause that harm in this particular plaintiff (specific causation). Many plaintiffs struggle to demonstrate that a particular quantity of exposure has occurred and then, even if they have demonstrated a sufficient level of exposure, that it could have caused their illness. In other words, plaintiffs fail to demonstrate that the toxic agent has the potential to cause the health condition that is the foundation of their complaint. To meet their burden of proving this general causation, plaintiffs must introduce reliable scientific evidence that the specific toxic agent they were exposed to causes the specific ailment for which they seek compensation.

Gene expression data may provide a tool that can assist plaintiffs in showing this. The specificity of gene expression data will enable reasonable extrapolations from known toxicological impacts to the toxic agents and gene expression evidence in the plaintiff's case. For example, a plaintiff may be able to use similarities in gene expression patterns to argue that the toxic substance the plaintiff was exposed to is likely to have similar toxicological properties to another chemical known to cause the health effect in question. In other words, where there is a lack of data linking the specific chemical and health endpoints at issue in a specific case, toxicogenomic data may be able to provide an evidentiary bridge to link to more favorable data sets for similar chemicals or endpoints.

Toxicogenomic data may be able to provide direct evidence of specific causation. Currently, there is generally no way to reliably ascertain whether a toxic agent caused a particular illness in a specific individual, because there are usually other potential alternative factors that could have caused the same condition. As a result, the courts rely on crude statistical assumptions or methods such as differential diagnosis, which are highly uncertain and controversial. By providing chemical-specific biomarkers of exposure within a given individual, gene expression and other toxicogenomic data have the potential to provide, for the first time, individualized evidence of causation.

Gene expression data can also help quantify the plaintiff's exposure (i.e., it may provide a quantitative dosimeter of exposure). In an important case, *In re TMI Litigation* (1999), plaintiffs alleged radiation induced neoplasms as a result of ionizing radiation released during the Three Mile Island incident, which was a partial meltdown of a nuclear reactor in Middletown, Pennsylvania, on March 28, 1979. However, they lacked data quantifying their exposure from the radiation. They instead relied on "biological indicators of radiation dose" in the form of a chromosomal rearrangement known as a dicentric chromosome. The court held that the dicentric chromosomes did provide a valid and reliable dosimeter of exposure, but that they were not stable and hence unreliable fifteen years after the exposure. The court held that the evidence was admissible and scientifically reliable, but, because it was offered by the plaintiff's expert so long after exposure, it lacked the certainty of a professional judgment.

The *TMI* court did find that the measurements of chromosomal translocations using fluorescence in situ hybridization (FISH) would provide a "valid and reliable scientific methodology" to support the plaintiffs, but the plaintiffs failed to provide timely evidence using that method. Another plaintiff's expert adduced a causal connection between hypothetical quantities of radionuclides released during the accident and the plaintiffs' neoplasms but provided no evidence that the hypothetical releases had actually occurred. Without admissible evidence quantifying their exposure, the plaintiffs' case was dismissed. Notwithstanding the adverse outcome for the specific plaintiffs in this case, the court's decision sets a precedent that genetic biomarkers of exposure can be used to quantify exposures provided they are collected within a reasonable time of the exposure.

Gene expression data can also be used to assist defendants, who can rely on the absence of a characteristic genetic expression response to argue the lack of exposure or causation. If the plaintiff alleges an exposure to a particular toxin and we know that that toxin produces a characteristic toxicogenomic signature, then the absence of such a response in the plaintiff would be evidence against exposure and causation. This was the case in *Wells v. Shell Oil Co.*, where a worker alleged that he had contracted acute myelogenous leukemia (AML) from exposure to benzene at his worksite (Expert Testimony, 1998). The defendants successfully argued that benzene produces AML only with breaks in chromosomes 5 and 7 and that the plaintiff did not have those breaks. The impact of this expectation that plaintiffs link their alleged harm with evidence of damage to their genome at the chromosome site where the exposure is known to exert its effect could be enormous. It would likely become standard practice for plaintiffs to submit to tests of their genome either before they file their complaints or, at the behest of the defendant, shortly thereafter.

Gene expression data may help plaintiffs who seek funds for medical monitoring of their health subsequent to an exposure to a toxic substance. Some states do permit the recovery of costs for medical monitoring of exposed plaintiffs in limited circumstances. However, such claims are often rejected because medically effective screening tests are generally lacking. There is a reluctance to order monitoring when it is not clear that the monitoring will produce an actual benefit (i.e., identify changes in the plaintiff's condition that are relevant to the exposure). For example, in 2001 a West Virginia court rejected a claim made by the smoker plaintiffs for periodic medical surveillance using a new diagnostic lung test (a spiral CT scan; *In re Tobacco Litigation,* 2004). At least part of the explanation for this result lies in the uncertainty about the reliability of the test and the link between its results and the harm caused by the defendant. The capability to link medically significant gene expression changes with exposures attributed to the defendants will make medical monitoring a more plausible and therefore more common plaintiff remedy.

The increasing availability and accuracy of gene expression data will support arguments that employers who use toxic substances in their workplaces may have a duty to test their employees for exposure. The more reliable the tests (i.e., the better they track toxic exposures in workers), the stronger the argument that these tests do provide a demonstrable benefit to employees. Such tests are intrusive and a program of testing requires care in its implementation, but it would appear that the potential value of the data that the tests generate in support of early detection and treatment will spur support for their adoption. Indeed, the growing sentiment that the tests are a prudent measure may support the contention that there is a duty to test. In what may be a portent of things to come, a widow of a Dow Chemical worker who died of leukemia brought suit claiming that Dow was negligent for not conducting cytogenetic tests of its workers (Olafson, 2000). Her suit was buoyed by the fact that Dow had previously conducted such tests but discontinued them in 1980 in response to widespread criticism.

Several challenges and limitations will affect the adoption of gene expression data in toxic tort settings. A logistical challenge concerns the different microarrays that are currently in use. There is not yet a consensus about standards for microarrays, and there may be some initial difficulties comparing data from these different microarrays. These difficulties should work clear as the properties and comparable strengths of the several approaches manifest themselves, and significant progress has been made in this regard in the past few years.

Another challenge to gene expression data will arise from the different values of that data. Gene expression data will vary across different species, different tissues within a species, different developmental stages of a species, and different time courses. These differences are clearly relevant to the validation of the studies that rely on these different values to generate and test hypotheses. Over time the differences will even out as more studies will permit the collation of results across these differences and substantiate hypotheses that accommodate data value differences. However, that understanding will accumulate over time and early efforts to cite gene expression data may fail because the fact-finder (or the judge considering the admissibility of the evidence) is not persuaded the extrapolations are justified for use between species or between different tissues of the same species or between different time courses of the same tissue of the same species.

The most critical issue in the short term is the temporal variability and pattern of gene-expression changes (Marchant, 2002). Most gene expression data analyzed to date involve short-term responses to toxic insults, usually consisting of data collected within forty-eight hours of exposure (Freeman, 2004). It will be a difficult challenge to extrapolate these results to long-term, chronic exposures that are more typical for toxic tort plaintiffs. As the *TMI* litigation discussed above demonstrates, courts are likely to be skeptical of biomarker data collected beyond the time period that has been validated as producing reliable results. Because of this problem, toxicogenomic data will likely first be useful in toxic tort litigation involving acute exposures where biological samples are collected for analysis within a day or so of exposure. This will require potential plaintiffs to have the awareness to immediately contact lawyers who are attuned to the availability and limitations of gene expression data promptly after exposure to ensure timely samples are collected.

Related to this challenge are problems of data management, analysis, and presentation. The gene expression studies and their results are not designed to serve as evidence for tort litigation. Their designs are a function of more tightly circumscribed problems and hypotheses, all of which bear on the growing significance of gene expression data, but most of which are not coordinated as a single research program. The problem is that there are thousands and thousands of data points in these studies. How does one sort and coordinate this huge volume of data in order to understand its significance? The variability makes it difficult to phrase a unitary account about how the disparate pieces are in fact supporting the same theme. It is a familiar problem: a surfeit of information and a scarcity of means to systematize, cross-reference, and evaluate that information.

The cumulative challenge is identifying when the approach is ready for adoption. There is a growing recognition of the relevance of gene expression data. The issue is what criteria should be recognized to frame the threshold for sanctioning the use of that data in toxic tort cases. Given the way the common law tradition works, it is likely that the introduction and use of this data in toxic tort litigation will be incremental and piecemeal. Consistent with the virtues of an incremental adoption, it would be helpful if a combination of scientists and lawyers phrased the relevant issues that should be addressed as conditions precedent to the wide-scale use of gene expression data so that courts and the parties before them could better anticipate their use (Marchant, 2006).

Susceptibility Genes and Toxic Torts

The second category of genomic information that is important for toxic torts is susceptibility genes. Generally speaking, there are two types of susceptibility genes: those that increase the risk of disease in everyone with that gene (e.g., the breast cancer gene *BRCA1*) and those that increase the risk of disease only in the presence of a triggering exposure. For this second type, though the genes are associated with an altered risk of developing a disease, the presence of the gene alone is not sufficient to cause the disease. Whereas gene expression data focus on the relationship between exposure to a toxic substance and genetic evidence of that exposure, susceptibility gene research is focusing on the probabilities that a particular gene makes its possessor especially vulnerable to a disease, especially a disease triggered by a toxic substance. As with gene expression data, there are several potential applications of genetic susceptibility data in toxic tort litigation.

The first issue is specific causation. Many courts require plaintiffs to prove that exposure results in a doubling of the background risk, such that the exposure was "more likely than not" the cause of the harm. The question is relative risk for whom, the general population or an identifiable subpart of that population with a genetic susceptibility that has a higher relative risk from exposure than the general population. If we cannot identify those with special vulnerabilities, then we may be justified in considering them as part of the larger pool of subjects. However, if we can identify them and if we know their specific vulnerabilities, are we justified in ignoring that known vulnerability?

The district court in *In re Hanford Nuclear Reservation Litigation* (1998) required the plaintiffs to demonstrate a doubling of risk attributable to exposure. Although the court of appeals subsequently overturned this part of the district court's holding (*In re Hanford Nuclear Reservation Litigation*, 2002), the district court's treatment of genetic susceptibility data remains a leading example of how courts are likely to view such data. The plaintiff's expert in the *Hanford* case added a fivefold genetic susceptibility factor for radiation in calculating the "doubling dose," which is the level of exposure the plaintiff must demonstrate to satisfy the more likely-than-not standard of proof. The court rejected this attempt because it concluded, first, that there was no method to identify those who are at increased risk and, second, that not everyone is genetically susceptible. The implication of this decision is that genetic susceptibility can assist a plaintiff's causation proof, but only for plaintiffs who show that they actually carry the relevant susceptibility gene. As another example, some silicone breast implant plaintiffs alleged that a genetic variant conferred susceptibility to silicone in order to argue that they may have been harmed by silicone leaking from their implants despite epidemiologic studies that show no significant increase in disease associated with silicone breast implants in the general population (*Hall v. Baxter*, 1996; Marchant, 2001).

Another issue is whether product manufacturers have a duty to warn or recommend genetic testing for genetically susceptible product users. If it is clear that a particular class of individuals has a special vulnerability that is affected by the manufacturer's product and that class of individuals can be identified, assuming that the effect crosses a relevant threshold of significance, arguably there should be a duty to warn product users that they can be harmed by the use of the product. *Cassidy v. SmithKline Beecham Corp* (2003) is a class action suit that alleged the LYMErix vaccine contains a protein (OSPA) that produces autoimmune arthritis in individuals with *HLA-DR4k* genotype (which is approximately 30% of the population). The complaint alleged that drug manufacturers have a duty to warn drug users of susceptibility gene responses and to advise drug users to obtain genetic tests prior to a vaccination. The case eventually settled before going to trial, shortly after LYMErix was taken off the market (Marchant, 2001).

In another recent case, *Easter v. Aventis Pasteur* (2005), the plaintiffs alleged that thimerosal, a mercury preservative in the defendant's vaccines, caused their son's autism. The plaintiffs contended that "some children are genetically susceptible to mercury poisoning and cannot excrete or otherwise eliminate the mercury in the vaccine preservative" (p. 575). However, genetic testing revealed that their son did not have the pertinent genetic variant allegedly conferring susceptibility. As the court indicated, the plaintiffs could not prove that the autism was caused by thimerosal because their son did "not meet the genetic profile for children who . . . are at increased risk for developing autism by thimerosal" (p. 576). The genetic test results were decisive for a decision adverse to the plaintiffs, but genetic test results indicating that the child did carry the alleged susceptibility-conferred gene might have produced a very different outcome.

Defendants may be able to avail themselves of an idiosyncratic response defense in toxic tort litigation, arguing that they are not liable for products that harm only genetically hypersusceptible individuals. In *Cavallo v. Star Enterprises* (1996), the plaintiff alleged chronic health problems caused by vapors produced by an underground oil flume. The plaintiff testified that she was "highly susceptible" to these flumes. This hypersensitivity did not have the intended effect of buttressing her claim. Rather, the court held that the company had a duty to protect only against harms "that would be suffered by a normal person" (p. 1154). The company was not liable because its vapors did not harm most of those who were exposed to it.

This idiosyncratic response defense provokes several questions. How do we judge where to cut off responses as idiosyncratic? If it is as easy as drawing a line at a specific percentage of the population, what is the applicable percentage cutoff? Do we limit protections for those who fall into the most vulnerable 10 percent of the population? Should we be concerned about the most vulnerable 5 percent? 3 percent? 0.05 percent? How do we decide when a response counts? If a certain percentage of people are temporarily, but not permanently, harmed by their exposure, do they count for or against the defendant's liability? Is it the workforce that serves as the pool within which we measure idiosyncrasy or the general population in the area where the toxic substance is released? If we opt for the general population as the appropriate reference class, should young children and elderly people (i.e., those who may be especially vulnerable) be included?

One approach imposes an obligation on the producer of toxins to identify and remedy the consequences of exposure to that toxin. An alternative approach articulates the conditions for an assumption of the risk by susceptible individuals who persist in exposing themselves to toxins. For example, approximately 30 percent of the population carries a susceptibility gene (*GLU-69*) for chronic beryllium disease. EPA has very strict standards for beryllium, but those standards are not zero. Very low levels of exposure may harm susceptible individuals. Should individuals who live near beryllium-processing facilities be tested for their susceptibility to beryllium exposure? If they are tested, should they be relocated if they test positive? If they do not relocate because their relocation expenses are not paid for by the company (or with public funds), can we impute to them a judgment to assume the risk of their exposure to beryllium? Should we impose an obligation on companies to pay for testing, relocating, and medical monitoring? Should we instead provide accurate information to affected people (i.e., that they might be susceptible and should seek testing or, having tested positive, that they should identify alternative employment and housing), but defer to their judgment about how to respond to the information? Will our answer change depending on how large the number of affected people is or how risky the exposure is likely to be? Should we limit our recognition of assumption of the risk to instances where there are trade-offs between benefits and costs that would justify reasonable people in accepting a risk because they were receiving (or might receive) a substantial benefit (e.g., employment)?

Susceptibility genes may also benefit defendants by providing alternative explanations for what would otherwise appear to be tortious exposure to a toxic substance. There will likely be instances where a disease is overdetermined (i.e., there are two independent and sufficient causes), and a recovery for tortious conduct is undermined by the nontortious genetic cause. In *Severson v. KTI Chemical,* a pregnant mother was occupationally exposed to a solvent (MEK) and subsequently gave birth to a severely retarded child (Lehrman, 1994). The defendant argued that the child had fragile X syndrome and thus would have been severely retarded aside from any exposure that may have occurred at its worksite. The court ordered genetic testing of the child to assess this alternative genetic explanation of the child's condition. The test results eventually demonstrated that the child did not have the genetic condition alleged, and the case settled on favorable terms for the plaintiff. If the testing had discovered a genetic explanation for the child's condition, the end result would presumably have been favorable to the defendant (Marchant, 2000).

There will likely be instances where the conduct that we observe, which would otherwise justify a judgment about causal responsibility and liability, is countermanded by genetic evidence that provides a wholly sufficient and equally or more persuasive alternative explanation. A recent example is a case brought by plaintiffs alleging that lead paint caused a neurological deficit in their children, a claim that lead paint manufacturers successfully defended by contending that the families were afflicted with familial mild mental retardation, a genetic condition (Byrd, 2006).

Susceptibility genes may also fund reservations about liability when there is multiple causation (i.e., the plaintiff contributed to the harm that she suffers and that contribution is explained in terms of her susceptibility genes). For example, individuals with a variant of the metabolic gene *CYP2E1* are more susceptible to solvents such as trichloroethylene (TCE). The enzyme is induced by ethanol, increasing the risk. The level of alcohol consumption of the susceptible individuals clearly affects their response to exposure to TCE. Should this be considered when an individual claims an injury from TCE exposure in assessing liability or damages? Should alcohol consumption be considered only if it substantially exceeds normal patterns? Does it matter whether we regard the behavior that complicates the plaintiff's susceptibility as abnormal or as a vice? Would we establish different standards for the effects of chronic amphetamine use on genetic susceptibility than for the effects of long-distance running or time before a computer screen or sunbathing?

When defendants are found solely liable for damages to the plaintiff, they may seek to reduce the amount of damages they have to pay if the plaintiff has a genetic disposition to the same or other diseases. The argument is that the plaintiff would not have lived a normal life span, but rather a genetic disposition to the same or some other disease would have resulted in a shorter life, aside from the defendant's conduct. There are precedents for this approach (e.g., a plaintiff with HIV has a diminished life expectancy and that fact has been used to reduce judgment awards to plaintiffs with HIV; *Prettyjohn v. Goodyear,* 1992).

This strategy may have alarming consequences; it may lead to routine requests by defendants for genetic screening of plaintiffs. The motive to undertake such "fishing expeditions" would be particularly strong in cases where the plaintiff otherwise seemed likely to realize a substantial recovery. As the costs of genetic tests fall, defendants might routinely request that plaintiffs submit to them and argue that all identified genetic susceptibilities should be used to discount the damages awarded to the plaintiff. This application of knowledge about susceptibility genes is the clearest instance of statistical reductionism facilitated by the use of genomic information. Debates about judgments and settlements frequently resort to actuarial tables and statistical probabilities to identify a reasonable award for a particular plaintiff. Susceptibility genes might be misapplied as a complete statement of the plaintiff's life prospects. Susceptibilities that are relevant to a person's employment or nutritional and lifestyle choices might play out instead as a definitive statement of that life's course.

Susceptibility genes may also affect class certification. Certification in a class action suit requires a "predominance" of common issues within the class seeking certification. The genetic variation among the petitioners for class certification in a toxic tort action seeking recovery for personal injuries may seriously undermine the claim of those petitioners. The genetic heterogeneity in susceptibility to the defendant's product may be used to argue against the class certification. In *Mahoney v. R.J. Reynolds* (2001), certification of a class of Iowa smokers was denied in part because the differences within the class in genetic susceptibility to tobacco smoke required an individualized proof of causation. Differences in susceptibility among individuals may undermine all efforts to establish classes of individuals affected by toxic substances unless the classes are established according to the susceptibility genes of its members.

Conclusion

Toxicogenomic data will play a steadily increasing role in toxic torts. The relevance of the data to many important issues is readily apparent. Moreover, doctrinal templates already exist for many applications of genetic biomarkers in tort law. The impacts of the genomic information will potentially be enormous, but that impact will be delivered largely via familiar legal pathways. Genetic biomarkers will be useful to plaintiffs and defendants both, depending on the context. Like forensic DNA, the overall effect of toxicogenomics will be to help inculpate the guilty and exonerate the innocent. Genetic biomarkers will more accurately identify the causal sources of diseases and harms and so enable a more reliable attribution of responsibility for them.

Given this potential improved accuracy, there are likely strong incentives for early, perhaps premature use of the genomic data. There is great need to systematize the information currently available (and soon to be available) to better evaluate its usefulness in toxic tort situations. The primary purpose of genome research is not focused on toxic tort applications. The research is acutely relevant to toxic torts, but some translation and reformatting is required to highlight the pertinence (and the limitations) of the research for toxic torts.

There is also a compelling need to validate biomarker data for relevance and reliability. There are reasons to anticipate that standardization will quickly coalesce under the pressure of FDA and perhaps EPA approval requirements. It is important that this standardization occur promptly because the stakes are high, both with respect to the impact of the biomarker data on toxic torts (and other important applications) and for the consequences of multiple standards for various data producers whose results might be isolated and undervalued if their research protocols prove inconsistent with the eventually adopted standards. There are also potential complications arising from many small companies that are attracted to the potential markets for biomarker data but that do not adopt clear standards of practice or that fail to comply with vaguely recommended models of practice.

Biomarker data will be adopted consistent with governing legal norms and policies, but their adoption will have particularly noteworthy effects on those first affected before the use of biomarker data is widespread.

The particularization of harm that is enabled by gene expression and susceptibility-gene data supports the general theme that tort law aims to compensate parties for harms that they have suffered for which they are not responsible. However, the role of susceptibility in the determination of damages does undermine the tort policy that the negligent tortfeasor, or person doing the harm, takes the injured party as he finds him. The traditional negligent tortfeasor was not permitted to claim a modification of his liability for damages because the victim had a special vulnerability, a doctrine known as the "eggshell skull" rule. If you negligently strike a person with a thin skull, you cannot complain later that he wouldn't have suffered so much if he had had a thicker skull. This negligence tort policy has not been followed without exception (moreover, theories of strict liability have expanded their reach considerably in recent decades), and susceptibility genes may prove to be the means to broaden the exceptions.

Deterrence is another traditional justification for tort law, and the use of genomic data to reduce the defendant's liability for damages serves to reduce the deterrence effect and focus of the damage award. If the award is intended only to compensate the harmed party, then improved accuracy in the evaluation of the harm clearly serves the compensatory purpose. If the award is intended also to deter potential defendants, then an exclusive focus on the harm suffered undermines the deterrence purpose that arguably should also be considered in formulating a tort judgment. This may be a disservice to the role of deterrence is fashioning theories of tort, but it may also be a recognition of the diminished role of deterrence overall in tort law and the ascendance of strict liability in its wake.

Another substantial policy concern affected by genomic data is the role of the judge as gatekeeper and the appropriate thresholds for the admission of genetic evidence. *Daubert* sharply phrased the responsibility that is borne by judges to make substantive judgments about the probative value of evidence adduced in their courts. The complexity of genomic data and its possible manipulation to confuse rather than enlighten toxic tort proceedings may dissuade judges against its admissibility. Indeed, the judges may be reluctant to admit the evidence because they may have concerns about the jury's ability to comprehend it. As is often the case with scientific evidence, there are widespread concerns that lay decision makers may not be able to competently evaluate genomic data.

Juries are charged with deciding the facts in the cases before them, and we want to carefully consider whether they should be charged with making judgments about the validity of science. On the one hand, science is fact dependent and its conclusions are tentative. Also, reasonable people do disagree about the soundness and persuasiveness of particular scientific claims. On the other hand, we do not want to encourage bias or disinterest or incompetence as a sufficient rebuttal to scientific evidence. If the science presented to juries is probabilistic (as good science often is), the juries may misinterpret this equivocal quality as a failure to stake a claim to any legitimate consideration. Or they may equate probabilities with certainties and forsake balancing for inapt thresholds and unjustified certitudes. One wants to affirm a confidence in the ability of juries to rise to the occasion and appropriately sort through the complexities of the evidence. Yet there is at least anecdotal evidence that juries sometimes make egregious blunders because of abject misunderstandings of basic science.

Finally, profound issues of privacy and discrimination must be addressed whenever genomic data are involved. We have not yet assembled a comprehensive account of what privacy means or what protections we intend to provide for it (Solove, 2006). Its meanings depend on context, so that our intuitions are different when we are concerned with the limits of our body, or the sanctuary of the home, or important personal decisions, or intimate relations with others, or the use of communications devices, or the storage of personal effects, or the collection of data from us for government or business purposes (whether mandated or voluntary). We have not settled on a clear view of the ownership interest of the individual in her genome, and we have similarly not settled on her right to protect the contents of her genome from access by others.

Initiating a tort action may be deemed a waiver of whatever protections are otherwise afforded because the data available in the genome are an invaluable benefit to our estimation of whether a tort has in fact occurred and how we ought to compensate for the damage it caused. Many privacy concerns are raised by the use of genomic data and, though we may not be able to solve them before we face the fully formed challenge, we would benefit ourselves by at least anticipating some of the more obvious impacts.

Another important concern is genetic discrimination. As it becomes more obvious that susceptibility genes do reveal important information about behavioral probabilities, there will be a temptation to pursue a stark behaviorist model that reduces the value of human life to the strengths and vulnerabilities of each particular individual's genome. The eugenics movement initially sought to reduce the social and personal burdens of disease and deformity, but it was easily reformulated to serve a Social Darwinist agenda that justified the prerogatives of the prosperous and abuses of the disempowered. Genomic data could be misused to favor the genetic blessed. An employer might test all prospective employees, ostensibly to identify those who are susceptible to a toxin present at its worksite, but actually to identify those with, to the extent that they can be identified, genetic advantages. The employer may pursue a brighter, healthier workforce that will work more efficiently and incur less health and safety costs. The extremes of the movie *Gattaca,* in which genetic imperfections were socially and politically recognized as disqualifications, may not loom in the future, but more subtle uses of genomic data to help distinguish among especially able candidates for highly sensitive positions may come soon.

At the margins, small differences can matter greatly, and genomic data may be considered in tiebreaker situations. The use of genomic data to evaluate individuals may operate as a slippery slope, introduced in carefully guarded situations and slowly growing to a more general application. There are numerous possibilities for genomic data to have discriminatory impacts, both purposeful and coincidental, and it would be useful to raise the issue before it confronts us as an impending crisis.

ACKNOWLEDGMENTS

Preparation of this chapter was supported by Grant 1 R01 ES12577-01 from the National Institute of Environmental Health Sciences (NIEHS) and the National Human Genome Research Institute (NHGRI) of the NIH. The contents of this chapter are the responsibility of the authors and do not necessarily represent the official views of the NIEHS or the NIH.

REFERENCES

Byrd, S. 2006. Parents angered by defense in lead case. *Seattle Times* (July 14):A9.
Cassidy v. SmithKline Beecham, Corp No. 99-10423 WL 22216528 (Pa. Com. Pl. July 1, 2003).

Cavallo v. Star Enterprises, 100 F. 3d 1150 (4th Cir. 1996).

Easter v. Aventis Pasteur, 358 F. Supp. 2d 574 (E.D. Tex. 2005).

Expert Testimony. 1998. Jury returns verdict for oil company after testimony on missing disease marker. *Chemical Regulation Reporter (BNA)* 22:193.

Freeman, K. 2004. Toxicogenomics data: The road to acceptance. *Environmental Health Perspectives* 112: A678–85.

Hall v. Baxter Healthcare Corp., 947 F. Supp. 1387 (D. Or. 1996).

In re Hanford Nuclear Reservation Litigation, WL 775340 (E.D. Wash. 1998).

In re Hanford Nuclear Reservation Litigation, 292 F.3d 1124 (9th Cir. 2002).

In re TMI Litigation, 93 F.3d 613, 622 (3d Cir. 1999).

In re Tobacco Litigation, 215 W.Va. 476, 600 S.E.2d 188 (W.Va. 2004).

Lehrman, S. 1994. Pushing limits of DNA testing: Suit prompts study into whether a birth defect was inherited or caused by toxins. *The (San Francisco) Examiner* (June 5):A1.

Mahoney v. R.J. Reynolds, Civil No. 4-97-CV-10461, 204 F.R.D. 150 (S.D. Iowa. 2001).

Marchant, G.E. 2000. Genetic susceptibility and biomarkers in toxic injury litigation. *Jurimetrics* 41:67–109.

Marchant, G.E. 2001. Genetics and toxic torts. *Seton Hall Law Review* 31:949–82.

Marchant, G.E. 2002. Toxicogenomics and toxic torts. *Trends in Biotechnology* 20:329–32.

Marchant, G.E. 2006. Genetic data in toxic tort litigation. *Journal of Law & Policy* 14:7–37.

Olafson, S. 2000. Suit claims Dow shirked duty on cancer-testing of workers. *Houston Chronicle* (Aug. 12):33.

Prettyjohn v. Goodyear Tire & Rubber Co., No. Civ. A. 91-CV-2681, 1992 WL 105162 (E.D. Pa. April 29, 1992).

Solove, D.J. 2006. A taxonomy of privacy. *University of Pennsylvania Law Review* 154:477–564.

CHAPTER 7

Genomics and Environmental Justice

Some Preliminary Thoughts

GARY E. MARCHANT AND JAMIE A. GRODSKY

Environmental justice is concerned with the disparate impact of environmental exposures on particular communities or subsets of the population. Genetic research recently has identified variations in the human genome that may make some individuals more susceptible than others to certain environmental pollutants (Kelada et al., 2003; Marchant, 2003; Grodsky, 2005). Differential genetic susceptibility to environmental exposures would seem to trigger environmental justice concerns. Indeed, EPA's white paper on the role of genomics in environmental regulation specifically mentions environmental justice as one regulatory application of genomic data (EPA, 2004b, p. 22).

There are, however, important ways in which justice and fairness concerns regarding genetic susceptibility differ from the traditional paradigm of environmental justice (Marchant, 2003). First, whereas the traditional environmental justice model focuses on populations that receive disproportionate exposure to environmental pollutants, genetic susceptibility involves populations that may be similarly exposed but are at greater risk due to intrinsic factors that make a given exposure more dangerous. Second, environmental justice often focuses on geographically defined communities that are disparately affected, whereas individuals with genetic susceptibilities generally are interspersed throughout the population. Third, environmental justice often focuses on disparately affected groups defined by race or ethnicity. Genetic susceptibilities to environmental agents generally are distributed among different racial and ethnic groupings, although some gene variants may be found at higher frequencies in groups sharing a common geographic ancestry (discussed below).

These differences from the traditional environmental justice paradigm raise questions about the applicability of environmental justice policies to recent findings of genetic variation in susceptibility to pollutants. In considering this fit, it is critical to define the meaning and purpose of environmental justice, which we discuss first. Next, we highlight the extraordinarily complex problems posed when susceptibility to toxic hazards is correlated with concepts of race or ethnicity. Finally, we provide some preliminary thoughts on the relationship between genetic susceptibility and environmental justice.

Differing Visions of Environmental Justice

There are many different conceptions and definitions of environmental justice. The relevance of genetic susceptibility depends significantly on which conception of environmental justice is adopted. This chapter focuses on environmental justice as a regulatory concept as applied by agencies such as the U.S. Environmental Protection Agency (EPA). This conception of environmental justice may be narrower than the vision of many environmental justice advocates, scholars, and organizations who take a more holistic view of environmental justice as part of a broader program for social and racial justice (e.g., The First People of Color Summit, 1991; Bullard, 2005; Brulle and Pellow, 2006). Many scholars and advocates who embrace this comprehensive environmental justice paradigm have articulated deep concerns about the ethical, social, and political aspects of human genetic research; in particular, how such research relates to, affects, and involves communities of color (Morales, 2002; Sze and Prakash, 2004).

Our focus here is narrower, however, as we seek to understand how one type of genetic information, the discovery of genetic susceptibilities to environmental agents, may apply to and affect regulatory applications of environmental justice principles. Two key aspects relevant to this question are: (1) Which communities or groups are environmental justice policies intended to protect?, and (2) Does environmental justice focus on disproportionate exposure or disproportionate risk?

Which Groups Are Covered by Environmental Justice?

One critical distinction among the different visions of environmental justice centers on the groups that are the focus of environmental justice concerns. Many environmental justice scholars and proponents view environmental justice as having both a physical and sociopolitical dimension. The physical dimension is that a community may bear a disproportionate share of environmental exposures (substantive environmental justice) or that it may be denied equal opportunity to participate in environmental decisions relative to other communities (procedural environmental justice). The sociopolitical dimension is that certain communities may be politically and economically disadvantaged, thus lacking the ability to protect their interests adequately against public or private decisions that might adversely affect them. These disadvantaged communities may have endured other social inequities that exacerbate environmental inequities including housing discrimination, segregation, inappropriate land use controls, lack of educational and employment opportunities, inadequate health services, and financial disinvestment (Tyson et al., 1998). Under this conception, both disparate exposure or treatment and political or economic disadvantage must be present for an environmental justice problem to exist.

Accordingly, under this view, environmental justice is primarily a concern of those minority or low-income communities that lack political, economic, and legal power to resist unfair treatment. In contrast, a politically advantaged community, even if exposed to a disproportionate burden of environmental pollutants, would not present an environmental justice problem because that community presumptively would have political, educational, and economic tools to remedy the problem (Tyson et al., 1998). The Clinton administration's 1994 Executive Order on Environmental Justice takes this approach, focusing on minority and low-income populations (Executive Order, 1994). Specifically, the executive order requires a federal agency to identify and address "disproportionately high and adverse human health or environmental effects of its programs, policies, or activities on minority populations and low-income populations" (§1-103).

The Bush administration's EPA has put forth a more generic vision of environmental justice. EPA currently defines environmental justice as disparate exposure to *any* group in the population. The language used in rulemakings is as follows:

EPA seeks to achieve environmental justice, the fair treatment and meaningful involvement of *all people, regardless of race, color, national origin, or income,* in the development, implementation, and enforcement of environmental laws, regulations, and policies. To help address potential environmental justice issues, the Agency seeks information on *any groups or segments of the population* who, as a result of their location, cultural practices, or other factors, may have atypical, unusually high exposure to [chemical x], compared to the general population (EPA, 2006c, emphasis added).

Under this approach, any group or segment of the population that is disproportionately exposed to pollution may present an environmental justice problem. As an example, one of the handful of environmental justice complaints accepted by EPA for further review (although ultimately dismissed) claimed that the state of Arizona discriminated on the basis of race by failing to provide a middle-class, predominantly Caucasian community with the same procedural opportunities for opposing a new plant's location as had been provided to minority and low-income communities (Citizens Environmental Awareness League, 2001). Under this conception of environmental justice, the simple fact of disproportionate exposure or treatment may trigger an environmental justice problem, without consideration of the sociopolitical context of the controversy.

In 2004, the EPA's Office of Inspector General issued a report criticizing the agency's programmatic shift from its earlier focus on minority and low-income populations (EPA, 2004a). In response, the EPA underscored its position that environmental justice transcended minority and low-income communities:

The Agency does not accept the Inspector General's central and baseline assumption that environmental justice only applies to minority and/or low-income individuals. The EPA firmly believes that environmental justice belongs to all people, including those living in minority and/or low-income populations. All Americans, including minority and/or low-income residents, have a right to clean air, clean land, and clean water, and to have a meaningful say in the environmental decisions that affect them. These are basic rights that belong to all people, regardless of race or income. (EPA, 2004a)

EPA's 2005 draft "Environmental Justice Strategic Plan" again emphasized that environmental justice "is the fair treatment and meaningful involvement of all people regardless of race, color, national origin, or income" (EPA, 2005, p. 2). This position invoked strong opposition from many members of Congress, environmentalists, and civil rights groups who argued that environmental justice policies should give explicit priority to limiting discrimination and disparate impacts in communities of color and low income (Risk Policy Report, 2005).

This ongoing controversy about the focus of environmental justice is in part a reflection of the gap between the existing legal authority for environmental justice policies and the broader sociopolitical emphasis of the environmental justice movement. Legal enforcement of environmental justice policies is based primarily on Title VI of the Civil Rights Act of 1964, which has been construed by the courts to protect against discrimination or disparate treatment of any racial or ethnic group, whether it be the majority or a minority population. Moreover, whereas Title VI protects against racial discrimination, it does not prevent discrimination against low-income populations. As long as this gap between the legal authority and the sociopolitical goals of environmental justice persists, there is likely to be continued controversy over which groups should be the focus of environmental justice policies.

Admittedly, variations in genetic susceptibility to the effects of toxic substances would be more germane to a conception of environmental justice that transcends race, ethnicity, or economic disadvantage. This is because intrinsic genetic variations are not caused by sociopolitical factors but rather are the results of stochastic processes and the residues of historical evolutionary pressures in different regions of the world. It follows that enhanced environmental risk from genetic susceptibility alone would not present an environmental justice issue under the more traditional definition that requires both a physical and sociopolitical dimension.

Exposure versus Risk

A second threshold issue is whether environmental justice is concerned with disproportionate exposure or disproportionate risk. This issue dovetails somewhat with the question above, because socioeconomic factors may explain why one group might be disproportionately exposed to environmental pollutants. Most environmental justice claims to date have focused on disproportionate exposure. The current EPA definition of environmental justice, noted above, also focuses on exposure, applying to "any groups or segments of the population who . . . may have atypical, unusually high exposure . . . compared to the general population" (EPA, 2006c, p. 43,742). Yet, in other statements, EPA refers to the Clinton administration's executive order, stating that the goal of environmental justice is to identify and address "disproportionately high and adverse human health and environmental *effects* of its programs, policies, and activities on minority populations and low-income populations" (EPA, 2006b, p. 27,405). By referring expressly to "effects," these statements appear to focus on disproportionate risk or harm rather than exposure. One could argue that disproportionate exposure is just a more readily quantifiable surrogate for disproportionate risk, which is the ultimate and most critical measure with which environmental justice should be concerned.

Susceptibility and Risk

The reason this threshold question about disproportionate risk versus exposure is important is that genetic susceptibility may confer differential risk on certain individuals or groups in the absence of differential exposure. Of course, the end result is the same, as differential susceptibility and exposure may both result in enhanced risk of disease from environmental hazards. Yet, the manner in which these at-risk groups arrived at their susceptible state is different, and susceptibility may compound the effects of the differential exposure problem. But the overarching question is whether genetic susceptibility justifies the same regulatory response that should be available to individuals who are at a higher risk due to disproportionate pollutant exposure.

There are reasons to believe that variations in genetic susceptibility would not invoke the same societal concerns as do differential exposures. To the extent that environmental justice involves a sociopolitical dimension, we might have greater concerns for populations who are placed at risk due to political and economic disenfranchisement than for those from all walks of life who are at risk due to the genetic lottery. From an ethical perspective, it may be more problematic to allow risk to concentrate in discrete communities placed at risk by their disadvantaged status than to tolerate the same overall risk randomly scattered through the population. Moreover, traditional environmental justice programs focusing on disproportionate exposures of minority or low-income populations impose, at least implicitly, some accountability on risk creators and the regulatory agencies that license them. In contrast, the evolutionary dispersion of genetic variation in the population cannot be attributable to recent historical or social factors.

Susceptibility, Risk, and Regulatory Standards

One additional consideration should inform the discussion of the role of pollutant susceptibility in environmental justice programs. Although environmental regulations may already account for differences in susceptibility to environmental pollutants, at least for noncarcinogens, there is less protection for higher cumulative exposures. For example, EPA generally applies a tenfold safety factor in determining the reference dose or reference concentration for noncarcinogens. These concentrations are used to set regulatory levels for such substances. Where genetically susceptible individuals fall within a factor of ten of the population median in their susceptibility to a particular agent, environmental standards should protect them, obviating the need for additional protection under environmental justice programs (Marchant, 2003). In contrast, while plausible upper-bound exposure levels generally are assumed in environmental risk assessment, those standards typically focus on exposure to individual pollutants—or pollutants from a single source—and thus may not fully protect against disproportionately high cumulative exposure levels experienced by some disadvantaged communities. To the extent that existing risk assessment methods already account for differences in intrinsic susceptibility, the extra level of protection afforded by environmental justice programs may be best directed to communities differentially exposed.

Given these factors, broadly dispersed genetic susceptibility generally should not trigger the application of environmental justice programs. Yet environmental susceptibility may raise broader environmental justice concerns, as discussed in the final section of this chapter. Moreover, in some cases, selected gene variants conferring environmental susceptibility may concentrate in certain ethnic populations with a shared geographic heritage. In that case, susceptibility may implicate traditional environmental justice concerns. Before turning to that question, we first underscore foundational concerns that merit far greater attention in the future.

The Environmental Justice Paradox in the Genomic Age: Racial Categorization for Remedial Purposes and Scientific Dismantling of Racial Categories

Any discussion of genetic susceptibility and environmental justice implicates crucial foundational questions about the meaning and validity of the concept of race. Although "environmental justice" in the broader sense transcends race, the two enforceable legal bases for achieving environmental justice, Title VI of the Civil Rights Act and the Equal Protection Clause, presuppose group identification on the basis of race or ethnicity. As genetic research has renewed the debate over whether there is any biological basis for racial groupings, a critical set of questions is whether or when existing racial categories should be used for identifying health disparities and developing remedial measures in communities disproportionately burdened by environmental hazards. On the one hand, the use of such categories may reify unfounded notions of biological difference (Foster and Sharp, 2004; Ossorio and Duster, 2005) just at the time when genomics permits us to focus on patterns of genetic variation unencumbered by outmoded social labels. On the other hand, attention to racial categories may in some cases be justified for the temporary, remedial purpose of countering the effects of current or historical discriminatory practices (Ossorio and Duster, 2005). Due to the challenges involved in remedying disparate treatment without perpetuating harmful social divisions that should be eliminated, the environmental justice issue raises some of the most difficult and important questions for environmental law in the genomic age.

The findings of the Human Genome Project have generated renewed debate about the biological validity of particular historical categories, such as race and ethnicity (Foster and Sharp, 2004). A number of prominent scientists have argued that race is such a flawed, inexact concept that it should no longer be used in research or medicine (Ossorio and Duster, 2005). As one scientist has noted, "[a] strict definition of race among humans does not exist . . . There are no good biological criteria on a phenotypic level to determine the race of any individual, or even to determine with any precision how many races exist" (Garte, 2002, p. 421). This biological argument is consistent with longstanding claims of the social sciences, including anthropology and sociology, that race is primarily a cultural construct, with little or no biological significance (Lee, Mountain, and Koenig, 2001; Henig, 2004). Yet other scientists counter that ignoring race will retard progress in biomedical research, and that even if race is an inexact proxy for studying variation in disease mechanisms, it remains a useful research variable (Burchard et al., 2003).

By finding that all human beings share 99.9 percent of their DNA, the Human Genome Project created a strong argument for the genetic homogeneity of humans (Collins and Mansoura, 2001; Subramian et al., 2001). Although subsequent research has focused on the limited genetic differences among individuals and groups (Lee, Mountain, and Koenig, 2001; Foster and Sharp, 2004), presumptions about racial categories are contradicted by findings that allele frequency comparisons rarely map onto racial boundaries (Bamshad et al., 2004; Ossario and Duster, 2005). Current racial categories, in fact, represent highly heterogenous groups:

> On a genetic level, human variation is a smooth continuum with very little evidence for sharp racially defined heterogeneities. The availability of data on thousands of DNA polymorphisms from the various genome re-sequencing projects has clearly shown that the largest part of genetic variability within the human population is dues to differences among individuals within populations, rather than to differences between populations. (Garte, 2002, p. 421)

Following completion of the Human Genome Project, geneticists have been engaged in "cataloging, lumping, and splitting human genetic variation" (Ossorio and Duster, 2005, p. 126). In fact, we might view the postgenomic era as an era of redefining groups. Whole-genome research presents us with the opportunity to move beyond social labels such as "race'" and "ethnicity" and to study patterns of gene variation that transcend traditional social groupings (Foster and Sharp, 2004). Such direct observation of genetic variation might dictate new categories for making meaningful comparisons across human populations based on molecular difference (Lee, Mountain, and Koenig, 2001, p. 65; Garte, 2002, p. 424), providing the opportunity to describe human similarities and differences without reaffirming old prejudices. This possibility has been articulated in the area of biomedical research:

> Future clinical trials may be driven by the delineation of subpopulations using DNA polymorphisms as opposed to current imprecise classifications such as 'race,' 'ethnicity,' or skin color. Polymorphism-based stratification of populations is expected to reduce adverse reaction to drugs and facilitate the identification of genetic variants that confer resistance or predispositions to many diseases. In this regard, and if successful, genomic data . . . may contribute to the deconstruction of 'race' and other imprecise group definitions as currently applied. (Rotimi, 2004, p. S46)

The environmental justice issue raises complex policy challenges in the genomic age, as it may sometimes warrant the continued recognition of racial groupings that may lack scientific validity. The argument has been made that including race, at least as one variable among several demographic variables, may be important for combating the historical legacy and current effects of discrimination (Schwartz, 2001). Although genomic research is further questioning the biological basis of race, the social ramifications of disadvantage—past or present—persist. If certain socially defined groups have been disfavored, explicitly or implicitly, there is a logic for acknowledging these groups in responsive public policies. Race may be an appropriate variable in certain circumstances because "the social fact of racial stratification has biological consequences" (Ossorio and Duster, 2005, p. 119). In seeking to rectify burdens imposed on socially disadvantaged groups, environmental justice policy may sometimes need to take racial classifications into account—as the law of environmental justice already recognizes.

For example, it is widely known that certain racial groups in the United States receive lower quality health care, have disparate access to health care, and have poor overall health status compared with other groups (American College of Physicians, 2004). Because "it is indisputable that social perceptions of what a person is or is not influence the availability, delivery, and outcome of medical care" (Schwartz, 2001, p. 1392), amelioration of this problem may in some cases depend on the use of racial categories for data gathering and development of remedial policies

(Lee, Mountain, and Koenig, 2001; Winker, 2004). As pollutant exposure is a well-known contributor to health disparities, the same argument can be made for remedying the effects of disparate environmental exposures. Evidence of a clustering of risk factors in a particular racial or ethnic community—for example, susceptibilities resulting from cumulative exposures, inadequate nutrition, or other factors—could provide evidence of disparate risk and in some cases help support environmental justice claims.

The challenge is when and how such categories can be used without perpetuating inaccurate generalizations of biological difference (Ossorio and Duster, 2005). One pair of commentators summarized the dilemma as follows:

> As a prominent way of defining population membership over the past 500 years, race has been used to advantage some groups over others. For that reason, race should not, and cannot, be avoided in considerations of issues such as access to care, exposure to environmental hazards and preferences regarding clinical interventions. However, when used to define populations for genetic research, race has the potential to confuse by mistakenly implying biological explanations for socially and historically constructed health disparities. (Foster and Sharp, 2004, p. 790)

This problem is compounded when the susceptibility factors under study are believed to be genetically influenced. For example, while the Human Genome Project revealed that there is much more genetic variation within than between populations, a limited subset of genes contains variations that may differ appreciably in frequency among populations based on geographic ancestry. Historic differences in diet, the presence of infectious organisms, plant toxins, and certain other exposures may affect allele selection for certain genes involved in metabolism, detoxification, pest resistance, and immune defense (Garte, 2002, p. 423). Thus, as one scientist has noted, "while for most loci genetic differences do not exist for different races, and the statement that race is not of any biological significance is correct . . . , for a particular subset of genes, many with important biomedical function and significance, average allele frequency differences are in fact observed between populations originating in different geographic areas, or with different exposures, diets, or other factors" (Garte, 2002, p. 423). Because of such genetic differences, some groups sharing a common geographic ancestry may have—on average, but by no means in every case—greater or lesser susceptibility to disease from specific toxic substances. However, while any correlations between race and risk may potentially be relevant in supporting environmental justice claims, these same correlations could lead to discrimination in other contexts (Garte, 2002).

Hence, the broader policy dilemmas illuminated by environmental justice are as follows: Can we recognize existing racial labels in the effort to promote social justice, while at the same time preventing the use of such labels for discriminatory purposes? Conversely, as the tools of the new genomics allow us to search for patterns of genetic variation unencumbered by racial labels, can we avoid developing new, biologically based categories that may invite equal or greater discrimination in the future? And, finally, can we use possible intergroup differences in pollutant susceptibility to further environmental justice policies and law, without at the same time further reifying outmoded conceptions of racial categories?

The Relationship between Genetic Susceptibility and Environmental Justice

Even though differential genetic susceptibility to environmental pollutants should not, by itself, trigger environmental justice policies, at least under the socioeconomic definition of environmental justice, a higher frequency of some susceptibility alleles in certain groups could have environmental justice implications. For example, in its most recent draft criteria document for lead exposure required under the Clean Air Act, EPA identified data suggesting that certain genetic variants may confer increased susceptibility to the effects of lead and that these alleles may vary in frequency by ethnic and geographical background (EPA, 2006a).

If enhanced sensitivity is combined with higher environmental exposures to lead in certain communities of concern—along with poor nutrition that enhances lead toxicity—an argument could be made that these groups are being subjected to even higher and perhaps even more unacceptable risks compared with the general population. This may be the case even where existing health-based environmental standards are attained. In such circumstances, genetic data may add weight to arguments that greater protections—whether it be further tightening of national regulatory standards or more targeted interventions—are needed to achieve environmental justice.

However, such arguments invariably raise important concerns and objections. First, if, as a result of these alleged genetic differences, certain groups are perceived to be predisposed to pollution-induced harm, "genetic stigmatization" of such groups may result (Garte, 2002; Sze and Prakash, 2004). This could contribute to greater social disempowerment of certain communities, further exacerbating the conditions giving rise to environmental justice problems.

Second, the genetic component of enhanced risk could be used to support arguments that intrinsic factors within a vulnerable population, rather than the activity of polluters, are responsible (at least in significant part) for the greater risk in that population. Such arguments could be marshaled to reduce risk creators' responsibilities (legal or ethical) for addressing environmental justice concerns.

Third, some environmental justice advocates have expressed concern that any focus on genetic susceptibility may divert attention from preventing pollutant exposure and promoting environmental quality (Sze and Prakash, 2004). And the methods and procedures of genetic research in ethnically defined communities may not be sufficiently sensitive and beneficial to the communities at hand (Sze and Prakash, 2004). Health researchers have long been criticized for using study populations for research purposes without providing reciprocal benefits to the relevant communities (Warne, 2005). Environmental justice advocates have argued that genetic research should promote community participation at all stages (Sze and Prakash, 2004).

Despite widespread skepticism about genetic research by many environmental justice advocates, some proponents cite to the potential value of susceptibility data for "limiting exposures in overburdened communities" (Sze and Prakash, 2004). Environmental justice studies and programs have been criticized for focusing on disproportionate exposure rather than disproportionate risk; a focus on risk would evaluate the health effects of disproportionate exposures in conjunction with all relevant risk factors (Brulle and Pellow, 2006). It is risk, after all, that we are most concerned with, and if disproportionate exposures of low-income and minority communities do not result in unacceptable levels of risk, then claims for legal or regulatory redress will have much less force and viability.

The *Select Steel* case (EPA, 1998), the first Title VI complaint decided on the merits by EPA, is illustrative. The Agency concluded that although a minority community adjacent to a proposed steel plant would receive disproportionate shares of pollutant exposure compared with other communities, the complaint failed because the exposure level fell within applicable regulatory standards in the region. Because EPA standards were designed to establish presumptively "safe" levels of pollutant exposure, the community was presumed to be protected, without a broader examination of actual cumulative risk to the community and the panoply of contributory risk factors. Such examples demonstrate that environmental justice may need to consider disproportionate risk as well as disproportionate exposure levels.

Indeed, one goal of a new generation of environmental justice studies both within and outside EPA is to better characterize cumulative risk. Under the substance-by-substance approach of traditional chemical risk assessment, it is difficult if not impossible to estimate real-world risk arising from exposure to complex mixtures of pollutants present in communities of concern. Moreover, emerging studies strive to better incorporate other risk factors that exacerbate the health effects of pollutants, including lifestyle, nutritional status, and health care availability.

Theoretically, genetic susceptibility to environmental agents would fit within this holistic framework of cumulative risk analysis. If a particular gene variant were present at a higher frequency in a disadvantaged community at issue, this could constitute a relevant factor in the risk assessment for that community. Even if a susceptibility gene is not more prevalent in that population, it may still be relevant for demonstrating the presence of disproportionate risk. Unlike "disease susceptibility" genes such as the *BRCA* breast cancer genes that enhance risk of disease in the absence of any chemical exposure, environmental susceptibility genes increase risk only if the relevant environmental triggers are present (Olden and Guthrie, 2001). Thus, certain environmental susceptibility genes may present a problem only in communities that encounter the triggering environmental exposures—even where the gene variant is uniformly distributed throughout the general population. Moreover, environmental susceptibility genes often have dose-dependent effects that result in differential risk at some exposure levels but not others (Hietanen et al., 1997). Here again, a gene variant uniformly distributed among populations may result in higher levels of environmental risk for some.

Finally, a susceptibility gene for a relevant pollutant may be less prevalent in a community of concern than in the general population, hence providing that community with a greater measure of resilience. This would tend to diminish environmental justice concerns to the extent that it equalized overall risk among communities. Thus, these susceptibility alleles may result in different risk profiles—and varying environmental justice concerns—depending both on exposure levels and gene prevalence in a particular community.

Of course, the ultimate goal of environmental justice is to improve the health of the communities of concern. "A basic tenet of the [environmental justice] movement is that outcomes matter more than intent" (Sze and Prakash, 2004, p. 741). The additional information provided by pollutant susceptibility in a population may help elucidate the nature of the risks presented and contribute to developing more effective interventions (Tyson et al., 1998).

Conclusion

The discovery of gene variants conferring susceptibility to environmental agents should not have a major impact on environmental justice programs, as susceptibilities generally are distributed broadly among populations. In some instances, however, where genetic susceptibility and exposure levels combine to produce elevated risk in a community of concern, genetic susceptibility may be relevant to environmental justice claims. Of course, the limited role of genetic susceptibility in environmental justice regulatory programs does not mean that genetic susceptibility to pollutants is of limited concern. It only means that such concerns need to be addressed outside the environmental justice context. As a partial analogy, EPA recently specified additional safety factors in its carcinogen risk-assessment guidelines to better protect children who are more susceptible to certain carcinogens than adults. EPA's action to protect this susceptible group was based on the agency's public health protective mandate rather than an environmental justice rationale. In the same way, although additional measures may be needed to protect individuals genetically susceptible to environmental exposures, such measures should not be confused with environmental justice, which has its own unique focus and priorities.

ACKNOWLEDGMENTS

Preparation of this chapter was supported by Grant 1 R01 ES12577-01 from the National Institute of Environmental Health Sciences (NIEHS) and the National Human Genome Research Institute (NHGRI) of the National Institutes of Health (NIH). The contents of this chapter are the responsibility of the authors and do not necessarily represent the views of the NIH. We would like to thank the following individuals for reviewing the chapter in draft: Dean Frederick Lawrence, Professors Theresa Gabaldon and Sonia Suter of the George Washington University Law School and Nicholas Targ, formerly with EPA's Office of Environmental Justice and currently with Holland & Knight LLP.

REFERENCES

American College of Physicians. 2004. Racial and ethnic disparities in health care. *Annals of Internal Medicine* 141:226–32.

Bamshad, M., S. Wooding, B.A. Salisbury, and J.C. Stephens. 2004. Deconstructing the relationship between genetics and race. *Nature Reviews Genetics* 5:598–609.

Brulle, R.J., and D.N. Pellow. 2006. Environmental justice: Human health and environmental inequities. *Annual Review of Public Health* 27:103–24.

Bullard, R.D. 2005. *The quest for environmental justice: Human rights and the politics of pollution.* San Francisco, CA: Sierra Club Books.

Burchard, E.G., E. Ziv, N. Coyle, S. Lin-Gomez, H. Tang, A.J. Karter, J. Mountain, E.J. Perez-Stable, D. Sheppard, and N. Risch. 2003. The importance of race and ethnic background in biomedical research and clinical practice. *Journal of the American Medical Association* 348:1170–75.

Citizens Environmental Awareness League. 2002. Letter to Christine Whitman, Administrator, U.S. Environmental Protection Agency, Aug. 17, 2001.

Collins, F.S., and M.K. Mansoura. 2001. The Human Genome Project: Revealing the shared inheritance of all humankind. *Cancer* 92 Suppl.:221–25.

Executive Order 12898. 1994. Federal actions to address environmental justice in minority populations and low-income populations, 59 Fed. Reg. 7629 (February 11, 1994).

The First People of Color Environmental Leadership Summit. 1991. Principles of environmental justice. At www.ejnet.org/ej/principles.pdf.

Foster, M.W., and R.R. Sharp. 2004. Beyond race: Towards a whole-genome perspective on human populations and genetic variation. *Nature Reviews Genetics* 5:790–96.

Garte, S. 2002. The racial genetics paradox in biomedical research and public health. *Public Health Reports* 117:421–25.

Grodsky, J.A. 2005. Genetics and environmental law: Redefining public health. *California Law Review* 93:171–270.

Henig, R.M. 2004. The genome in black and white (and gray). *New York Times Magazine* (Oct. 10, 2004) 47–51.

Hietanen, E., K. Husgafvel-Pursiainen, and H. Vainio. 1997. Interaction between dose and susceptibility to environmental cancer: A short review. *Environmental Health Perspectives* 105 (Suppl. 4):763–66.

Kelada, S.N., D.L. Eaton, S.S. Wang, N.R. Rothman, and M.J. Khoury. 2003. The role of genetic polymorphisms in environmental health. *Environmental Health Perspectives* 111:1055–64.

Lee, S.S., J. Mountain, and B.A. Koenig. 2001. The meanings of "race" in the new genomics: Implications for health disparities research. *Yale Journal of Health Policy, Law, and Ethics* 1:33–75.

Marchant, G.E. 2003. Genomics and toxic substances: Part II—Toxicogenetics. *Environmental Law Reporter* 33:10641–67.

Morales, J.F. 2002. *Genomic justice: Environmental justice biotechnology policy.* New York: Public Interest Biotechnology.

Olden, K., and J. Guthrie. 2001. Genomics: Implications for toxicology, *Mutation Research* 473:3–10.

Ossorio, P., and T. Duster. 2005. Race and genetics: Controversies in biomedical, behavioral, and forensic sciences. *American Psychologist* 60(1):115–28.

Risk Policy Report. 2005. EPA faces pressure to overhaul environmental justice policy. Washington, DC: U.S. Environmental Protection Agency.

Rotimi, C.N. 2004. Are medical and nonmedical uses of large-scale genomic markers conflating genetics and "race"? *Nature Genetics* 36:S43–47.

Schwartz, R.S. 2001. Racial profiling in medical research. *New England Journal of Medicine* 344:1392–93.

Subramian, G., M.D. Adams, J.C. Venter, and S. Broder. 2001. Implications of the human genome for understanding human biology and medicine. *Journal of the American Medical Association* 286:2296–2307.

Sze, J., and S. Prakash. 2004. Human genetics, environment, and communities of color: Ethical and social implications. *Environmental Health Perspectives* 112:740–45.

Tyson, F.L., K. Cook, J. Gavin, C.E. Gaylord, C. Lee, V.P. Setlow, and S. Wilson. 1998. Cancer, the environment, and environmental justice. *Cancer* 83:1784–92.

U.S. Environmental Protection Agency. 2004a. *Agency statement on the Inspector General's Report on EPA's Environmental Justice Implementation.* Washington, DC: Author.

U.S. Environmental Protection Agency. 2004b. *Potential implications of genomics for regulatory and risk assessment applications at EPA.* Washington, DC: Author.

U.S. Environmental Protection Agency. 2005. "Environmental justice strategic plan: Working draft." Washington, DC: Author.

U.S. Environmental Protection Agency. 2006a. Air quality criteria for lead: Second external review draft. EPA/600/R-5/144aB. Washington, DC: Author.

U.S. Environmental Protection Agency. 2006b. Ocean dumping; de-designation of ocean dredged material disposal site and designation of new site near Coos Bay. *Federal Register* 71:27396–405.

U.S. Environmental Protection Agency. 2006c. Organophosphate cumulative risk assessment; notice of availability. *Federal Register* 71:43740–41.

U.S. Environmental Protection Agency (Office of Civil Rights). 1998. *Investigative report for Title VI administrative complaint file no. 5R-98-R5* (Select Steel Complaint). Washington, DC: Author.

U.S. Environmental Protection Agency (Office of Inspector General). 2004. *EPA needs to consistently implement the intent of the executive order on environmental justice.* Report No. 2004-P-00007. Washington, DC: Author.

Warne, D. 2005. Genetic research in American Indian communities: Sociocultural considerations and participatory research. *Jurimetrics: Journal of Law, Science and Techonology* 45:191–203.

Winker, M.A. 2004. Measuring race and ethnicity: Why and how. *Journal of the American Medical Association* 292:1612–14.

CHAPTER 8

Setting Air Quality Standards in the Postgenomic Era

GARY E. MARCHANT

The sequencing of the human genome revealed that humans are more genetically homogeneous than previously appreciated. Any two humans differ on average only once in every thousand DNA base pairs, representing a striking 99.9 percent genetic alikeness (Venter et al., 2001). Notwithstanding this overall genetic homogeneity, one category of genes that are highly variable ("polymorphic") between individual humans are those coding for enzymes involved in the metabolism of foreign substances entering our bodies, including infectious agents, foods, drugs, and chemicals. Such variations likely represent the evolutionary vestige of trade-offs in seeking the optimal adaptation to the various environments, diseases, and diets that are present in different parts of the world (Nebert, 2000; Kalow, 2002).

In the past few years, considerable progress has been made in understanding the genetic basis of human variability in susceptibility to environmental exposures. Genes have been identified and mapped affecting susceptibility to virtually every major environmental pollutant (Marchant, 2003). The Environmental Genome Project, sponsored by the

National Institute of Environmental Health Sciences, identified a working list of more than 550 genes affecting variable response to environmental exposures and is in the process of characterizing variants of those genes (Wakefield, 2002; Wilson and Olden, 2004). These genetic variants affect all aspects of the body's handling of foreign substances, including metabolism, detoxification, DNA repair, receptors, and cell cycle controls.

The genes affecting variable susceptibility to environmental agents generally have several important features in common. First, unlike disease susceptibility genes such as the *BRCA1* and *BRCA2* breast cancer predisposition genes, which increase risks for everyone who has the gene, most environmental susceptibility genes increase risks only when both the gene and the corresponding environmental agent are present. This relationship between the gene and the agent has been described as being "similar to that of a loaded gun and its trigger. A loaded gun by itself causes no harm; only when the trigger is pulled is the potential for harm released or initiated. Likewise, one can inherit a predisposition for a devastating disease, yet never develop the disease unless exposed to the environmental trigger(s)" (Olden and Guthrie, 2001, pp. 3–4). Environmental susceptibility genes are generally neither sufficient nor necessary to cause environmentally induced disease; they merely increase the risk.

Second, the effect for the individual of any environmental susceptibility gene is rather modest, as most of the genes seem to increase risk by at most a fewfold over background rates, compared with some disease genes that generally increase risks much more dramatically (Caporaso and Goldstein, 1995; Garte et al., 2001). From a population perspective, however, many of these environmental susceptibility genes are important because they are very prevalent and thus may increase or decrease population risk substantially (Kelada et al., 2003).

Third, genetic susceptibility to environmental agents is likely to account for an increasing proportion of environmentally induced illnesses as environmental exposures are progressively reduced by regulatory and other initiatives. Some commentators have suggested that, following the major reductions that have been made in exposures to many environmental pollutants, the remaining adverse health impacts from residual pollutant levels are likely to be heavily or even almost exclusively concentrated in people with genetic and other susceptibilities to the relevant pollutants (Eaton et al., 1998; Olden and Guthrie, 2001). Many genetic susceptibilities to environmental pollutants are most significant at lower exposure levels, because higher exposure levels are likely to overwhelm defense mechanisms even in people with the most resilient genotypes.

Fourth, genes explain only some of the differences in individual susceptibility to environmental agents. Other genes and other environmental exposures, health conditions, age, and nutrition can also affect susceptibility, and moreover these types of susceptibility are likely to interact in complex ways with genetic susceptibilities. The result is that each individual, through the combination of his or her own mix of intrinsic and extrinsic factors, will be uniquely susceptible (or nonsusceptible) to the myriad of environmental agents to which we are all exposed. These types of susceptibility-susceptibility interactions make the study of genetic susceptibilities, and in particular the attempt to quantify the increased risk associated with such genetic susceptibilities, very complex and challenging.

As the scientific investigation of genetic susceptibilities to environmental agents advances, so too does the potential to use these susceptibility data in regulatory decision making. One of the first and most likely applications of genetic susceptibility data in environmental regulation may be the setting of national ambient air quality standards (NAAQS) (Marchant, 2003; Grodsky, 2005; Kramer et al., 2006). As discussed below, NAAQS are required to protect the most susceptible subgroups in the population, and thus the setting and revision of such standards generally focuses on susceptible subgroups. The NAAQS are also the nation's most important environmental regulations, providing the greatest health benefits and largest compliance costs of any environmental regulatory program (U.S. Environmental Protection Agency [EPA], 1999). These standards thus provide an important case study for considering how genetic susceptibility data might be used in standard-setting.

The NAAQS program is described in more detail below, including the requirement that the agency focus on protecting the most susceptible subgroups. The next section then summarizes the evidence for genetic susceptibilities to air pollutants such as ozone and particulate matter (PM) that are subject to NAAQS. The fourth section examines the evidentiary issues that will need to be addressed in incorporating genetic susceptibility data into the NAAQS standard-setting process. The fifth section addresses the normative issues that will be presented by the challenges of trying to protect the most genetically susceptible individuals. Finally, I discuss the tensions that genetic susceptibility data may create for the current NAAQS program and suggest some alternative approaches for protecting public health from ambient air pollutants.

The NAAQS Program

No provision of U.S. environmental statutes has focused greater attention on susceptible subgroups of the population than section 109(b)(1) of the Clean Air Act (CAA), which requires EPA to set NAAQS for common air pollutants such as ozone and PM. This statutory provision directs the EPA administrator to set NAAQS at a level that is "requisite to protect the public health" with "an adequate margin of safety." The U.S. Supreme Court upheld EPA's construction of this sparse statutory directive that the agency must set the NAAQS at a level that protects, with an adequate margin of safety, against "adverse effects" without any consideration of the costs or feasibility of attaining the standards (*Whitman v. American Trucking Associations*, 2001).

Although the statutory language of section 109 does not refer explicitly to susceptible subgroups, the Senate Report accompanying the 1970 legislation establishing the NAAQS program required EPA to set the standards at a level "which will protect the health of any group in the population" (U.S. Congress, 1970, 10). The D.C. Circuit has likewise construed section 109 and its legislative history to require EPA to set NAAQS "at a level at which there is an absence of adverse effect on . . . sensitive individuals," and therefore "if a pollutant adversely affects the health of these sensitive individuals, EPA must strengthen the entire national standard" (*American Lung Association v. EPA*, 1998, p. 389, quotations omitted).

Consistent with this directive to protect sensitive individuals, EPA has promulgated NAAQS that are intended to protect identifiable susceptible subgroups within the population. Not surprisingly, the level needed to protect sensitive subgroups becomes the determinative factor in setting air quality standards, and EPA's risk assessment and regulatory analysis tend to focus primarily on such susceptible subgroups. For example, in *Lead Industries Association v. EPA* (1980, p. 1141), the court endorsed EPA's position that "protection of the most sensitive groups within the population had to be a major consideration in determining the level at which the air quality standards should be set." In past NAAQS

standard-setting decisions, the sensitive subgroups that have been identified and used to base the standards have included asthmatic children
(ozone), individuals with preexisting respiratory and cardiovascular disease (PM), elderly people (PM), and children (PM).

As early as 1981, the president of the Conservation Foundation,
William Reilly, who would later become the administrator of EPA, recognized the looming dilemma posed by differential susceptibility to air
pollutants:

> The [CAA] incorporates the notion of threshold values of pollutants, levels
> below which there are presumed to be no adverse health effects, and re-
> quires that standards be set on the basis of the threshold, with a margin of
> safety. But the concept of a threshold becomes increasingly difficult to deal
> with scientifically when we try to reconcile it with what we know about
> the heterogeneity of the population. As the definition of the sensitive pop-
> ulation to be protected is increasingly refined, the threshold level becomes
> increasingly tighter, inevitably approaching zero. . . . Hence, in a heteroge-
> neous population it is unlikely that, for any pollutant, there will be a sin-
> gle scientifically defensible threshold applicable to all people. Instead there
> will be a series of thresholds for different sensitive populations and a thresh-
> old of zero for some people.
>
> In the absence of a scientifically definable threshold, the decision mak-
> ers responsible for establishing a standard are inescapably forced to make
> social, not scientific, judgments. Any standard above zero might cause in-
> jury to some people. But a zero standard might wreak economic havoc—a
> zero level for almost any of the major air pollutants would virtually halt
> industrialization. (Reilly, 1981)

As will be discussed below, this statement sagely predicted the
dilemma that will be created by the identification of individuals within
the population who are genetically susceptible to ambient air pollutants.

Genetic Susceptibility to Criteria Air Pollutants

For many years it has been known that people respond differently to
air pollutants such as ozone and PM (Kleeberger and Ohtsuka, 2005;
Kramer et al., 2006). Some of this variation in responsiveness is likely
due to extrinsic factors such as socioeconomic status, previous exposures,
and aspects of the physical environment in which exposure occurs such

as temperature and altitude (Kleeberger, 1995). Intrinsic factors such as age, gender, and preexisting disease also explain some of the variation. Yet, even when these factors are controlled, significant interindividual variation in response to air pollutants still exists in healthy subjects. For example, in one study healthy male subjects exposed to 0.40 parts per million (ppm) ozone exhibited a decline in pulmonary function—measured as forced expiratory volume in one second—that ranged from 3 to 48 percent in different subjects, and these differences were reproducible over the ten-month duration of the study (McDonnell, 1996). Other studies have examined inflammatory responses in the lung rather than changes in lung function in response to controlled ozone exposures and again have found significant variation between subjects (Aris et al., 1993). Nongenetic susceptibility factors such as age, height, baseline pulmonary function, allergies, or smoking history appear to have a minimal or negligible impact on this interindividual variation in response to ozone (McDonnell et al., 1993). This interindividual variation in ozone responsivity in normal healthy human subjects, in which all other known risk factors have been accounted for, under controlled exposure conditions provides "presumptive evidence of genetic predisposition" in response to air pollution (Kleeberger, 1995; Kleeberger et al., 2000). No correlation appears to exist between the lung functional changes and the inflammatory effects of ozone exposure, suggesting that the two responses may be regulated by different genetic pathways (Kleeberger, 1995).

Further evidence of a genetic role in differential susceptibility to air pollutants is provided by animal models. Different inbred strains of laboratory rodents differ markedly in their response to exposure to ozone or PM under carefully controlled laboratory conditions, suggesting that genetic differences are primarily responsible for this interstrain variation in susceptibility (Kleeberger, 1995; Leikauf et al., 2000; Savov et al., 2004; Kleeberger and Ohtsuka, 2005). Specific genetic loci have been identified that appear to be responsible at least in part for the interstrain differences in susceptibility (Kleeberger et al., 2000). A recent review of the animal data on genetic susceptibility to ozone exposure by EPA scientists in the criteria document prepared for considering possible regulatory changes to the ozone standard concluded that mice studies "illustrate that genetic background is an extremely important determinant of susceptibility" to ozone, but, "at this point, corresponding human polymorphisms have not yet been identified as being associated with differing human sensitivities" (EPA, 2006, pp. 5-26, 5-27). Similarly, the criteria document for PM concludes that "genetic susceptibility to the effects of PM are becoming increasingly apparent as various strains of rodents are characterized for strain-specific responses," but "the extent to which genetic susceptibility plays a role in humans remains to be determined" (EPA, 2004, p. 7-223).

In one particularly significant human study, changes in biomarkers of lung inflammation were studied in healthy human volunteers performing mild physical exercise while exposed indoors for two hours to ozone levels (0.1 ppm) typically encountered in cities with high ozone levels (Corradi et al., 2002). Biomarkers of lung inflammation and oxidative stress were significantly elevated only in individuals carrying a combination of the wild type gene for NAD(P)H:quinone oxidoreductase ($NQO1$) and the null genotype for glutathione-S-transferase M1 ($GSTM1$). An earlier study had found that outdoor ozone levels ranging from 0.032 to 0.103 ppm induced changes in lung function and blood proteins only in individuals with the same $NQO1wt$ and $GSTM1null$ genotypes (Bergamaschi et al., 2001). These findings suggest that individuals carrying this genotype combination are more susceptible to ozone pollution than are other genotypes and indeed raises the possibility that adverse effects from at least short-term exposures to ozone may be largely restricted to this vulnerable genotype.

Another potential source of genetic susceptibility to air pollutants includes individuals with genetically determined or genetically influenced respiratory diseases that increase susceptibility to air pollution. For example, individuals with a genetic condition called α_1-antitrypsin deficiency are prone to developing chronic obstructive pulmonary disease. Although smoking is the primary environmental risk factor for the development of this disease in α_1-antitrypsin-deficient individuals, particulate and other environmental exposures are also believed to contribute to development of lung disease in such susceptible populations (Sandford and Silverman, 2002). Similarly, many genetic variants have been identified that appear to predispose an individual to developing asthma, which in turn makes the individual more susceptible to adverse health effects from air pollution exposures (Kleeberger and Peden, 2005; McCunney, 2005; Peden, 2005). An even more complex genetic-environmental interaction has been suggested whereby in utero exposures to respiratory toxins such as environmental tobacco smoke increase the risk of genetically susceptible individuals subsequently developing asthma (Kabesch, 2006).

These existing data indicate that there are significant genetic susceptibilities to ambient air pollutants in the general population. The issue
presented is then whether and how this information can and should be
used to better protect genetically susceptible individuals. An editorial in
the prestigious British medical journal *The Lancet* noted, "We now have
ways to identify individuals susceptible to air pollution and, because this
sensitivity appears to be regulated by genetic and dietary factors, new
approaches are emerging that might help protect these individuals from
ambient pollution" (Kelly and Sandström, 2004, p. 95).

Evidentiary Issues in Standard-Setting

The growing body of evidence suggesting genetic susceptibilities in
the human population to common air pollutants raises the possibility
that data on these susceptibilities may eventually be considered in setting air quality standards. Indeed, EPA has already discussed genetic susceptibilities in its regulatory documents but has yet to base standards on
these susceptibilities. For example, in its staff paper on PM, EPA stated
that "there is some new suggestive evidence on genetic susceptibility to
air pollution, but no conclusions can be drawn at this time" (EPA, 2005,
p. 3-36). Likewise, in its 2006 criteria document for ozone, EPA concluded that "recent studies have shown that an individual's innate susceptibility to [ozone] may be linked to the genetic background of an
individual" (EPA, 2006, p. 6-29). EPA has to date not based NAAQS on
genetic data, and there are a number of threshold evidentiary issues that
would need to be satisfactorily addressed before genetic susceptibility
could be used to define a susceptible subgroup on which to base an
NAAQS.

An initial issue is whether genetically susceptible individuals were
intended to be included within the protection given to sensitive subgroups by the statute. There is no official or standard definition of "susceptibility" for purposes of setting air quality standards, and different
unofficial definitions have been offered or assumed. Some key differences
in the various definitions of susceptibility include whether only intrinsic host factors (e.g., health, age, genetics) should be considered or
whether extrinsic factors such as exposure levels are also relevant. Another possible issue is whether susceptibility should be defined on an individual or population basis (Parkin and Balbus, 2000). The Senate report

that is part of key legislative history of the CAA gives as examples of sensitive subgroups that must be protected persons with asthma and emphysema (U.S. Congress, 1970, p. 10). Other statements in that same Senate report, however, suggest that susceptibility should be construed more broadly than existing respiratory diseases would be. For example, the report states that protection from air pollution "must extend beyond 'normal' segments of the population to effects on the very young, the aged, the infirm, and other susceptible individuals" (p. 7). There is no obvious reason or evidence that genetically susceptible individuals should be excluded from the catchall category "other susceptible individuals."

This understanding is consistent with EPA's statements and definitions of "susceptible" groups recognized by the courts. In promulgating an air quality standard for lead in the late 1970s, for instance, EPA staff stated that the statute is intended to protect people at high risk from air pollutants due to either "inherent susceptibility" or unique exposure situations. EPA defined "inherent susceptibility" as "a host characteristic or status that predisposes the host to a greater risk of heightened response to an external stimulus or agent" (EPA, 1977, p. 13-11). Genetic susceptibility would clearly fit within this definition. In more recent NAAQS rule makings, EPA has discussed the possible existence of genetically susceptible subgroups but has so far concluded that such susceptibilities are not sufficiently characterized to be used for standard-setting (EPA, 2005, 2006).

Another set of issues relates to the type and number of studies needed to demonstrate a genetically defined subgroup that is sufficiently validated to be used for standard-setting. Environmental health studies generally fall into three categories: (1) human studies, (2) animal studies, and (3) in vitro assays. EPA principally relies on human studies in setting NAAQS, with animal and in vitro studies playing only a secondary, supporting role. In discussing the possibility of genetic susceptibilities in its most recent criteria document for PM, for example, EPA noted that "a few studies have begun to demonstrate that genetic susceptibility can play a role in the response to inhaled particles" but declined to base the standards on these studies because they were animal studies involving "extremely high" exposures in comparison to ambient PM levels to which humans are exposed (EPA, 2004, p. 7-133). Valid human studies will therefore likely be needed before an NAAQS can be based on genetic susceptibility data.

Human data can consist of large-scale retrospective epidemiology studies (such as a cohort or case control study), or smaller clinical challenge studies. Epidemiologic studies are generally much more expensive and time consuming to conduct, and no large-scale human epidemiology studies examining genetic susceptibilities to air pollutants have been reported to date. A small number of laboratory challenge studies directly examining human genetic susceptibility to air pollutants have been reported. In previous NAAQS rule makings, EPA has primarily relied on larger epidemiology studies, but in some cases (e.g., 1997 ozone standard revision) EPA relied primarily on clinical human studies. Thus, an NAAQS based on genetic susceptibility could possibly be based on smaller human challenge studies, but larger epidemiology studies that examine genotype and pollutant susceptibility would provide a much stronger rationale for setting a standard based on genetic susceptibility.

A related issue is the number of confirmatory studies needed to support a standard based on genetic susceptibilities. EPA generally does not base an NAAQS on a single study. In adopting a fine PM standard for the first time in 1997, EPA was severely criticized for relying primarily on only a few studies directly evaluating the health impacts of fine particulates. When identifying susceptible subgroups on which to base the standard in past NAAQS rule makings, EPA often uses the term *numerous* to describe the number of studies that have established the susceptible subgroup (e.g., EPA, 2004, p. 9-83). The studies need not be unanimous in identifying the susceptible group, but the weight of the evidence must support the decision. When the evidence is equivocal, however, EPA will not rely on such evidence in selecting a susceptible group on which to base the standard.

Replication and validation will be key requirements for confirming any genetic susceptibility to air pollutants sufficiently to be used in regulatory decisions. Many initial studies reporting an association between a genetic variant and susceptibility to a particular disease or exposure often do not stand up in subsequent replication studies. Nebert (2005) identified thirty factors that can complicate attempts to associate a genetic variant with a particular trait. Given the difficulty of confirming putative genetic associations, EPA and its science advisors are likely to insist on strong confirmation of any genetic variation conferring susceptibility to air pollutants before accepting such a link for regulatory purposes. In its 2006 criteria document for ozone, EPA concluded that "a number of potential [ozone] susceptibility genes have been identified," but "the validity of these markers and their relevance in the context of prediction to population studies need additional validation" (EPA, 2006, pp. 6-29, 8-65).

Another set of questions relates to how well the susceptible subgroup must be characterized. In the 1997 adoption of the fine PM standard, EPA conceded it did not know the mechanism by which fine PM caused the significant mortality the agency associated with exposure to it, but that lack of information should not preclude setting a standard. Thus, knowing the mechanism of susceptibility does not appear to be essential for standard-setting. In other words, the knowledge that a gene or set of genes confers a susceptibility to a regulated pollutant should be sufficient to base a standard on that susceptible subgroup without furthering characterizing or identifying the specific genes involved.

The next factor is the magnitude of susceptibility conferred by the gene or genes. Genetic susceptibility will be relevant for standard-setting only if it identifies more sensitive individuals than do any other types of susceptibility due to preexisting disease, age, or other factors, because otherwise those greater susceptibilities should be the focus of the standard. Genetic susceptibilities to environmental pollutants appear to be most salient at low concentrations, because high-level exposure tends to overwhelm protective mechanisms and saturate enzyme activity regardless of genotype (Vineis and Martone, 1995). Thus, the relative importance of genetic susceptibilities is likely to increase as pollutant levels get lower, suggesting that genetic susceptibilities may become increasingly important from a regulatory perspective as standards are progressively lowered over time. No analyses are currently available that examine the relative magnitude of genetic versus other types of susceptibilities with respect to vulnerability to harm from air pollutants. Presumably, such analyses would be necessary and must show that genetically susceptible individuals constitute the most susceptible subgroup, before genetic susceptibilities can be used in setting standards. EPA's most recent version of the criteria document for PM gives the following explanation for not using genetic susceptibility in setting the standard: "The extent to which genetic susceptibility plays as significant a role in the adverse effects of ambient PM as does age or health status remains to be determined" (EPA, 2004, p. 7-133).

It will also be necessary for EPA to be able to quantify the risk in genetically susceptible individuals. EPA does use risk assessment in setting NAAQS, although the agency does not consider itself strictly bound to follow the risk-assessment strictly. Rather, risk assessment is a tool that can assist the agency in setting a standard. Nevertheless, if EPA lacks sufficient data to even make a credible estimate of the risk to genetically susceptible individuals, it will likely conclude that the data are inadequate to base the standard on genetic susceptibility. In its 1978 rule making to establish a lead ambient air quality standard, EPA based the standard on children (ages one to five) as the relevant sensitive population, but various commentators suggested that EPA should focus instead on subgroups of children within that larger group with enhanced risk due to genetic conditions or other factors (EPA, 1978a). EPA acknowledged "the higher risk status of such groups" but declined to base the standard on these susceptible subgroups of children because it lacked adequate information "for estimating a threshold for adverse effects [for such subgroups] separate from that of all young children" (EPA, 1978a, p. 46,252).

Defining a genetically susceptible subgroup will also be problematic. EPA has in the past characterized a sensitive subgroup as a "defined population" with "significantly higher probability of developing a condition, illness, or other abnormal status" from pollutant exposure (EPA, 1977, p. 13-11). However, the idea of discrete subcategories of the population with unique risk profiles is increasingly obsolete when differences in genetic susceptibility are now combined with differences in susceptibility due to disease conditions, nutritional status, other environmental exposures, age, and other factors. The likely interactive effects of many different genes and environmental factors modulating susceptibility to air pollutants will complicate the task of defining a susceptible subgroup to use for standard-setting. Given this multitude of factors affecting susceptibility to pollutants, it is likely that each individual will be uniquely susceptible to a given pollutant along a continuum of susceptibility based on his or her individual medley of intrinsic and extrinsic factors affecting susceptibility (Grodsky, 2005). The concept of identifiable subcategories of the population on which to focus the standard is therefore, at best, a very crude assumption. With respect to genetic susceptibilities, EPA is likely to define a subclass based on one or at most two genes that studies show have a clear impact on susceptibility, but the group of people sharing the susceptible genotype is likely to include a range of susceptibilities because of modifying genetic and environmental influences.

This raises the question of whether EPA is required to establish a standard that will fully protect the health of every single individual within the susceptible subgroup. The legislative history of section 109 is somewhat cryptic on this question:

> The Committee emphasizes that included among those persons whose health should be protected by the ambient standard are particularly sensitive citizens such as bronchial asthmatics and emphysematics who in the normal course of daily activity are exposed to the ambient environment. In establishing an ambient standard necessary to protect the health of these persons, reference should be made to a representative sample of persons comprising the sensitive group rather than to a single person in such a group. Ambient air quality is sufficient to protect the health of such persons whenever there is an absence of adverse effect on the health of a statistically related sample of persons in sensitive groups from exposure to the ambient air. An ambient air quality standard, therefore, should be the maximum permissible ambient air level of an air pollution agent or class of such agents (related to a period of time) which will protect the health of any group in the population. For purposes of this description, a statistically related sample is the number of persons necessary to test in order to detect a deviation in the health of any person within such sensitive group which is attributable to the condition of the ambient air (U.S. Congress, 1970, 10).

On the one hand, by requiring protection of "any group in the population" based on "a representative sample" rather than "a single person in such group," this legislative history could be read as focusing on susceptible groups rather than on individuals and thus not requiring protection of the most susceptible individual within any such group. On the other hand, by requiring a sample large enough to detect an effect in "any person" within the group and then mandating an "absence of adverse effect" in that sample, the provision could also be read as requiring the protection of the most susceptible individual in the population. As one commentator noted, "this definition could reasonably be interpreted to mean that the single most sensitive individual of the most sensitive group is the benchmark of an adequate health standard" (Friedman, 1981, p. 8).

In the few cases where EPA has addressed this issue explicitly, the agency has in fact not attempted to protect the most sensitive individuals within susceptible subgroups. In revising the ozone air quality standard in 1979, for example, EPA and its scientific experts focused "not only on the most sensitive population group, but also on a very sensitive portion of that group (specifically, those persons who are more sensitive than 99 percent of the sensitive group, but less sensitive than 1 percent of that group)" (EPA, 1979, p. 8215). In other words, the most sensitive 1 percent of the most susceptible subgroup would not be protected by the standard. In promulgating its lead air quality standard in 1978, EPA likewise set a level that would protect 99.5 percent of children, who had been designated the most susceptible subgroup (EPA, 1978a, p. 46,249).

A related issue is if EPA is required to set the standards at the levels required to protect the most susceptible "groups," does it matter how big the susceptible subgroup is? Some genes conferring susceptibility are likely to be present in the population at frequencies of 1 percent or more, and thus would be comparable in size to susceptible groups used in previous NAAQS rule makings. But it is also possible that genetic research will identify genes or gene combinations that are very rare but may present extraordinary high levels of susceptibility to a particular air pollutant. To posit an extreme hypothetical, what if a particular gene combination conferring unusually high risks to air pollution were present in only one thousand people in the entire United States? Or one hundred? Or ten? It seems increasingly implausible that a national standard could be based on such a small group as its size progressively shrinks. Yet, under EPA's past precedents, the size of the susceptible group is relevant only for determining how high to set the margin of safety, with a larger margin appropriate for a larger susceptible group. Until now, however, the agency's precedents suggest that any susceptible subgroup must be protected, no matter how large or small.

Normative Issues

Identifying and characterizing genetic variations conferring susceptibility to pollutants will present daunting policy, economic, and ethical challenges for environmental decision making. Protecting 99 or 99.5 percent of the individuals most genetically susceptible to air pollutants has the potential to impose enormous costs on the nation and may even be economically infeasible. Yet, the Supreme Court recently reaffirmed that the CAA precludes any consideration of costs or feasibility in promulgating standards that will adequately protect public health, including susceptible subgroups (*Whitman v. American Trucking*, 2001). As the genetic basis of susceptibility differences to air pollutants is better characterized, EPA may be forced to adopt standards that could impose unprecedented regulatory costs on society, if it adheres strictly to the statutory mandate to protect susceptible subgroups regardless of cost.

There are reasons to believe that such standards would not be technologically or politically feasible. The 1997 revisions to the ozone and PM NAAQS were the most expensive environmental regulations ever adopted. EPA has recently proposed even more stringent revisions of these two standards, which likely will push the limits of what is practicable. The standards would likely need to be made substantially more stringent still to protect all genetically susceptible subgroups. To consider a specific example, people who are carriers of the serum α_1-antitrypsin deficiency are at increased risk of developing emphysema from pollutant exposure. Approximately 3 percent of Caucasians carry this allele (Eaton et al., 1998). An NAAQS standard would almost surely need to be set at zero (or at least background levels) to fully protect this susceptible subpopulation. Similarly, recent data suggest that individuals carrying a combination of two different gene variants, which occur in combination in as much as a third of the population, experience effects from ozone exposure at levels that do not appear to affect people with other genotypes (Bergamaschi et al., 2001). The ozone standard would presumably need to be significantly tightened to protect this susceptible subpopulation.

Standards approaching background levels, if enacted, would likely require closing many industrial facilities and imposing draconian restrictions on use of motor vehicles and other polluting equipment. Such restrictions would like be politically impossible to impose. On the other hand, it would also be politically infeasible to expressly decide that we cannot afford to protect some members of the population from harm to pollution because of no fault of their own; they were born with a particular susceptibility. As Carl Cranor wrote, "do we want to suggest that the most susceptible people in the community do not have sufficient moral standing to warrant protection, or that their standing to be protected is not equal to the healthy among us?" (Cranor, 1997, p. 245). Developing concepts of "genetic equity" imposes a responsibility on society to take additional measures to protect the most genetically susceptible in order to provide them the same health protections other citizens receive (Harris and Sulston, 2004).

EPA has already had to face such issues (at least subtly) in deciding to set the ozone standard in the late 1970s at a level that would protect 99 percent of the most sensitive subgroup, rather than the most sensitive individual within that subgroup. EPA stated, somewhat defensively, that "it would be incorrect to interpret this [determination] as an indication of an utilitarian judgment to trade off the interests of 1 percent of a sensitive group against the interests of society as a whole" (EPA, 1978b, p. 9). EPA went on to say that "by redefining the threshold in terms of 0.005 or 0.05 [rather than 0.01] of the most sensitive group we *can* say that roughly half as many or five times as many people will be effected. So the somewhat arbitrary choice of 1 percent is not unimportant. But this kind of choice must be made" (p. 9). The further development and validation of data on genetic susceptibility to air pollutants is likely to bring these difficult issues to the forefront of NAAQS decision making.

The unfortunate reality is that we probably cannot afford to provide full protection to the most susceptible genotypes in the population, and indeed such protection may not even be possible. Certainly, we face similar "tragic choices" in other contexts, such as the rationing of expensive medicines and medical treatments, limits on the provision of police and fire protection services, and inadequate protection of people with life-threatening allergies to products such as peanuts. But, in all of these contexts, just as will be the case with genetic susceptibilities to environmental pollutants, there are enormous political and moral impediments to explicitly facing this reality and making decisions based on it. Genetic susceptibility information may be in that rare category of unwanted information that people would be more comfortable not knowing (Kavka, 1990), but once they have the information, they cannot ignore it and are forced to make difficult choices based on it.

Alternative Approaches

The emerging data on genetic susceptibility to air pollutants are likely to challenge if not disrupt the current regulatory framework for setting air quality standards. One alternative approach would be to impose some type of cost-benefit or cost-effectiveness criteria in setting NAAQS standards. EPA has consistently advocated for thirty years, and the courts have upheld, the position that costs should not and cannot be considered in setting air quality standards. Critics of the present program insist that it is impossible to set air quality standards for nonthreshold air pollutants at any nonzero level without giving some weight to costs and that EPA in fact does implicitly consider costs is setting air quality standards (Coglianese and Marchant, 2004). Whatever the merits of this cost debate, there does not seem to be any political feasibility to amend the statute to explicitly require consideration of costs in setting the standards, in large part of the queasiness described above to expressly address the fatal trade-offs that often get resolved implicitly. In other words, even if consideration of costs was permissible, making explicit decisions to decline to protect identifiable susceptible groups because it would be too expensive would be politically difficult if not impossible.

If some type of cost-balancing is politically infeasible, how else might the statute be modified to better address the challenges created by genetic susceptibilities to air pollutants? One approach might be to adopt a two-tier approach to air quality protection. The first tier would be the adoption of nationwide ambient standards similar to the NAAQS that attempt to protect most of the general population. These primary standards would be supplemented in the second tier with targeted interventions aiming to protect susceptible individuals left inadequately protected by the ambient standards. This two-tier approach is consistent with Geoffrey Rose's classic formulation of the need to address public health needs at both the population and individual level simultaneously (Rose, 1985).

This two-tier strategy recognizes that there are two major types of strategies for reducing exposure to air pollution, which can be employed separately or together (Kunzli et al., 2003). "Primary strategies" seek to reduce ambient concentrations of air pollutants, whereas "secondary" strategies seek to reduce the exposure of sensitive individuals to air pollutants without affecting overall ambient levels. Secondary strategies have been suggested as a strategy to protect the susceptible group of children, which is a clearly identifiable subpopulation that is often concentrated in certain locations (e.g., schools, playgrounds, day care centers, etc.). Thus, location-based secondary strategies such as filtering air in schools or limiting vehicles near schools or playgrounds may be effective protective strategies. Another secondary strategy would be to reduce outdoor activity on high-pollution days. The current air quality program already implicitly provides for such susceptible individuals with the Air Quality Index program. Notwithstanding the legal myth that the NAAQS protect all susceptible subgroups with an adequate margin of safety, the

EPA provides a warning system, including a warning on some high-pollution days that the air is "unhealthy for sensitive groups." The purpose of this warning system is to alert susceptible individuals to try to minimize exertion and outdoor exposures on such days.

It will not be as easy to provide this type of targeted protection for genetically susceptible individuals, however, both because they will be much harder to identify or self-identify than, for example, children. Moreover genetically susceptible subgroups do not aggregate in specific locations such as schools or playgrounds. Nonetheless, targeted interventions may be useful for providing protection for genetically susceptible individuals. Indeed, a primary benefit of identifying genetic susceptibilities to environmental agents is the potential such knowledge creates to develop more targeted interventions to better protect the health of susceptible individuals (Tyson et al., 1998).

One such secondary strategy could include providing dietary supplements (e.g., magnesium, potassium, antioxidants such as vitamins C and E) to genetically susceptible individuals, which some evidence suggests may provide a protective effect from the oxidative stress induced by air pollution (Kunzli et al., 2003). In particular, one study found that asthmatic children with a gene (*GSTM1null*) that confers genetic susceptibility to ozone pollution benefited from oral antioxidant supplementation (vitamins C and E), whereas children without the genetic susceptibility received no apparent benefit from such antioxidants (Romieu et al., 2004). Pharmaceutical and other nutritional interventions may be available in the near future that can selectively protect individuals with susceptible genotypes from damage from air pollutants (Peden, 2005; Kirkham and Rahman, 2006).

Of course, targeting genetically susceptible individuals with antioxidant treatment or some other intervention would require somehow identifying those susceptible individuals. One could instead apply the targeted treatment to identifiable at-risk populations (e.g., children and elderly people) or to people with symptoms of adverse effects from air pollution, with the goal of trying to ensure treatment of the most at-risk genetically susceptible individuals embedded within those larger susceptible groups. But such measures would be overinclusive if the targeted treatment benefited only individuals who carried the susceptible genotype. Such overinclusive interventions could be unduly expensive and provide no benefit (or perhaps even harm) to the majority of the overinclusive targeted groups who do not carry the relevant susceptibility gene.

The alternative is to identify those individuals who carry the susceptibility genotype and then target the intervention specifically to those susceptible individuals. Such a program would require genetic testing of most or all of the general population to identify the genetically susceptible individuals. Such a testing program would raise a litany of difficult ethical and legal issues (Sharp, 2003), including:

- Who would pay for the testing program?
- What types of risks relating to privacy and discrimination would be created by such a large-scale testing program, and how could such risks be minimized?
- How would information be conveyed and how would confidentiality be assured?
- Would testing be done through physicians or other health professionals in an organized campaign, or would it instead be a voluntary program, including possibly the availability of direct-to-consumer genetic testing over the Internet?
- What would be the psychological and social consequences of identifying asymptomatic individuals as "at risk" for harm from air pollution (Scott et al., 2005)?
- Will at-risk individuals comply with the recommended interventions such as antioxidant supplementation or pharmaceutical treatment?

These issues are not easily resolved but would have to be addressed before any intervention program specifically targeted at genetically susceptible individuals could be implemented. Whether it will be worth the expense and risks to attempt a population-based genetic screening program for susceptibility to air pollutants or any other environmental agent will depend on the proportion of people harmed by air pollution that are in genetically susceptible subgroups. Such a program will likely be politically and economically feasible and justified only if a substantial portion of the people at risk from air pollution fall into genetically susceptible subgroups that would receive significant health benefits available only from targeted interventions.

Conclusion

Findings of genetic susceptibilities to common air pollutants are likely to present one of the first opportunities for integration of genetic susceptibility data into environmental regulatory decision making. As discussed in this chapter, use of such genetic information will present two broad categories of implementation issues. The first set involves evidentiary issues about what types of data are useful, how well they must be replicated and validated, and what the data must demonstrate to have a practical and legal effect on regulatory outcomes. The second set includes a wider range of policy, economic, social, and ethical issues relating to the collection and use of genetic information. Both sets of issues present formidable challenges to the real-world use of genetic susceptibility data in environmental regulation. Nevertheless, attempting to overcome these challenges is warranted by the overriding goal of trying to protect the health of individuals in an economically feasible manner.

ACKNOWLEDGMENTS

Preparation of this chapter was supported by Grant 1 R01 ES12577-01 from the National Institute of Environmental Health Sciences (NIEHS) and the National Human Genome Research Institute (NHGRI) of the NIH. The contents of this article are the responsibility of the author and do not necessarily represent the official views of the NIEHS or the NIH.

REFERENCES

American Lung Ass'n v. EPA, 134 F.3d 388 (D.C. Cir. 1998).

Aris, R.M., D. Christian, P.Q. Hearne, K. Kerr, W. Finkbeiner, and J. Balmes. 1993. Ozone-induced airway inflammation in human subjects as determined by airway lavage and biopsy. *American Review of Respiratory Disease* 148:1363–72.

Bergamaschi, E., G. De Palma, P. Mozzoni, S. Vanni, M.V. Vettoni, F. Broeckaert, A. Berard, and A. Mutti. 2001. Polymorphism of quinone-metabolizing enzymes and susceptibility to ozone-induced acute effects. *American Journal of Respiratory and Critical Care Medicine* 163:1426–31.

Caporaso, N., and A. Goldstein. 1995. Cancer genes: Single and susceptibility: Exposing the difference. *Pharmacogenetics* 5:59–63.

Coglianese, C., and G.E. Marchant. 2004. Shifting sands: The limits of science in setting risk standards. *Pennsylvania Law Review* 152:1255–1360.

Corradi, M., R. Alinovi, M. Goldoni, et al. 2002. Biomarkers of oxidative stress after controlled human exposure to ozone. *Toxicology Letters* 134:219–25.

Cranor, C.F. 1997. Eggshell skulls and loss of hair from fright: Some moral and legal principles that protect susceptible populations. *Environmental Toxicology and Pharmacology* 4:239–45.

Eaton, D.L., Farin, F, Omiecinski, C.J., and Omenn, G.S. 1998. Genetic susceptibility. In *Environmental and Occupational Medicine, edited by* W.N. Rom. 3rd ed., 209–21. Boston: Little, Brown.

Friedman, R.D. 1981. *Sensitive populations and environmental standards.* Washington, DC: Conservation Foundation.

Garte, S., L. Gaspari, A.K. Alexandrie, et al. 2001. Metabolic gene polymorphism frequencies in control populations. *Cancer Epidemiology, Biomarkers and Prevention* 10:1239–48.

Grodsky, J.A. 2005. Genetics and environmental law: Redefining public health. *California Law Review* 93:171–270.

Harris, J., and J. Sulston. 2004. Genetic equity. *Nature Reviews Genetics* 5:796–800.

Kabesch, M. 2006. Gene by environment interactions and the development of asthma and allergy. *Toxicology Letters* 162:43–48.

Kalow, W. 2002. Both populations and individuals are evolutionary targets: Pharmacogenomic and cultural indicators. *Pharmacogenomics Journal* 2:12–13.

Kavka, G.S. 1990. Some social benefits of uncertainty. In *The philosophy of the human sciences, edited by* P.A. French, T.E. Uehling, and H.K. Wettstein 311–26. Notre Dame, IN: University of Notre Dame Press.

Kelada, S.N., DL. Eaton, S.S. Wang, N.R. Rothman, and M.J. Khoury. 2003. The role of genetic polymorphisms in environmental health. *Environmental Health Perspectives* 111:1055–64.

Kelly, F.J., and T. Sandström. 2004. Air pollution, oxidative stress, and allergic response. *The Lancet* 363:95–96.

Kirkham, P., and I. Rahman. 2006. Oxidative stress in asthma and COPD: Antioxidants as a therapeutic strategy. *Pharmacology & Therapeutics* 111:476–94.

Kleeberger, S.R. 1995. Genetic susceptibility to ozone exposure. *Toxicology Letters* 82/83:295–300.

Kleeberger, S.R., and Y. Ohtsuka. 2005. Gene-particulate matter-health interactions. *Toxicology and Applied Pharmacology* 207:S276–81.

Kleeberger, S.R., and D. Peden. 2005. Gene-environment interactions in asthma and other respiratory diseases. *Annual Review of Medicine* 56:383–400.

Kleeberger, S.R., S. Reddy, L.Y. Zhang, and A.E. Jedlicka. 2000. Genetic susceptibility to ozone-induced lung hyperpermeability. American Journal of Respiratory Cell and Molecular Biology 22:620–27.

Kramer, C.B., A.C. Cullen, and E.M. Faustman. 2006. Policy implications of genetic information on regulation under the Clean Air Act: The case of particulate matter and asthmatics. *Environmental Health Perspectives* 114:313–19.

Kunzli, N., R. McConnell, D. Bates, et al. 2003. Breathless in Los Angeles: The exhausting search for clean air. *American Journal of Public Health* 93:1494–99.

Lead Industries Ass'n v. EPA, 647 F.2d 1130 (D.C. Cir.), *cert. denied,* 449 U.S. 1042 (1980).

Leikauf, G.D., S.A. McDowell, K. Gammon, S.C. Wesselkamper, C.I. Bachurski, A. Puga, J.S. Wiest, J.E. Leikauf, and D.R. Prows. 2000. Functional genomics of particle-induced lung injury. *Inhalation Toxicology* 12:59–73.

Marchant, G.E. 2003. Genomics and toxic substances: Part II—Toxicogenetics. *Environmental Law Reporter* 33:10641–67.

McCunney, R.J. 2005. Asthma, genes, and air pollution. *Journal of Occupational and Environmental Medicine* 47:1285–91.

McDonnell, W.F. 1996. Individual variability in human lung function responses to ozone exposure. *Environmental Toxicology and Pharmacology* 2:171–75.

McDonnell, W. F., K.E. Muller, P.A. Bromberg, and C.M. Shy. 1993. Predictors of individual differences in acute response to ozone exposure. *American Review of Respiratory Disease* 147:818–25.

Nebert, D.W. 2000. Drug-metabolizing enzymes, polymorphisms, and interindividual response to environmental toxicants. *Clinical Chemistry and Laboratory Medicine* 38:857–61.

Nebert, D.W. 2005. Inter-individual susceptibility to environmental toxicants: A current assessment. *Toxicology and Applied Pharmacology* 207:S34–42.

Olden, K., and J. Guthrie. 2001. Genomics: Implications for toxicology, *Mutation Research* 473:3–10.

Parkin, R.T., and J.M. Balbus. 2000. Can varying concepts of susceptibility in risk assessment affect particulate matter standards? *Journal of Air and Waste Management Association* 50:1417–25.

Peden, D.B. 2005. The epidemiology and genetics of asthma risk associated with air pollution. *Journal of Allergy and Clinical Immunology* 115:213–19.

Reilly, W.K. 1981. Foreword. In *Sensitive Populations and Environmental Standards,* edited by R.D. Friedman. Washington, DC: Conservation Foundation.

Romieu, I., J.J. Sienra-Monge, M. Ramirez-Aguilar, H. Moreno-Macias, N.I. Reyes-Ruiz, B. Estela del Rio-Navarro, M. Hernandez-Avila, and S.J. London. 2004. Genetic polymorphism of GSTM1 and antioxidant supplementation influence lung function in relation to ozone exposure in asthmatic children in Mexico City. *Thorax* 59:8–10.

Rose, G. 1985. Sick individuals and sick populations. *International Journal of Epidemiology* 14:32–38.

Sandford, A.J., and E.K. Silverman. 2002. Chronic obstructive pulmonary disease 1: Susceptibility factors for COPD the genotype-environment interaction. *Thorax* 57:736–41.

Savov, J. D., G.S. Whitehead, J. Wang, G. Liao, J. Usuka, G. Peltz, W.M. Foster, and D.A Schwartz. 2004. Ozone-induced acute pulmonary injury in inbred mouse strains. *American Journal of Respiratory Cell and Molecular Biology* 31:69–77.

Scott, S., L. Prior, F. Wood, and J. Gray. 2005. Repositioning the patient: The implications of being 'at risk'. *Social Science & Medicine* 60:1869–79.

Sharp, R. 2003. Ethical issues in environmental health research. *Environmental Health Perspectives* 111:1786–88.

Tyson, F.L., K. Cook, J. Gavin, C.E. Gaylord, C. Lee, V.P. Setlow, and S. Wilson. 1998. Cancer, the environment, and environmental justice. *Cancer* 83:1784–92.

U.S. Congress. 1970. S. Rep. No. 91-1196, 91st Cong., 2d Sess.

U.S. Environmental Protection Agency. 1977. Air Quality Criteria for Lead. Washington, DC: Author.

U.S. Environmental Protection Agency. 1978a. National primary and secondary ambient air quality standards for lead; final rulemaking, *Federal Register* 43: 46246.

U.S. Environmental Protection Agency. 1978b. A method for assessing the health risks associated with alternative air quality standards for ozone. Quoted in R.D. Friedman *Sensitive populations and environmental standards* (Washington, DC: Conservation Foundation, 1981).

U.S. Environmental Protection Agency. 1979. Revisions to the National Ambient Air Quality Standards for Photochemical Oxidants; final rulemaking. *Federal Register* 44:8202.

U.S. Environmental Protection Agency. 1999. The benefits and costs of the Clean Air Act 1990 to 2010: EPA Report to Congress. At www.epa.gov/air/sect812/copy99.html.

U.S. Environmental Protection Agency. 2004. Air quality criteria for particulate matter, vol. 2. At http://cfpub2.epa.gov/ncea/cfm/recordisplay.cfm?deid=87903.

U.S. Environmental Protection Agency. 2005. Review of the National Ambient Air Quality Standards for Particulate Matter: Policy assessment of scientific and technical information—Staff Paper. At www.epa.gov/ttn/naaqs/standards/pm/data/pmstaffpaper_20051221.pdf.

U.S. Environmental Protection Agency. 2006. Air quality criteria for ozone and related photochemical oxidants. At http://cfpub.epa.gov/ncea/cfm/recordisplay.1cfm?deid=149923.

Venter, J.C., M.D. Adams, E.W. Myers, et al. 2001. The sequence of the human genome. *Science* 291:1304–51.

Vineis, P., and T. Martone. 1995. Genetic-environmental interactions and low-level exposure to carcinogens, *Epidemiology* 6:455–57.

Wakefield, J. 2002. Environmental genome project: Focusing on differences to understanding the whole. *Environmental Health Perspectives* 110:A757–59.

Whitman v. American Trucking Associations, Inc., 531 US 457 (2001).

Wilson, S.H., and K. Olden. The environmental genome project: Phase I and beyond. *Molecular Interventions* 4:147–56.

PART III

OCCUPATIONAL
HEALTH
PERSPECTIVES

CHAPTER 9

Genetics and Workplace Issues

PAUL A. SCHULTE

Attention to genetic issues in the workplace is a relatively recent occurrence (Schulte, 1987; Office of Technology Assessment [OTA],
1990). Historically, genetic factors have not been considered to any extent in occupational safety and health research, practice, regulation, or
litigation. This was, in part, due to the overwhelming and relatively dis-
cernible effects of exposure to occupational hazards and to the absences
of technology that could assess genetic factors. Various changes have led
to increased attention to genetic factors in the workplace. These factors
include development of the technology and science related to the human
genome, improved control of some of the most egregious chemical and
physical hazards (high doses) in the workplace (increasing the likelihood
that gene-environment interactions may have an impact), and the rapidly
increasing costs of health care, which fosters an environment for consideration of genetics as causal factors of occupational diseases.

The scientific and technological developments from the various
genome projects have provided the opportunity for investigators to study
the genetic components of disease more easily and in greater depth. Us-

ing polymerase chain reaction amplification and DNA microarray technologies, researchers can obtain minute amounts of DNA and analyze
them for a vast number of genes. Scientists are now beginning to be able
to explore the genetic components of disease in general and of environmental and occupational disease in particular (Christiani et al., 2001).
The increasing control of exposure to most occupational chemical and
physical hazards has increased the likelihood that differential personal
factors, such as genetics, may play more of a role in disease causation.
One reason for that could be that enzyme systems involved in activation
or detoxification of chemicals may have been saturated when exposures
were high but may be still active at lower exposures (Vineis, 1992). Polymorphism in the genes that code for these enzymes may influence a person's risk for disease, once exposed.

Increased health care costs serve as the backdrop against which many
workplace issues currently occur (Council on Ethical and Judicial Affairs,
1991). Moreover, a small percentage of workers may account for the majority of health care costs of an employer (Light, 1992). Thus, there may
be motivation for the employers to consider genetic risk factors along
with other risk factors in job actions such as hiring, placement, and ter-
mination. It may be, however, that the largest impact of genetics in the
workplace will not be from work-related diseases but rather from non-
work-related diseases that an employer will have to pay for in insurance
premiums or in self-insurance costs or from employee absence or reduced
productivity. In addition, employers may be motivated to look for genetic
or other non-work-related risk factors in legal disputes over claims of
work-relatedness of disease (Poulter, 2001).

Regardless of the reason for increased attention to genetics in the workplace, the underlying fact is that all diseases have a genetic component.
That is, that etiology (the reason for disease), mechanism, pathogenesis,
treatment, and prognosis are all influenced by the action of somatic (non-
hereditary cells) or germ (hereditary) cell genes (Khoury, 2003). It is now
increasingly common practice to identify genetic components of disease
in general medical research and practice (Crooke, 1996; Grody, 2003). It
has long been known that there is a range of variability in human response to occupational hazards, particularly chemical hazards. Genetic
factors contribute to the variability and consequently may be useful to
consider in research and in control of hazards (Neumann and Kimmel,
1998). Growing knowledge about the role of genetic factors promises the

development of sensitive, early-warning indicators of exposure or risk and the identification of characteristics on which to base workplace interventions (Perera, 2000; Christiani et al., 2001). For the most part, these advances are yet to be realized. In fact, although genetic information about disease is inherently important, it is yet to be demonstrated whether it will mean much in investigating genetic factors to improve the ultimate understanding and control of occupational disease.

In this chapter, genetics related to the workplace will be considered in three categories of use: research, practice, and regulation or litigation (Table 9.1). To further explore these categories, I will consider them with respect to inherited genetic factors and acquired genetic effects—a common classification scheme for genetic risks. Inherited genetic effects pertain to somatic and germ cell DNA transmitted through mitosis or meiosis, respectively. These are the processes of cell division that involve the formation of either new body cells (mitosis) or new reproductive cells in the gonads (meiosis). Acquired genetic effects involve modification of genetic material over time and can include genetic damage or genetic expression resulting from workplace or environmental exposures. When measured in a biological specimen, either type of information can be considered a genetic biomarker (Ashford et al., 1990).

The line between inherited genetic factors and acquired genetic damage and effects can be blurry in some areas, particularly those related to gene expression status, such as observed by the technologies of transcrip-

TABLE 9.1
Uses of Genetic Information in the Workplace

Use	Type of genetic information	
	Inherited genetic factors	Acquired genetic effects
Research	Gene-environment interactions	Effects of exposure
	Mechanistic insight	Linkage to disease
	Population characterization	Early warning
	Predictive value	Mechanistic insight
Practice	Disease diagnosis	Genetic monitoring
	Preventive services	Intervention evaluation
	Genetic screening	Risk profiling
	Risk management	Risk management
Regulation or litigation	Risk assessment	Risk assessment and management
	Workers' compensation	Premarket testing
	Tort litigation	Workers' compensation cases
	Standard-setting	Tort litigation
		Standard-setting

tomics, proteomics, toxicogenomics, and metabolomics (the study of metabolic response to environmental exposures, drugs, and diseases). Gene expression is a series of biochemical steps resulting in the production of a specific protein by a specific gene. It is also part of the underpinning of metabolomics. The term "inherited genetic factors" indicates knowledge about the structure and function of the gene and how that gene compares with similar ones in other species. Often this knowledge can be used for the genetic characterization of cell lines or disease tissue leading to molecular classification of the disease (Golub et al., 1999; Nuwaysir et al., 1999; Hanash, 2003). The products of genes (the transcriptomes, proteomes, and metabolomes) involve not only the gene but also the exogenous (environmental) and endogenous (internal) stressors that up- or down-regulate the gene as it responds. For heuristic purposes, these are included in the broad category of "acquired genetic effects." In many cases, these effects are purely adaptive or homeostatic and are not pathological. In other words, a gene may code for a protein (enzyme) that will respond to an environmental stress. The response may be a normal adaptation and not indicative of disease. In short, the distinction between "inherited genetic factors" and "acquired genetic factors" is that the former is what a person is born with and the latter is what occurs during life.

The definition of genetic information includes not only the results of genetic tests but also a variety of elements in a medical record. The medical record of a worker can include family history, history of disease with known strong genetic etiologies, and results of physical examinations and common laboratory tests. This type of information is often routinely reported by workers on job applications, health questionnaires for jobs, insurance applications, and workers' compensation forms. Such information could be used discriminatorily and should be treated like other sensitive medical information (Rothstein, 1999).

Inherited Genetic Factors
Research

Despite the strong causal associations that have been detected in many occupational studies, there remains a differential distribution of diseases among workers that cannot be accounted for by differences in exposure, work practice, or lifestyle. Genetic factors are likely to be responsible for some of this distribution (Neumann and Kimmel, 1998). It is clearly accepted that practically no disease is determined solely by either genes or environment. In the early history of occupational epidemiology, genetic influences were considered only with respect to confounding by race and sex. Today as many occupational exposures are being controlled to lower levels, the importance of genetic factors as sources of variability in risk estimates is increasing. This is not to imply that occupational etiologies will be replaced with genetic etiologies, rather that genetic factors, which might confound exposure-disease associations, are being included as relevant variables in study designs and analyses.

Five major methodological approaches have been commonly used in the use of occupational disease involving genetic factors. These are (1) adjustment for confounding by race, ethnicity, and sex in epidemiologic studies; (2) case studies of occupational diseases in genetically susceptible workers; (3) cross-sectional studies of the prevalence of disease among genetically differentiated groups; (4) case control studies of the association of genetic characteristics and disease; and (5) family studies of disease aggregations (Schulte, 1987).

These approaches coupled with the scientific advances brought about by the sequencing of the human genome and by advances in molecular biology, such as the polymerase chain reaction and the use of restriction enzymes to identify gene variants, have begun to transform research questions and study designs and analytic approaches in occupational health (Shostak, 2003). This transformation focuses more on studies of gene-environment interactions, which aim to describe how genetic and environmental occupational factors jointly influence the risk of developing disease (Kelada et al., 2003; Hunter, 2005). The study of gene-environment interactions (1) allows for better estimates of population-attributable risk of genetic and occupational factors, (2) strengthens associations between occupational risk factors and disease, (3) provides insight into mechanisms of action, and (4) provides new opportunities for intervention and prevention (Hunter, 2005).

In addition to the approaches mentioned earlier, new analytic and methodological techniques are being used. These include case-only designs, genome-wide association studies, Mendelian randomization, and neural networks (Vineis et al., 2004; Hunter and Kraft, 2007). Case-only designs use only a sample of people with a particular disease. This approach allows for testing whether there is interaction, the coparticipation of two or more factors, in the same causal mechanism leading to disease. That the case-only approach allows for assessing the interaction of genetic and environmental factors in only a series of cases, but with no comparison group (Vineis et al., 2004). Genome-wide association studies are case-control studies involving entire or major parts (e.g., 500,000 polymorphisms) of a genome (Hunter and Kraft, 2007). Mendelian randomization (the use of genotype-disease associations to make inferences about environmental causes of disease) involves exploiting the random assignment of genes as a means of reducing confounding in exposure-disease associations (Khoury et al., 2005). Neural networks (an approach to modeling complex relationships) may allow for the identification of multiple genetic risk factors (gene-gene interactions) in relatively small sample sizes (Ritchie et al., 2003).

New high-throughput technologies, such as DNA and gene microarrays, and automated work stations capable of extracting, amplifying, hybridizing, and detecting DNA sequences will present a number of benefits and issues in studying genetic and environmental variables (Christiani et al., 2001). The benefits include the ability to study large numbers of genes, practically the entire human genome, in one study or experiment and to have access to data banks containing further information on genomic DNA. The primary attendant issue with this technology includes heightened difficulties in analyzing and interpreting such large amounts of data (Ermolaeva et al., 1998).

The underlying rationale of most research involving genetic and occupational risk factors is determining the extent to which the genetic factors may modify the exposure-effect relationship. That is, will the risk of disease attributable to an occupational exposure be decreased, unchanged, or increased among individuals with a particular genetic characteristic (Le Marchand and Wilkens, 2008)? For the most part, this may be because the gene in question codes for an enzyme or receptor involved in the activation, metabolism, or detoxification of the occupational exposure. This genetic factor is generally not a risk for disease without the exposure. In contrast, some genes may be risk factors for the same disease that the occupational exposure is and, thus, the two may be additive (Vineis et al., 2004). In addition, there may be variation in genetically coded repair capabilities in people for mutations or damages.

Ultimately, the focus of occupational genetic research should be conditioned by criteria for the importance of the research to answer questions with workplace relevance. As Millikan (2002) noted: "If epidemiologists only direct their efforts toward a comprehensive search for the genetic underpinnings of every discrete health outcome and ignore environmental exposures and attributable risks, they will miss opportunities to prevent disease" (p. 477).

For research on the role of genetics in occupational disease to be useful and informative, the validity of the genetic information needs to be assessed or confirmed. Validity can pertain to the assay used to evaluate genetic polymorphisms and also to the population characteristics that influence the prevalence and distribution of a polymorphism. Only when the underlying validity questions have been assessed can a genetic assay be used effectively to study occupational exposure-disease associations. Genetic research that focuses on one or a few genes may be overly simplistic (Staley, 2003). There are many genes that might affect risk in the event of an exposure. Ultimately, the research needed regarding genes or gene expression will need to take a systems biology approach (Toyoshiba et al., 2004). Such an approach requires much investment and experimentation. However, with the emergence of technologies that enable collection of comprehensive genomic data sets it may be possible obtain system level understanding (Kitano, 2002; Hunter and Kraft, 2007).

Also on the horizon is the possibility of research on the genetic basis of behavior and on psychological characteristics and their role in workplace injuries and accidents. This is a highly controversial area, even more than research on physiological effects of genetic factors (Bouchard and McGue, 2003; Hobert, 2003). Understanding the behavior of workers and employers is an important part of identifying occupational safety and health risk factors, but applying behavioral genetics to that factor will raise many ethical, legal, and social issues (Nuffield Council on Bioethics, 2002). Moreover, focusing on behavior of workers fails to account for the responsibilities of employers to provide safe and healthy workplaces.

Rights of Participants in Research

How workers are recruited into occupational genetic studies can involve serious ethical and social issues (Schulte and Sweeney, 1995). These issues hinge on what potential subjects are told about the study and whether they can truly give informed consent. If subjects are deceived or coerced in to participating in a study or are given false expectations (e.g., "We can tell if you are sick or well") with respect to the value of the study to the participant, ethical principles are violated. For example, a researcher could coerce a potential subject directly (e.g., "You may lose your job if you don't participate") or by implication. Communicating false expectations or using pressure is patently dishonest and unethical. It is unlikely that such deception or coercion would be overt; rather, it would be more subtle and difficult to detect.

A broad spectrum of opinion exists about what obtaining informed consent entails and when it is achieved (Clayton et al., 1995; Samuels, 1996; Hunter and Caporaso, 1997; Schulte, Hunter, and Rothman, 1997). Some believe that for genetic data (biomarkers) for which the meaning is not known at the time of the study, a subject or worker in an occupational study cannot give truly informed consent (Samuels, 1996). This implies a much higher standard of interpretation for genetic biomarker information than for other information routinely obtained by questionnaires, environmental monitoring, or record linkage. Until there is determination of predictive value and course in the natural history, such genetic biomarkers are clearly only research variables with no clinical meaning, and participants should be made aware of this. The extent to which a biomarker has been validated (i.e., quantitatively linked to risk of disease at the group or individual level) should be clearly described to potential research participants.

With regard to informing participants of risks, general practice has been to identify only medical risks; however, it has been argued that truly informed consent should include reference to nonmedical risks that might affect participants. For example, a person might need to be informed that the mere acknowledgment on an employment or insurance application that the subject had a biological or "genetic test" in a research study may result in risk of denial of employment or insurance, although this may be less of an issue with the passing of the Genetic Information Nondiscrimination Act of 2008. Participants in occupational genetic studies consent to provide the specimens and corollary demographic and risk factor information and, hence, cooperate in the specified research. The participant generally does not consent or imply consent to distribution of the data in a way that identifies him or her individually to any other parties, such as employers, unions, insurers, and so on (Schulte et al., 1997).

Interpreting and Communicating the Results of Occupational Genetic Research: A Case Study

Critical in research are issues in interpretation and communication of results. These issues are illustrated by a case study of an occupational genetic investigation involving hospital workers exposed to ethylene oxide, which is used to sterilize hospital equipment and materials and has been classified as a human carcinogen by the International Agency for Research on Cancer (1994). A study was conducted to assess the relationship between the glutathione-S-transferase theta 1 (*GSTT1*) null variant (a gene that will detoxify the active form of ethylene oxide) and hydroxyethyl valine (HEV) hemoglobin adducts, surrogates for DNA adducts and, hence, cancer risks (Yong et al., 2001). The study showed a twofold higher risk of HEV adducts in exposed workers with the *GSTT1* null genotype than in those with the wild type (at least one copy of the gene). The researchers were faced with the question of what to tell the study participants who were found to have the *GSTT1* null genotype during the research.

Three issues regarding interpreting and communicating results in this study merit consideration. First, making a decision about what to tell particpants is a manifestation of the problem that epidemiologic information pertains to the group and not to any particular person. Thus, there is a need to extrapolate and make assumptions about individual risks. Second, when the risk factors were modeled, the variability (R^2) of HEV adducts for workers with the *GSTT1* null genotype was 4 percent compared with 28 percent for smoking (tobacco smoke contains ethylene) and 30 percent for workplace exposure to ethylene oxide exposure. Thus, the genetic factor, while statistically significant, may not play an important role in risks for ethylene oxide exposure because it explained a relatively small proportion of the adduct variability. Third, while this study was apparently the first to find the link between *GSTT1* and HEV hemoglobin adducts in ethylene oxide-exposed workers, it was a small transitional study. The results of many initial or transitional studies of gene-environment interactions have not been replicated due to the use of small sample size or samples of convenience with little control for bias (Bogardus, Concato, and Feinstein, 1999). Consequently, although there was laboratory support from in vitro studies (Fost et al., 1991, 1995) without epidemiologic corroboration linking exposure and disease, the results were tentative.

Thus, investigators informed participants of what they knew; namely, "The absence of the gene may be related to a person's risk of cancer if exposed to ethylene oxide, but this is not certain." At the time this study was being conducted, there was relatively little or no guidance regard-

ing informed consent available specifically for population-based or occupational studies of low-penetrance gene variants like *GSTTI*. Subsequently, a Centers for Disease Control and Prevention multidisciplinary
group (Beskow et al., 2001) using expert opinion, as well as federal regulation, the National Bioethics Advisory Commission's report on research
involving human biological materials (National Bioethics Advisory Commission [NBAC], 1999), and the relevant literature suggested that participants not be told of information that has no direct clinical relevance.
However, occupational studies differ from population-based studies in
the sampling frame used and the types of intervention available. In occupational settings "clinical relevance" could be defined as whether participants could take reasonable preventive or medical action based on the
results. In the workplace, these reasonable actions could include implementation of various engineering, administrative, or behavioral controls
(Weeks, Levy, and Wagner, 1991). Nonetheless, although the findings of
this epidemiologic study were not deemed to be clinically relevant, the
investigators had informed participants of the results as part of a prior
informed consent agreement. While informing the participants of these
results was appropriate, the larger issue is that in population studies of
low penetrant genes, informing participants of results should be based
on clinical relevance.

Practice
Prevention and Diagnosis

Genetic tests have been shown to be useful for various nonoccupational diseases in diagnosing disease, assessing individual risk, and providing preventive services (Burke et al., 2002; Grody, 2003). Thus these
tests are becoming a part of general medical practice. The extent to which
they will permeate practice related to the workplace and workers is not
known, nor is whether such approaches will be useful for preventing or
controlling occupational disease. If genetic tests are to be useful in occupational health, a process of evidence-based integration of data will be
needed to develop of guidelines for disease prevention and health services, similar to that which has been suggested for general clinical and
public health practice (Centers for Disease Control and Prevention, 2007).

In the future, the practice of occupational medicine may occur against
the backdrop of individualized or personal medicine. At the least this

may involve the need to consider an individual's genetic profile in the context of risk and prevention regarding occupational exposures. The pressures to consider genetics and occupational exposures may grow as pharmacogenetic assessments become more common in medical practice (Rothstein, 2003). The question that arises is who actually makes the decisions based on the individual genetic profile: the worker, the employer, or both.

Employment Decisions

The capacity of the human body to respond to chemical exposure and physical agents varies from one individual to another. To some extent this is due to genetic characteristics which, in principle, could become part of employment testing known as genetic screening.

Four objectives of genetic screening have been identified: (1) to ensure appropriate placement at the job site, (2) to exclude job applicants with increased susceptibility to disease, (3) to set limit values for more susceptible subgroups, and (4) to provide individual health counseling (Van Damme et al., 1995). In general, pre- and postemployment nongenetic testing is a relatively common practice in selection and placement in the workplace. Susceptibility, however, is the result of a variety of genetic and nongenetic factors. Despite the profound advances in understanding the human genome, there are still no genetic tests that have been fully validated for use to screen perspective employees for occupational disease. Moreover, much controversy surrounds the practice of genetic screening including such issues as the poor predictive value of the tests (Van Damme et al., 1995; Holtzman, 2003). Genetic polymorphisms may be unevenly distributed in the population among different ethnic groups. Thus, racial or ethic discrimination could be a consequence of inappropriate use of genetic screening, which might be aimed at excluding workers at employment examination (Van Damme et al., 1995). In the practice of occupational medicine, genetic information has been used selectively, mostly as derived from medical history and used in job placement or in diagnosis (American Management Association [AMA], 1999; Staley, 2003).

Genetic information may be obtained in three stages during the employment process: (1) preemployment, preoffer; (2) postoffer, preplacement; and (3) postemployment, postplacement. However, the Americans with Disabilities Act (ADA) prohibits medical inquiries including genetic inquiries and tests prior to extending a conditional job offer. At other times, use of genetic information must be "job-related" and consistent with "business necessity." These two criteria are defined by the Equal Employment Opportunity Commission to mean that an employer has a reasonable belief based on objective evidence that (1) an employee's ability to perform essential job functions will be impaired by a medical condition or (2) an employee will pose a direct threat to other employees or customers because of a medical condition (U.S. Equal Employment Opportunity Commission [EEOC], 2000).

One way of obtaining genetic information is through screening, which examines the genetic makeup of employees or job applicants for certain inherited traits. The actual use of genetic assays or tests of workers in job offering or placement is believed to be rare, but the available data to assess such activity are weak. According to a 1999 survey of the American Management Association, 6.7 percent of companies tested and used genetic information to hire applicants, 7.3 percent to reassign employees, and 1.7 percent to dismiss or retain employees (AMA, 1999; Schill, 2000). The accuracy or generalizability of this survey has not assessed, and it is not clear to what extent these statistics are actually representative of the true use of genetic information.

Genetic screening has been assessed by the European Group on Ethics in Science and New Technologies (EGE; 2003), which concluded that the use of genetic screening in the context of the medical examination, as well as the disclosure of results of previous genetic tests, is not ethically acceptable. Furthermore, EGE found that, to date, there is no proven evidence that the existing genetic screening tests have relevance or reliability in the context of employment. Generally, genetic screening tests still have uncertain predictive value (EGE, 2003).

Genetic screening could focus on occupational-related and nonoccupational-related disease or susceptibility. There is no Occupational Safety and Health Act standard that requires genetic testing for occupational susceptibility. Such testing has been described as running contrary to the spirit and intent of the act, which requires a safe and healthy workplace for all workers (see Schill, 2000). Nonetheless, genetic information is increasingly used in understanding and diagnosing of disease. Some proponents of genetic screening argue that, in a competitive business environment, employers should have the opportunity to use technical innovations, such as genetic screening, to select employees, or may, in fact, have the responsibility to use it (Seltzer, 1998; French, 2002). Genetic factors are already indirectly considered in job decisions to the extent that they affect abilities, skills, and knowledge. Ostensibly, organizations would use genetic screening to avoid placing hypersusceptible workers in hazardous jobs (OTA, 1990). With these potential benefits, some have argued that companies may have an obligation to screen (Seltzer, 1998).

Genetic screening information may be useful to inform potential employees of job risks, if that information is not available to employers in individually identifiable form. This was illustrated in a pilot screening program in a company where beryllium was machined. The employer developed the program for prospective employees because of concern for the debilitating lung condition, chronic beryllium disease, in workers with beryllium exposure. Research had shown that in addition to beryllium exposure, a certain genetic characteristic, $HLA\text{-}DPB^{E69}$ was also a risk factor. Moreover, beryllium sensitization could occur regardless of dose and had occurred even in relatively well-controlled areas. The employer established the screening program so that job applicants could receive their individual results. The predictive value of the screening test was poor, and a negative test was not an assurance for lack of risk because other variants on chromosome 6, which were not tested for, also were risk factors (Weston, 2002). There are no published data on the results of the program or the issues that arose. The program was stopped after a few years. While, in principle, it seems useful that prospective employees would benefit from information about potential risks, the attendant problems are without impact. In such a test there would be many false positive findings, and many people would make employment decisions based on flawed information. Second, it is a slippery slope from voluntary anonymous screening to mandated screening of individually identifiable applicants by prospective employers. In this case with the test for $HLA\text{-}DPB^{E69}$ many workers not at increased risk would be discriminated against. In contrast, if the test had a high (>90%) predictive value an employer may have an argument for the right to use it in employee selections.

The occupational safety and health community has identified a hierarchy of controls for preventing occupational disease and injuries (Halperin and Frazier, 1985). Genetic screening is not part of the hierarchy of control. It involves evaluating employees prior to employment. There is, however, a history of medical evaluation as part of job placement decision making. The addition of genetic screening to the process of job placement has the potential to reverse the emphasis in the hierarchy of controls from changing the environment to changing (excluding) the workers (Schulte and Halperin, 1987).

Various authoritative and scholarly groups have identified criteria for the use of genetic screening tests (Van Damme et al., 1995; American College of Occupational and Environmental Medicine [ACOEM], 1994; ACOEM, 1995; NBAC, 1999). In addition to the ADA requirements that tests be job-related and consistent with business practice, as well as other civil rights stipulations in legislation, there are the issues of the validity and utility of the tests as well as ethical, legal, and social safeguards. In short, an adequate evidence base is needed before the use of a genetic screening test in the unique case such testing might be useful. Until such a base is established, the test would not be ready for use in a worker population. In 1994, the American College of Occupational and Environmental Medicine concluded in that "until extensively validated by researchers, tests should be considered a form of human investigation." This means that until validated, the test is useful only in research and not in practice.

Although currently no genetic tests have been validated for assessing the increased risk of susceptibility to workplace hazards, it is anticipated that such tests will eventually become available. Whether these tests would be socially approved is still in question. The Genetic Nondiscrimination Act of 2008 will prohibit discrimination with respect to employment and health insurance.

Regulation and Litigation

One of the first workplace areas where genetic information has been used is workers' compensation. There is no legal prohibition against including any medical or genetic tests in the independent medical examination that is routine in workers' compensation cases (Rothenberg et al., 1997). In addition, informed consent for such testing is not required. By extension, genetic information may also be used as proof of causation in toxic injury litigation. However, analysis of the role of genetic factors in multiple cause cases requires statistical and mechanistic data about how the combination of genetic and toxic risks causes disease (Poulter, 2001).

The use of genetic information in a workers' compensation matter is illustrated by a case involving railroad track workers who filed compensation claims, under the Federal Railway Act (that does not have a no-fault-based compensation system), for carpal tunnel syndrome due to repetitive motion stress in their track work. Without their knowledge or consent, the employer tested them for a deletion in chromosome 17, involving a protein, peripheral myelin protein-22 (*PMP22*). This is not a test for carpal tunnel syndrome, but for "hereditary neuropathy with liability to pressure palsies," which may have a manifestation that includes carpal tunnel syndrome. The issue here is that, beyond the ethical and legal aspects at the time of use, there was an inadequate knowledge base (most particularly an absence of epidemiologic data) on which to make a decision to incorporate such a test (Schulte, 2004). Although there is extensive information on the work-relatedness of carpal tunnel syndrome, there is less information on the role of hereditary factors. For the most part, the role of hereditary factors for carpal tunnel syndrome was assessed in family studies, however, on a population basis, the *PMP22* deletions are rare. It would therefore be unlikely that there would be any individuals in the group of 20 railroad workers tested that had this deletion.

This is an example of inappropriate and premature testing—that is, testing for a genotype that had not been validated at the population level. Specifically, the predictive value, absolute, relative, and attributable risks had not been assessed. Also of relevance to work-related cases, the question of whether society should use genetic testing for susceptibility genotypes to apportion causation is unresolved. In fact, under the Federal Railway Act, non–work-related causes may be considered in compensation cases. This question raises the issue of whether immutable traits beyond a worker's control should be factored into a claim of work-relatedness of a disease. In some jurisdictions (various states such as Iowa, Wisconsin, New York, and New Hampshire), consensual genetic testing is allowed in compensation cases. In the United States, most workers' compensation statutes permit medical testing, including genetic testing, to ascertain the medical condition of the claimant and the potential work-relatedness of the claim (Schulte, 2004). However, many U.S. organizations do not generally condone genetic testing without informed consent (ACOEM, 1994).

There are no examples in occupational safety and health regulations where genetic information is required. Numerous state laws, laws in development, and Federal Executive Order No. 13145 in 2000 (Clinton, 2000) have called for safeguards or prohibitions from such use (Rothenberg et al., 1997). In 1995, the Equal Employment Opportunity Commission updated the Compliance Manual for the Americans with Disabilities Act (ADA) to define "disability" to apply to those who are subject to discrimination on the basis of genetic information. However, the worker must be able to prove that the employer regards them as "disabled." This interpretation has not been tested in court (Rothenberg et al., 1997), but recent judicial decisions may call into question the Equal Employment Opportunity Commission's interpretation. (See Rothstein in this book.)

Genetic advances push at the historic boundaries of the Occupational Safety and Health Act of 1970. The act mandates standards and rules to assure "that to the extent feasible employees will not suffer material impairment of health or functional capacity." This raises the question of whether workers who could be defined by certain genetic polymorphisms as "hypersusceptible" should have special protections. The implementation of these protections raises a host of questions and issues regarding privacy, discrimination, and responsibility (Bergeson, 2003).

One component of the regulatory process is the practice of risk assessment, the quantitative identification of risks at given levels of exposure. Risk assessment is one of the activities related to regulation and litigation that may use genetic information (Neumann and Kimmel, 1998). Risk assessment involves the evaluation of exposure and response data to identify levels of risk and safety where limits can be set. The use of genetic data may help to better understand the risks of various levels of exposure. Genetic susceptibility information has been used in risk-assessment models to determine the impact of the role of metabolic polymorphisms on risk estimates (Bois, Krowech, and Zeise, 1995; El-Masri, Bell, and Portier, 1999). To gauge the impact of genetic markers on risk assessment, El-Masri, Bell, and Portier (1999) conducted a simulation study of cancer risk estimates for exposure to dichloromethane. The risk estimates from statistical models were 23 percent to 30 percent higher when an effect-modifying polymorphism (*GSTT1*) was not included. Susceptibility biomarkers may reflect variation in exposure, kinetics, and effects and are, therefore, important to consider in risk assessments. Mechanism-based modeling has the potential to decrease uncertainties across and within species and exposure scenarios and to quantify pathways and complex relationships within gene networks.

The establishment of a recommended level of exposure with some margin of safety is an important aspect of quantitative risk assessment. In the occupational field, the historic approach involved the use of uncertainty factors to account for cross-species and interindividual variability. More recently, the benchmark has been the 1 in 1,000 level of risk described by the Supreme Court in the *Industrial Union Department, AFL-CIO v. American Petroleum Institute* 448 US 607 (1980), which is commonly known as the *Benzene* decision. Genetic factors could be used to address uncertainties and provide more precise risk assessments and identify specific subgroups with different risks.

Acquired Genetic Effects
Research

There is an extensive scientific literature assessing the impact of environmental hazards on genetic material (Albertini et al., 2000; Albertini, 2001a; Jones et al., 2002; Bonassi et al., 2004; Hagmar et al., 2004). For the most part, this has involved assessment of cytogenetic effects (e.g., effects on chromosomes), changes in various reporter genes (e.g., glycophorin–A [GPA] and hypoxanthine phosphorsibosyltransferase [HPRT]), and mutations and the formation of DNA and protein adducts following exposure to electrophilic chemicals or ionizing radiation (Schulte and DeBord, 2000; Albertini, 2001b). In addition gene function can be altered by more than just changes in DNA sequences. A wide variety of illnesses, behaviors, and other health indicators have some level of evidence linking them with epigenetic mechanisms. These are any process that alters gene activity without changing the DNA sequence (Southerland and Costa, 2003; Weinhold, 2006). The objectives of much of this research were to determine whether genetic damage did occur and whether it could lead to harmful health effects. The forerunners of this type of research included studies of the Japanese atomic bomb survivors.

More recent studies of workers exposed to various genotoxic chemicals have demonstrated that high frequencies of chromosomal aberrations indicated increase risk of cancer in groups of healthy people (Bonassi et al., 2004; Hagmar et al., 2004). The newer DNA and expression technologies, including toxicogenomics, transcriptomics, proteomics, and metabolomics are means to assess acquired genetic effects (Christiani et al., 2001; Waters, Olden, and Tennant, 2003; Toyoshiba et al., 2004; Wang et al., 2005). These approaches allow for the assessment of the expression of many thousands of genes before and after exposure. Implicit in these approaches is the assumption that effects of xenobiotics can be detected in expression of genes. The ability to analyze and interpret the vast amounts of data that arises from the studies will be critical in using this technology. Such interpretation is quite difficult because many factors affect gene expression, and adaptive or homeostatic responses need to be distinguished from pathologic ones.

An investigation of workers exposed to welding fumes is illustrative of the type of studies that use microarray expression technologies. The study compared exposed workers (pre- and postexposure) compared with nonexposed controls. The investigators found that genes with altered response clustered in biological processes related to oxidative stress, intracellular signal transduction, cell cycle, and programmed cell death (Wang et al., 2005). A similar type of study of automobile emissions inspectors and waste-incineration workers involved 1,152 genes. The expression profiles showed that the expression of genes and proteins involved in oxidative stress was up-regulated in both groups of workers compared with controls. Additionally, proteomic analysis revealed that several proteins such as transthyretin, sarcolectin, and haptoglobin were highly up- or down-regulated, and the investigators concluded that these could serve as biological markers in future research (Kim et al., 2004). Thus, patterns of genes can be detected that may reflect specific exposures.

If a microarray pattern can be validated as a biomarker of effect, it may be used as an independent or dependent variable in etiologic or intervention research, and as evidence of harm in workers' compensation or tort litigation. These patterns could also be used in standards as biological exposure indices.

The acquisition of effects on the genome also involves change in gene expression that does not involve DNA. This is known as "epigenetics" (Southerland and Costa, 2003; Weinhold, 2006). A broad spectrum of diseases and environmental exposures has some evidence that links them with epigenetics. However, there is need for more mechanistic research before epigenetics can be used widely in population studies, practice, or regulation (Wade and Archer, 2006; Weinhold, 2006).

Practice

Ascertaining acquired genetic damage information in occupational safety and health practice would generally occur in the form of genetic monitoring. This is the periodic examination of employees to evaluate modification of their genetic material (e.g., chromosomal damage or evidence of increased occurrence of molecular mutations) that might have occurred during the course of employment and exposure to workplace substances (OTA, 1990). In principle, genetic monitoring is similar to other types of health effects or exposure monitoring that is conducted in the workplace (for example, monitoring for lead in blood; Van Damme et al., 1995). However, the fact that genetic monitoring involves somatic genetic effects often leads to its being considered as a somewhat different form of monitoring. In fact, genetic monitoring is generally no different from other forms of biological monitoring and should have the following criteria met before use: an acceptable level of sensitivity and specificity; the acceptance by the population being monitored; an established linkage to exposure or disease; protections for privacy and confidentially; notification to participants of results; and a plan for addressing abnormal results. At present, the results of genetic monitoring can only be interpreted on a group level; they have not been validated as individual risk predictors (Van Damme et al., 1995). If high-throughput expression technologies become candidates for use in genetic monitoring, the issues of standardization, validation, and interpretability will have to be overcome because these will be much greater than with a single test.

Medical removal is a critical workplace issue that is related to any type of medical monitoring, including genetic monitoring. Medical removal is moving the worker to another job location where the exposure is lower or absent. It has been argued that medical removal should be accompanied with continued pay at the rate before the removal (Ashford et al., 1990). Medical removal is not meant to replace exposure controls through engineering means.

Regulation and Litigation

Currently, no U.S. regulations require genetic monitoring of workers. In part, this is because questions arise about whether genetic monitoring indicates just exposure or a potential health problem or compensable injury (Schulte and DeBord, 2000). No genetic monitoring test has been fully validated to assess an individual's risk (Van Damme et al., 1995).

The various expression array technologies also can be applied to human or animal cell cultures that have been exposed to xenobiotics

(Waters et al., 2003; Toyoshiba et al., 2004; Wang et al., 2005). This approach could be used to screen chemicals prior to introduction into commerce.

The gene expression technologies have been viewed as potentially providing useful data for risk assessment (Simmons and Portier, 2002). However, there are numerous questions, as summarized by Freeman, regarding the use, by regulating agencies, of data from microarray experiments (Freeman, 2004). These include

- How does a regulator deal with risk-assessment data that scientists are often unable to interpret—data that some companies are anxious to submit and others to withhold?
- How does this same regulator evaluate information that is produced without a universally recognized standard for laboratory protocols or data formats?
- Should companies submit all information voluntarily without knowing whether regulators will be able to understand it, whether they will use it, and if they do, exactly how?
- What if data that cannot be interpreted now are later shown to indicate toxicity, perhaps at a low level that could not be detected in animal testing? The critical issue in using genomics data is that, if and when such data are interpretable with respect to population risks, what will be the regulatory focuses if sensitive subgroups are identified? Will controls be required to protect these groups? Or will risk-management strategies, such as communications, be applied (Freeman, 2004)?

In the short-term, transcriptomics and proteomics will probably be of most value for the hazard identification aspect of risk assessment (Faustman and Omenn, 1996; Morgan et al., 2002). However, if gene expression technology is to enter the mainstream of the risk-assessment process, protocols for assays to confirm selected biochemical responses will need to be developed as regulatory requirements (Morgan et al., 2002).

Development and Use of Occupational Genetic Biomarker Information

There is a continuum of stages between the discovery and use of genetic biomarker information in public health in general and in occupational safety and health, particularly (Figure 9.1). This continuum is multidirectional. While discoveries of genetic biomarkers in the labora-

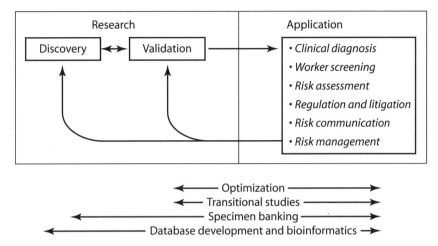

Figure 9.1. Continuum for the development and use of occupational genetic biomarkers

tory are driving factors, there is also an impetus for research provided by problems that arise in applications of genetic information. However, for genetic biomarkers to be successfully developed there is a critical need for laboratory and population validation. Laboratory validation pertains to characteristics of the marker and the assay. Population validation pertains to its prevalence and distribution in the population and in the predictive value of the marker. The developmental process for a validated useful biomarker may entail various studies to optimize the use of the assay and to assess its characteristics in various populations. These have been referred to as transitional studies (Schulte et al., 1997; Albertini, 2001). Knowledge of the relationship between exposure, genetic susceptibility, and disease is still limited, and further epidemiologic research aiming to clarify these relationships is needed (Van Damme and Casteleyn, 2003). Collection of biologic specimens (DNA) is usually costly; consequently, much of the specimen is often saved in biological specimen banks (or biobanks) following the initial study for other uses. Additionally, the results of analyses of DNA samples are often saved in human genetic databases. The establishment of human specimen banks and genetic databases raises complex questions about their ethical, legal, and social implications (Arnason, Nordal, and Arnason, 2004). Of particular relevance to the workplace setting is determining who will have access to the information and specimens, and for what purpose.

Ultimately, genetics should be integrated into public and occupational health. It should not be treated as exceptional but should be handled like other sensitive medical information and used as other disciplinary tools are used—when needed (Schulte, 2004; Khoury et al., 2005). Until that integration occurs, there may be a need for specific safeguards that address the real and perceived power of genetic information.

Safeguards against Improper Use of Genetic Information

The power of genetic information, both inherited factors and acquired indications of effects, must be carefully considered before use in the workplace (Ashford et al., 1990). Uncertainty over the meaning and relevance of a single metabolic gene or combinations of genes can be the basis of ethical controversy (Lemmons, 1992; Van Damme et al., 1995; Schulte et al., 1999; Grody, 2003; Holtzman, 2003). If there were certainty that a particular genetic characteristic had an exact risk, then the basis might exist for a deliberative societal response. Genetic information derived from biological specimens adds an element of "individual results" to epidemiological studies. However, until genetic markers are validated as individual risk predictors, their use should be restricted.

Van Damme et al. (1995) concluded that the availability of a genetic test should neither automatically enhance the assumption of its usefulness nor allow its application in the absence of clear objectives and without evaluation of its relevance and consequences in a particular context. There is no federal legislation that explicitly and completely protects against genetic discrimination in the workplace or in individual insurance coverage.

Information on acquired genetic effects is less controversial and may be more useful in monitoring exposed workers. While such approaches may have issues that need to be considered, they do not have the same degree of concern as that is involved with inherited genetic factors.

Occupational safety and health researchers, practitioners, and policy specialists should consider the wide range of deleterious effects of using genetic information without proper safeguards (Rothstein, 2000; Burke et al., 2002; McCunney, 2002; Holtzman, 2003; Brandt-Rauf and Brandt-Rauf, 2004). These safeguards include protecting the autonomy of workers in making decisions about their genetic information and providing for the confidentiality and security of genetic information. To a large extent, the passage of the Genetic Information Nondiscrimination Act will provide some protection against using genetic information in employment and insurance decisions. Meanwhile genetic knowledge will continue to pervade medical science and public health, and judicious use should result in practical advances for workers.

ACKNOWLEDGMENTS

From the National Institute for Occupational Safety and Health, Centers for Disease Control and Prevention. The findings and conclusions in this report are those of the author and do not necessarily represent the views of the National Institute for Occupational Safety and Health. The author is grateful for comments on earlier versions of this chapter from Gayle Debord, Myron Harrison, Muin Khoury, and David Christiani.

REFERENCES

Albertini, R.J. 2001a. Developing sustainable studies on environmental health. *Mutation Research* 480–481:317–31.
Albertini, R.J. 2001b. HPRT mutations in humans: Biomarkers for mechanistic studies. *Mutation Research* 489:1–16.
Albertini, R.J., D. Anderson, G.R. Douglas, et al. 2000. IPCS guidelines for the monitoring of genotoxic effects of carcinogens in humans. International Programme on Chemical Safety. *Mutation Research* 463:111–72.
American College of Occupational and Environmental Medicine. 1994. *Genetic screening in the workplace.* At www.jserranomd.medem.com/.
American College of Occupational and Environmental Medicine. 1995. ACOEM position on the confidentiality of medical information in the workplace. *Journal of Occupational and Environmental Medicine* 37:594–96.
American Management Association. 1999. *Workplace testing: Medical testing.* Annual research report. New York: Author.
Ashford, N.A., C.J. Spadafor, D.B. Hattis, and C.C. Caldart. 1990. *Monitoring the worker for exposure and disease.* Baltimore: Johns Hopkins University Press.
Arnason, G., S. Nordal, and V. Arnason (eds.). 2004. Blood and data—Ethical, legal, and social aspects of human genetic databases. Reykjavik: University of Iceland Press.
Bergeson, L.L. 2003. Toxicogenomics and the workplace: What you need to know. *Manufacturing Today* Jan/Feb:8–9.
Beskow, L.M., W. Burke, J.F. Merz, et al. 2001. Informed consent for population-based research involving genetics. *Journal of the American Medical Association* 286:2315–21.

Bogardus Jr., S.T., J. Concato, and A.R. Feinstein. 1999. Clinical epidemiological quality in molecular genetic research: The need for methodological standards. *Journal of the American Medical Association* 281:1919–26.

Bois, F.Y., G. Krowech, and L. Zeise. 1995. Modeling human interindividual variability in metabolism and risk: The example of 4-aminobiphenyl. *Risk Analysis* 15:205–13.

Bonassi, S., A. Znaor, H. Norppa, and L. Harmar. 2004. Chromosomal aberrations and risk of cancer in humans: An epidemiologic perspective. *Cytogenetic and Genome Research* 104:376–82.

Bouchard Jr., T.J., and M. McGue. 2003. Genetic and environmental influences on human psychological differences. *Journal of Neurobiology* 54:4–45.

Brandt-Rauf, P., and S. Brandt-Rauf. 2004. Genetic testing in the workplace: Ethical, legal, and social implications. *Annual Review of Public Health* 25:139–53.

Burke, W., D. Atkins, M. Gwinn, et al. 2002. Genetic test evaluation: Information needs of clinicians, policy makers, and the public. *American Journal of Epidemiology* 156:311–18.

Centers for Disease Control and Prevention. 2007. Genetic testing. At www.cdc.gov/genomics/gtesting.htm.

Christiani, D.C., R.R. Sharp, G.W. Collman, and W.A. Suk. 2001. Applying genomic technologies in environmental health research: Challenges and opportunities. *Journal of Occupational Environmental Medical* 43:526–33.

Clayton, E.W., K.K. Steinberg, M.J. Khoury, et al. 1995. Informed consent for genetic research on stored tissue samples. *Journal of the American Medical Association* 274:1786–92.

Clinton, W.J. 2000. To prohibit discrimination in federal employment based on genetic information. Federal Executive Order No. 13145, 65 Fed. Reg. 6,877.

Council on Ethical and Judicial Affairs, American Medical Association. 1991. Use of genetic testing by employers. *Journal of the American Medical Association* 266:1827–30.

Crooke, S.T. 1996. New drugs and changing disease paradigms. *Nature Biotechnology* 14:238–41.

El-Masri, H.A., D.A. Bell, and C.J. Portier. 1999. Effects of glutathione transferase theta polymorphism on the risk estimates of dichloromethane to humans. *Toxicology and Applied Pharmacology* 158:221–30.

Ermolaeva, O., M. Rastogi, K.D. Pruitt, et al. 1998. Data management and analysis for gene expression arrays. *Nature Genetics* 20:19–23.

European Group on Ethics in Science and New Technologies. 2003. *Opinion on the ethical aspects of genetic testing in the workplace.* Opinion No. 18. Brussels: Author.

Faustman, E.M., and G.S. Omenn. 1995. Risk assessment. In K. Klaassen, ed., *Casarett and Doull's toxicology, the basic science of poisons,* pp. 75–88. New York: McGraw Hill.

Fost, U., E. Hallier, H. Ottenwalder, H.M. Bolt, and H. Peter. 1991. Distribution of ethylene oxide in human blood and its implications for biomonitoring. *Human and Experimental Toxicology* 10:25–31.

Fost, U., M. Tornqvist, M. Leutbecher, F. Granath, E. Hallier, and L. Ehrenberg. 1995. Effects of variation in detoxification rate on dose monitoring through adducts. *Human and Experimental Toxicology* 14:201–3.

Freeman, K. 2004. Toxicogenomics data: The road to acceptance. *Environmental Health Perspectives* 112:A618–85.

French, S. 2002. Genetic testing in the workplace: The employer's coin toss. *Duke Law and Technology Review:* 0015.

Golub, T.R., D.K. Slonim, P. Tamoya, et al. 1999. Molecular classification of cancer: Class discovery and class prediction by gene expression monitoring. *Science* 286:531–37.

Grody, W.W. 2003. Ethical issues raised by genetic testing with oligonucleotide microarrays. *Molecular Biotechnology* 23:127–38.

Hagmar, L., U. Stromberg, S. Bonassi, I.L. Hansteen, L.E. Knudsen, C. Lindholm, and H. Norppa. 2004. Impact of types of lymphocyte chromosomal aberrations on human cancer risk: Results from Nordic and Italian cohorts. *Cancer Research* 64:2258–63.

Halperin, W.W., and T.M. Frazier. 1985. Surveillance for the effects of workplace exposure. *Annual Review of Public Health* 6:419–32.

Hanash, S.M. Disease proteomics. *Nature* 422:226–32.

Hobert, O. 2003. Introduction: Behavioral genetics—The third century. *Journal of Neurobiology* 54:1–3.

Holtzman, N.A. 2003. Ethical aspects of genetic testing in the workplace. *Community Genetics* 6:136–38.

Hunter, D.J. 2005. Gene-environment interactions in human diseases. *Nature Reviews Genetics* 6:287–98.

Hunter, D.J., and N. Caporaso. 1997. Informed consent in epidemiologic studies involving genetic markers. *Epidemiology* 8:596–99.

Hunter, D.J., and P. Kraft. 2007. Drinking from the fire hose—Statistical issues in genomewide association studies. *New England Journal of Medicine* 357:436–39.

International Agency for Research on Cancer. 1994. Some industrial chemicals. *IARC Monographs on the Evaluation of Carcinogenic Risks to Humans.* Vol. 60. Lyon, France: Author.

Jones, I.M., H. Galick, P. Kato, et al. 2002. Three somatic genetic biomarkers and covariates in radiation-exposed Russian cleanup workers of the Chernobyl nuclear reactor 6–13 years after exposure. *Radiation Research* 158:424–42.

Kelada, S.N., D.L. Eaton, S.S. Wang, et al. 2003. The role of genetic polymorphisms in environmental health. *Environmental Health Perspectives* 111:1055–64.

Khoury, M.J. 2003. Genetics and genomics in practice: The continuum from genetic disease to genetic information in health and disease. *Genetics in Medicine* 5:261–68.

Khoury, M.J., R. Davis, M. Gwinn, M.L. Lindegren, and P. Yoon. 2005. Do we need genomic research for the prevention of common diseases with environmental causes? *American Journal of Epidemiology* 161:799–805.

Kim, M.K., S. Oh, J.H. Lee, H. Im, Y.M. Ryu, E. Oh, J. Lee, E. Lee, and D. Sul. 2004. Evaluation of biological monitoring markers using genomic and proteomic analysis for automobile emission inspectors and waste incinerating workers exposed to polycyclic aromatic hydrocarbons or 2,3,7,8,-tetrachlorodecibenso-p-dioxins. *Experimental Molecular Medicine* 36:396–410.

Kitano, H. 2002. Systems biology: A brief overview. *Science* 295:1662–64.

Le Marchand, L., and L.R. Wilkins. 2008. Design considerations for genomic associated studies: Importance of gene-environment interactions. *Cancer Epidemiology, Biomarkers, & Prevention* 17:263–67.

Lemmens, T. 1997. What about your genes? Ethical, legal, and policy dimensions of genetics in the workplace. *Politics and the Life Sciences* 16:57–75.

Light, D.W. 1992. The practice and ethics of risk-rated health insurance. *Journal of the American Medical Association* 267:2503–8.

McCunney, R.J. 2002. Genetic testing: Ethical implications in the workplace. *Occupational Medicine: State of the Art Reviews* 17:665–72.

Millikan, R. 2002. The changing face of epidemiology in the genomics era. *Epidemiology* 13:472–80.

Morgan, K., H.R. Brown, and G. Benavides, et al. 2002. Toxicogenomics and human disease risk assessment. *Human and Ecological Risk Assessment* 8:1339–53.

National Bioethics Advisory Commission. 1999. Report and recommendations of the National Bioethics Advisory Commission. Vol. 1 of Research involving human biological materials: Ethical issues and policy guidance. Rockville, MD: Author. Neumann, D.A., and C.A. Kimmel, eds. 1998. *Human variability in response to chemical exposures: Measures, modeling and risk assessment.* Washington, DC: International Life Sciences Institute/ILSI Press.

Nuffield Council on Bioethics. 2002. *Genetics and human behaviour: The ethical context.* London: Author.

Nuwaysir, E.F., M. Bittner, J. Trent, J.C Barrett, and C.A. Afshari. 1999. Microarrays and toxicology: The advent of toxicogenomics. *Molecular Carcinogenesis* 24:153–59.

Office of Technology Assessment. 1990. *Genetic Monitoring and Screening in the Workplace.* Washington, DC: Government Printing Office.

Perera, F.P. 2000. Molecular epidemiology: on the path to prevention. *Journal of the National Cancer Institute* 92:602–12.

Poulter, S.R. 2001. Genetic testing in toxic injury litigation: The path to certainty or blind alley? *Jurimetrics* 41:211–38.

Ritchie, M.D., B.C. White, J.S. Parker, L.W. Hahn, and J.H. Moore. 2003. Optimization of neural network architecture using genetic programming improves detection and modeling of gene-gene interactions in studies of human diseases. *BMC Bioinformatics* 4:28.

Rothenberg, K., B. Fuller, M. Rothstein, et al. 1997. Genetic information and the workplace: Legislative approaches and policy changes. *Science* 275:1755–57.

Rothstein, M.A. 1999. Why treating genetic information separately is a bad idea. *Texas Review of Law & Politics* 4:33–37.

Rothstein, M.A. 2000. Ethical guidelines for medical research on workers. *Journal of Occupational and Environmental Medicine* 42:1166–71.

Rothstein, M.A., ed. 2003. *Pharmacogenomics: Social, ethical, and clinical dimensions.* Hoboken, NJ: Wiley-Liss.

Samuels, S.W. 1996. A moral history of the evolution of a caste of workers. *Environmental Health Perspectives* 104S:991–98.

Schill, A.L. 2000. Genetic information in the workplace: Implications for occupational health surveillance. *American Association Occupational Health Nurses Journal* 48:80–91.

Schulte, P.A. 1987. Simultaneous assessment of genetic and occupational risk factors. *Journal of Occupational Medicine* 29:884–91.

Schulte, P.A. 2004. Some implications of genetic biomarkers in occupational epidemiology and practice. *Scandinavian Journal of Work, Environment and Health* 30:71–79.

Schulte, P.A., and D.G. DeBord. 2000. Public health assessment of genetic information in the occupational setting. In M.J. Khoury, W. Burke, and E.J. Thomson, eds., *Genetics and public health in the 21st century: Using genetic information to improve health and prevent disease.* New York: Oxford University Press.

Schulte, P.A., and W.E. Halperin. 1987. Genetic screening and monitoring in the workplace. In J.M. Harrington, ed., *Recent advances in occupational health,* pp. 135–54. Edinburgh: Churchill Livingstone.

Schulte, P.A., D. Hunter, and N. Rothman. 1997. Ethical and social issues in the use of biomarkers in epidemiological research. In P. Toniolo et al., eds., *Applications of biomarkers in cancer epidemiology* (pp. 313–18). Lyon, France: International Agency for Research on Cancer.

Schulte, P.A., G.P. Lomax, E.M. Ward, and M.J. Colligan. 1999. Ethical issues in the use of genetic markers in occupational epidemiologic research. *Journal of Occupational Environmental Medicine* 41:639–46.

Schulte, P.A., and M.H. Sweeney. 1995. Ethical considerations, confidentiality issues, rights of human subjects, and uses of monitoring data in research and regulation. *Environmental Health Perspectives* 103S:69–74.

Seltzer, J. 1998. The Cassandra complex: An employer's dilemma in the genetic workplace. *Hofstra Law Review* (Winter):411.

Shostak, S. 2003. Locating gene-environment interaction: At the intersections of genetics and public health. *Social Science and Medicine* 56:2327–42.

Simmons, P.T., and C. Portier. 2002. Toxicogenomics: The new frontier in risk analysis. *Carcinogenesis* 23:903–5.

Southerland, J.E., and M. Costa. 2003. Epigenetics and the environment. *Annals of the New York Academy of Science* 983:151–60.

Staley, K. 2003. Testing in the workplace. Buxton, England: GeneWatch.

Toyoshiba, H., T. Yamanaka, H. Sone, F.M. Panham, N.J. Walker, J. Martinez, and C.J. Portier. 2004. Gene interaction network suggests dioxin induces a significant linkage between aryl hydrocarbon receptor and retinoic acid receptor beta. *Environmental Health Perspectives* 112:1217–24.

U.S. Equal Employment Opportunity Commission. 2000. Policy guidance on Executive Order 13145: To prohibit discrimination in federal employment based on genetic information. Notice No. 915.002. Washington, DC: Author.

Van Damme, K., and L. Casteleyn. 2003. Current scientific, ethical and social issues of biomonitoring in the European Union. *Toxicology Letters* 144:117–26.

Van Damme, K., L. Casteleyn, E. Heseltine, A. Huici, M. Sorsa, N. van Larabeke, and P. Vineis. 1995. Individual susceptibility and prevention of occupational diseases: Scientific and ethical issues. *Journal Occupational and Environmental Medicine* 37:91–99.

Vineis, P. 1992. Uses of biochemical and biological markers in occupational epidemiology. *Revue d'épidémiologie et de santé publique* 40 Suppl.1: 563–69.

Vineis, P., et al. 2004. Issues of design and analysis in studies of gene-environment interactions. In P. Buffler, J. Rice, R. Baan, and M.B. Boffetta, eds., *Mechanisms of carcinogenesis: Contributions of molecular epidemiology,* pp. 417–36. Lyon, France: International Agency for Research on Cancer.

Wade, P.A. and T.K. Archer. 2006. Epigenetics: Environmental instructions for the genome. *Environmental Health Perspectives* 114:A140–A141.

Wang, Z., D. Neuburg, C. Li, L. Su, J.Y. Kim, J.C. Chen, and D.C. Christiani. 2005. Global gene expression profiling in whole-blood samples from individuals exposed to metal fumes. *Environmental Health Perspectives* 113:233–41.

Waters, M.D., K. Olden, and R.W. Tennant. 2003. Toxicogenomic approach for assessing toxicant-related disease. *Mutation Research* 544:415–24.

Weeks, J.L., B.S. Levy, and G.R. Wagner, eds. 1991. *Preventing occupational disease and injury.* Washington, DC: American Public Health Association.

Weinhold, B. 2006. Epigenetics: The science of change. *Environmental Health Perspectives* 114:A160–A167.

Weston, A.A. 2002. Racial differences in prevalence of a supratypic HLA-genetic marker immaterial to pre-employment testing for susceptibility to chronic beryllium disease. *American Journal of Industrial Medical* 41:457–65.

Yong, L.C., P.A. Schulte, J.K. Wiencke, M.F. Boeniger, L.B. Connally, J.T. Walker, E.A. Whelan, and E.M. Ward. 2001. Hemoglobin adducts and sister chromatid exchanges in hospital workers exposed to ethylene oxide: effects of glutathione S-transferase T1 and M1 genotypes. *Cancer Epidemiology Biomarkers Prevention* 10:539–50.

CHAPTER 10

Advances in Human Genome Epidemiology

Implications for Occupational Health and Disease Prevention

MARC WEINSTEIN

The convergence of information technology and biology helped accelerate the mapping of the human genome, creating the possibility that advances in knowledge about human biology may follow the same exponential trajectory witnessed in information technology. Uncertain, however, is whether this accelerated rate of growth will translate into a comparable increase in the speed of development of new diagnostic tools and clinical therapies. Despite this uncertainty, human genome epidemiology has already deepened our knowledge of gene-environment interactions and this, in turn, has important ethical, legal, and social implications.

This is particularly true in occupational health where two sets of factors could create pressure to use information about individual susceptibility to modify employment practices. The first relates to the size and nature of the occupational health risk pool. The second relates to how the current legal and regulatory environment in the United States de facto permits environmental exposures and the use of personal data that is not tolerated elsewhere in American society. This chapter considers both forces and concludes by identifying key issues that should be addressed when considering policy choices related to genetic privacy and occupational health.

Public Health Implications of Advances in Human Genome Epidemiology

Describing the central role that epidemiological methods will have in the era of genomic research, Khoury, Little, and Burke (2004) note three essential contributions of human genome epidemiology: First, there is the discovery of new gene-disease associations through linkage analyses, family association studies, and other methodologies that constitute the core of traditional genetic epidemiology. Second is the determination of population prevalence of alleles, which is the domain of molecular epidemiology. Finally, there are the contributions of applied epidemiology that attempt to assess the value of genetic information in the diagnosis and prevention of disease. Because human genome epidemiology is in its early stages, most recently published articles have reported on gene prevalence and gene-disease associations. Fewer articles have been published on the how this new knowledge can be integrated into clinical practice and public health policy. An analysis of abstracts of published papers in the area of human genome epidemiology in 2001 showed that 82 percent of the 2,401 published articles reported on the population prevalence of gene variants and gene-disease associations, 15 percent reported on gene-gene and gene-environment interactions, and only 3 percent focused on the evaluation of genetic tests and population screening (Khoury, Little, and Burke, 2004). Over time, as advances in human genetics continue there will likely be a greater emphasis in this last area.

It is important to note that these advances could promise a new era of individualized medicine and a paradigm shift in epidemiological methods themselves. Traditionally, epidemiology, the scientific cornerstone of public health, has focused on the identification of determinants of health and disease across relatively large populations. These epidemiological studies provide insights into general risk factors for various diseases and help to identify particularly vulnerable demographic groups or lifestyle choices. By contrast, much of human genome epidemiology seeks to understand individual predisposition to disease and environmental triggers of disease, through the identification of gene-disease and gene-environmental interactions and then through the identification of individuals with the alleles that make them susceptible to disease. As our understanding of these associations becomes more advanced, and our understanding of the gene-gene and gene-environment interactions becomes more nuanced, epidemiologists will be able to characterize risk in smaller and smaller populations. Identification of individual risk, particularly as it relates to environmental exposures, is a logical extension of human genome epidemiology.

Without questioning the basic scientific value of genetic research, Rockhill, Kawachi, and Colditz (2000) are skeptical about the public health value of individualized risk assessment. Drawing on the seminal work of Geoffrey Rose (1981), they note that most chronic diseases arise from the mass of the population with risk factor values close to the average, and as a result, most risk factors have poor positive predictive power. In other words, some individuals with low risk factors will acquire a disease, while the majority of individuals with high risk factors will not. Although advances in human genome epidemiology promise better individual risk assessment, the reality is that most common diseases, such as breast cancer, typically have a small genetic component. Because disease risk association is typically a continuum, public health practitioners are often faced with an arbitrary demarcation between high- and low-risk exposures, and "population attributable fractions for many chronic diseases can be inflated only by defining risk factors in such a way that nearly the entire population is labeled 'exposed'" (Rockhill, Kawachi, and Colditz, 2000, p. 176).

The practical implication of this is that for many diseases, more can be done to reduce risk through general public health initiatives than through pursuing genetic research. Because only 5 percent of all cancers are thought to have a strong genetic component, the emphasis on genomic research could distract energy and resources from general prevention strategies (Vineis, Schulte, and McMichael, 2001). Rose favors a population-wide approach that attempts to move the entire distribution of risk factors, including the high-risk tail, in a favorable direction thereby reducing the risk of the entire population (Rose, 1992). Beyond this, those advocating a population approach are concerned that the focus on individual susceptibility could detract policy makers from addressing general exposure levels that could impact entire populations and will lead to other problems, including the genetic labeling of hypersusceptible individuals with concomitant psychosocial costs.

Which view is correct? Does human genome epidemiology hold the promise of individualized medicine that will provide individuals with valuable guidance in disease prevention? Or is does it constitute a potential threat to the general population approaches to health promotion that have been the foundation of modern public health policies?

There may not be a universal answer to those questions. Rather, the value and appropriateness of individual risk assessment depends on both the penetrance of a genetic allele (the likelihood that the allele will be expressed as a disease) and the size of the population or risk pool (Table 10.1). For example, the northwest quadrant of Table 10.1 represents instances where there might be a subpopulation whose members are at a substantially elevated disease risk, either because of family history (e.g., Huntington disease) or environmental exposure (e.g., localized environmental or occupational exposure), *and* cases where researchers have identified a high penetration allele with a readily identifiable biomarker. In these cases, particularly if successful therapies are developed, individualized risk assessment and medicine could have an important role in disease prevention and treatment. By contrast, the risk distribution for most cancers follows the pattern described by Rose (1992) and fits into the southeast quadrant of Table 10.1. This describes our current understanding of most diseases. In these instances, genetic polymorphisms have generally low levels of penetration and only provide an incomplete etiology of a disease in a small percentage of its occurrence. Moreover, the distribution of these polymorphisms is not easily predicted among members of the general population. This pattern describes most disease risk, and given the poor positive predictive power of allele-associated biomarkers

TABLE 10.1
Characterizing Risk Assessment

Penetrance of biomarker	Size of risk pool	
	Small	Large
High	High value for individualized risk assessment	Some value for prescriptive advice for subpopulations
Low	No value for human genome epidemiology	Value for traditional approaches to epidemiology

and the prohibitive cost of general population screening, current public policy health promotion initiatives (e.g., lifestyle changes and screening for at-risk demographic groups) may still be the most effective way to reduce the incidence of these diseases.

This concept is further illustrated in Figure 10.1, which maps genetic markers for three diseases with respect to their penetrance and the relative size of the population class. In the case of Alzheimer disease, a variant allele (E4) of the apolipoprotein *APOE* has been associated with the onset of the disease in individuals between the ages of fifty and eighty. However, this genetic association has low penetrance and poor positive predictive power. The frequency of *APOE*E4* may be as high 40 percent in individuals with Alzheimer disease, but 15 to 20 percent of unaffected

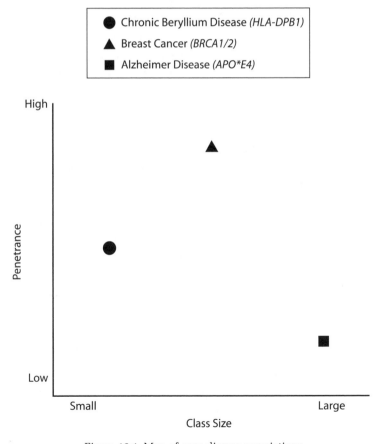

Figure 10.1. Map of gene-disease associations

individuals also have the *APOE*E4* polymorphism (Mayeux, 2004). In other words, many people who have the *APOE*E4* polymorphism will never develop Alzheimer disease, and many people without that allele *will* develop Alzheimer disease.

By contrast, consider a hereditary form of breast cancer that constitutes between 5 and 10 percent of breast cancer cases in the United States. Women who are carriers of *BRCA1/2* mutations have about an 80 percent chance of developing breast cancer by age 70, though population studies indicate that the allele frequency in the general population is estimated to be only .0013 and .0017, respectively (Antoniou et al., 2000). However, this low prevalence of the *BRCA1/2* in the population does not accurately reflect the size of the risk pool. The likelihood of presence of the *BRCA1/2* allele increases dramatically when there has been breast cancer among first- and second-degree relatives, particularly among women of Ashkenazi Jewish ancestry. For this reason, even though there is not a primary genetic factor for most breast cancer, there is an identifiable and relatively small subpopulation for whom screening for the *BRCA1/2* polymorphisms is likely to be appropriate. Therefore, in the case of breast cancer there may be a role for genetic screening for the women who are identifiably at higher risk of carrying the allele. But for the vast majority of women, nongenetic screening (e.g., mammograms) and lifestyle recommendations (e.g., weight loss promotion among postmenopausal women) are the appropriate public health responses.

The importance of gene-environment interactions can also be seen in the case of chronic beryllium disease (CBD). This granulomatous lung disease occurs in 1 to 6 percent of exposed workers and is associated with an allelic substitute of Glu^{69} in the *HLA-DPB1* gene. Wang et al. (1999) report that 97 percent of individuals with CBD have some form of Glu^{69} substitution, but anywhere from 30 to 45 percent of exposed workers *without* CBD also have the Glu^{69} substitution. Because beryllium exposure occurs in the occupational setting, the effective size of the risk pool is readily identifiable and small. At the same time, the presence of Glu^{69} substitution is not a perfect predictor of which workers will develop CBD. One challenge for occupational health researchers and advocates is whether to consider genetic screening for CBD susceptibility despite the relatively high number of false positives likely to result from relatively low penetrance of the *HLA-DP1* gene. With respect to our map of gene-disease association, CBD is mapped in the western frontier of the matrix, because the risk pool is relatively small.

The serious risk resulting from beryllium exposure and the success in identifying the Glu[69] marker create some difficult policy dilemmas and highlight the distinctive challenges that occupational health poses to the application of human genome epidemiology. While the low sensitivity of the Glu[69] marker would normally rule out its utility in disease prevention for population-wide exposure, the relatively small and identifiable size of the workforce exposed to beryllium has brought workforce screening for beryllium sensitivity to the forefront of policy considerations in applying genetic research to the occupational setting. This persistent interest comes at a time when the Occupational Safety and Health Administration (OSHA) has rejected reduction in the permissible exposure limit (PEL) of beryllium for private sector workers from a level set in 1949, despite the Department of Energy's decision to reduce the PEL by a factor of ten in 1998 (Michaels, 2005).

Interest in the Glu[69] marker, despite its low penetrance is largely consistent with the model of risk assessment illustrated in Figure 10.1. Workers exposed to beryllium constitute a population that can be readily tested and monitored, and they constitute a small percentage of the U.S. workforce. As human genome epidemiology research reveals more higher-penetrance biomarkers of gene-environmental interactions, pressure will be stronger to use these markers for workplace screening.

Institutional Environment
Health Risk Management and Prevalence in Occupational Settings

The regulation, enforcement, and practice of occupational health in the United States provide additional incentives and, possibly, credibility for the use of genetic markers in employment. American employers enjoy considerable prerogatives in the employment relationship, despite the patchwork of regulations and statutes designed to prevent discrimination in employment. This and the lack of national political commitment to improved occupational safety and health has generally meant that there has been weak and inconsistent enforcement of occupational safety and health standards. At the same time, the limited sanctions faced by employers are occasionally punctuated by large class action suits (e.g., asbestos). This threat of civil litigation does ensure some level of concern about potential liabilities related to occupational exposures. However, for reasons that are ultimately related to the incentive structures resulting from the institutional environment governing the employment relationship, American companies are likely to opt for removing or refusing to employ susceptible individuals rather than investing in engineering controls to reduce overall exposures. In this context, the ability to identify hypersusceptible individuals through genetic screening could be attractive to employers.

This is particularly true because occupational illnesses, though difficult to quantify, constitute a serious health risk for American workers. One broadly cited estimate attributes sixty thousand deaths and one million illnesses annually to occupational exposures (Leigh et al., 2000). Despite these troubling figures, there are no OSHA-regulated exposure limits for most chemicals used in American workplaces. Of the three thousand chemicals produced in quantities of more than one million pounds annually, OSHA enforces PELs for fewer than five hundred. The National Institute for Occupational Safety and Health, an independent research branch of the Centers for Disease Control, recommends PELs for 667 chemicals, and the American Conference of Governmental Industrial Hygienists recommends PELs for an even larger number (Cullen, 2002). However, only OSHA has legally enforceable PELs, and these PELs are limited and unlikely to change in the current political environment. The resistance to the establishment of new PELs has been so effective that only two new OSHA standards have been introduced in the past ten years (Michaels, 2005).

Ironically, resistance to new PELs and the limited number of chemicals for which they are available may in part be a result of the OSHA General Duty Clause, which requires employers to provide "a place of employment which is free from recognized hazards that are causing or likely to cause death or serious physical harm to employees" (Section 5(a)(1) of the Occupational Safety and Health Act). The General Duty Clause would seem to require employers to provide sufficient protections from occupational hazards to workers, but the precise obligation under the General Duty Clause is to provide protection from "recognized" hazards. There is no requirement for employers or others to aggressively identify new risks. Whether by design or as an unintended consequence, the General Duty Clause creates disincentives for employers and industry groups to uncover hazards heretofore unrecognized. This, along with the common concern about costs associated with new engineering controls to reduce occupational exposures, has created an environment in which it is difficult to achieve consensus on what constitutes a recognized hazard. Business interests have increasingly and routinely backed research and researchers that cast doubt on findings suggesting the need to establish new and more stringent PELs for thousands of chemicals routinely used in the workplace (Markowitz and Rosner, 2002).

In this context, genetic screening of hypersensitive individuals may seem like a viable option and extension of "preventive" law to occupational health in the new era of human genome epidemiology. The inability of OSHA to keep pace with the introduction of new substances and new information and research about existing chemicals has arguably created a gap between what is legally permissible and what constitutes a safe workplace environment. While the exclusive remedy doctrine common to most worker compensation schemes limits the ability of workers to sue employers for negligence, lawsuits can be pursued when there has been gross negligence or when the employee was a subcontractor and could sue the owner of the worksite for negligence. This legal opening and the prevalence of chemicals with likely but unknown occupational risks mean that in many instances, employees often seek economic redress through the court system. This threat of individual or class action lawsuits has created a risk-averse bias among some employers even as the weak regulatory system allows exposure to chemicals with unknown health consequences. This has led many companies to establish corporate policies with PEL restrictions below those set by OSHA. In other instances, it has led to the development of "preventive law," in which employers attempt to remove the possibility of lawsuits through restrictive hiring and personnel practices (Draper, 2003).

Early Employer Attempts to Use Genetic Information in Workplace Setting

One manifestation of preventive law is that when faced with the prospect of expensive lawsuits, companies have demonstrated an increasing interest in developing screening policies aimed at identifying individuals who have a greater risk from occupational exposures and injuries and who, as a result, may be more likely to file a workers' compensation claim. In the preoffer stage of employee selection, the screening techniques generally consist of computer-based or traditional pen-and-pencil tests that employ sophisticated psychometric analysis to identify candidates who may be more prone to occupational injury or more likely to press worker compensation claims associated with an occupational injury. In the postoffer and preplacement phases of employee selection, some employers and third-party vendors have developed highly refined "fitness-for-work" criteria. These criteria carefully navigate Americans with Disabilities Act and affirmative action guidelines, providing special attention to conditions that do not prevent major life activities and adhere to job-relatedness criteria. Given the generally high cost of engineering controls to reduce the risk of occupational disease and the uncertainty of future lawsuits, workplace screening options are particularly attractive to U.S. employers.

In light of the trend to use more stringent employee screening, it should not be surprising that U.S. employers have already attempted incorporate research from human genome epidemiology. These limited initial attempts to use genetic biomarkers have been successfully challenged—not because of core principles involved regarding employer prerogative, but because other aspects of employment law were violated (Weinstein, Widenor, and Hecker, 2005).

In the case of *Norman-Bloodsaw v. Lawrence Berkeley Laboratories.* (1998) job applicants challenged Lawrence Berkeley Laboratories' practice of testing African American job applicants for sickle cell anemia trait, a genetically linked disorder with a higher rate of incidence in the African American population. The court ruled that there was no legitimate need to exclude workers with sickle cell anemia trait, as it did not have any recognizable affect on workers' ability to do their jobs, and because the screen had a disparate impact on a protected class of individuals. Although this ruling was a victory for job applicants, it did not rule out the use of biomarkers that might indicate disease susceptibility, particularly if the subpopulation of affected individuals does not constitute a legally protected class of workers.

In *Avary v. Burlington Northern and Santa Fe Railroad* (BNSF), a railroad worker was tested without his knowledge for a genetic marker purported to indicate a predisposition for hereditary neuropathy with liability to pressure palsy (HNPP)—a carpal-tunnel-like condition. In this case, the distinctive structure of workers' compensation in the railway industry provided BNSF the incentive to take this unusual measure. Whereas in most industries workers' compensation provides a no-fault exclusive remedy, in the railway industry a third-party apportions liability and benefits for each workplace injury. In others words, if BNSF could demonstrate that a worker was genetically predisposed to carpal tunnel syndrome, then it would be argued the worker, not the company, would be liable for the injury. The legal challenge to the company, however, was on the basis that BNSF did not request informed consent. The case was quickly settled in a 1999 consent decree, in which BNSF agreed not to consider test results and not to do further testing (U.S. Equal Employment Opportunity Commission, 2001). However, there was no determination made as to whether BNSF would have been able to move forward with the testing had they obtained the required informed consent.

Whatever chilling effect these two cases have had on the use of genetic information could be mitigated by future advances in toxicogenomics and a 2002 Supreme Court ruling in *Chevron U.S.A. Inc. v. Echazabal.* This case provides a legal foundation for an employer to deny employees a position if they constitute a risk to themselves. Such a situation may arise for individuals with a genetic susceptibility to an occupational exposure. Specifically, in this 2002 ruling, the Court determined that Chevron could deny Mario Echazabal employment because his exposure to the workplace environment might pose a direct threat to his health. Echazabal, a long-time employee of a Chevron contractor, applied for a job directly with Chevron at its refinery in El Segundo, California, in 1992 and 1995. On both occasions, Chevron extended Echazabal job offers contingent on his passing a physical examination. The results of the examinations revealed that Echazabal had chronic active hepatitis C, which was asymptomatic and never precluded him from performing his work in his capacity as a subcontracted employee. Instead, Chevron's denial of employment was based on its physicians' conclusion that Echazabal should not be exposed to hepatoxic chemicals used in the refinery. In February 1996, Chevron wrote to Irwin Industries, the subcontractor that employed Echazabal on Chevron's site, requesting that he be removed from the refinery or placed in a position that did not expose him to hepatoxins.

Although the case did not consider a genetic marker, it provides an analogue for issues that could arise as human genome epidemiology identifies new biomarkers indicating genetic susceptibility to environmental exposures. A prospective employee would not be covered by the Americans with Disabilities Act, because the condition is asymptomatic and does not prevent the applicant from major life activities. And, as might be the case with disease susceptibility marker, no burden is placed on the employer to make special accommodations for the applicant. Rather, the Court accepted Chevron's contention that it had job-related or business necessity reasons for rescinding its initial job offer to Echazabal, specifically noting the company's desire to avoid time lost to sickness, excessive turnover from medical retirement or death, litigation under state tort law, and the risk of violating the national Occupational Safety and Health Act of 1970 (*Chevron*, 2002). The Court did remand the case to the Ninth Circuit to consider whether Chevron's determination was based on an individualized inquiry, as required by EEOC ADA Title I regulations. More important, the Court recognized an employer's right to determine whether occupational exposure would constitute an employee's threat to self and the right to deny employment as a result of that determination.

Conclusion

The occupational health regulatory environment, risk aversion among employers, and the Supreme Court ruling may provide the scientific and legal basis for employers to use the findings of toxicogenomic research in the prevention of occupational disease. What has been missing to date is the discovery of sensitive biomarkers of alleles indicating which employees are likely to have an adverse physical reaction to environmental exposures. Whether advances in human genome epidemiology will ever yield identification of such biomarkers remains an open question, though recent rapid advances in human genome research suggest the plausible anticipation of important discoveries.

Despite the seeming logic of selectively using future discoveries from toxicogenomics in the prevention of occupational disease, considerable changes in the current regulatory environment will be needed before occupational health advocates will accept such applications. First and foremost, the move toward individual risk assessment cannot be seen as coming at the expense of equally or more important efforts to promote a generally safe work environment. In addition to more effective enforcement of existing standards, workers and their advocates will need to see how new findings from toxicogenomics research are translated into updated and new PELs that will be subject to OSHA enforcement.

Beyond this, as new biomarkers of gene-environment interaction are discovered, some consideration should be given to the creation of a compensation fund that would provide income protection to workers who are identified in a postoffer or posthire employee screening effort as being hypersusceptible to occupational disease. Bohrer (2002) suggested that such a fund would pay for itself, because in the long run, placing workers on paid leave would be less expensive than bearing the costs associated with a workers' compensation claim. Bohrer's proposal, though well intentioned, has at least one limitation. In the current regulatory environment, many legitimate cases are ineligible for workers' compensation insurance due to the difficulty of establishing such a claim. Therefore, the cost of a compensation fund for hypersusceptible workers could turn out to be higher than the money saved by a reduction in workers' compensation claims. This also underscores the need to make important progress in occupational health before a new and more ambitious effort to integrate the findings of human genome epidemiology into the mainstream of occupational health efforts is undertaken.

REFERENCES

Antoniou, A.C., S.A. Gayther, J.F. Stratton, B.A.J. Ponder, and D.F. Easton. 2000. Risk models for familial ovarian and breast cancer. *Genetic Epidemiology* 18:173–90.

Bohrer, R. 2002. Genes and the just society: A Rawlsian approach to solving the problem of genetic discrimination in the toxic workplace. *San Diego Law Review* 39:747–67.

Chevron U.S.A. Inc. v. Echazabal, 536 U.S. 73 (2002).

Cullen, L.2002. *A job to die for.* Monroe, ME: Common Courage Press.

Draper, E. 2003. *The company doctor.* New York: Russell Sage Foundation.

Khoury, M., J. Little, and W. Burke. 2004. *Human genome epidemiology: A scientific foundation for using genetic information to improve health and prevent disease.* New York: Oxford University Press.

Leigh, P.J., S. Markowitz, M. Fahs, and P. Landrigan. 2000. *Costs of occupational injuries and illness.* Ann Arbor: University of Michigan Press.

Markowitz, G., and D. Rosner. 2002. *Deceit and denial: The deadly politics of industrial pollution.* Berkeley: University of California Press.

Mayeux, R. 2004. Apolipoprotein E and Alzheimer disease. In *Human genome Epidemiology:* A scientific foundation for using genetic information to improve health and prevent disease, edited by M. Khoury, J. Little, and W. Burke, 365–82. New York: Oxford University Press.

Michaels, D. 2005. Doubt is their product. *Scientific American* (June):96–101.

Norman-Bloodsaw v. Lawrence Berkeley Laboratories. (135 F.3d 1260, 1272, 9th Cir. 1998).

Rockhill, B., I. Kawachi, and G.A. Colditz. 2000. Individual risk prediction and population-wide disease prevention. *Epidemiological Review* 22:176–80.

Rose, G. 1981. Strategy of prevention: Lessons from cardiovascular disease. *British Medical Journal* 292:1847–51.

Rose, G. 1992. *The strategy of preventive medicine.* New York: Oxford University Press.

U.S. Equal Employment Opportunity Commission. 2001. EEOC settles ADA suit against BNSF for genetic bias. At www.eeoc.gov/press/4-18-01.html.

Vineis, P., P. Schulte, and P. McMichael. 2001. Misconceptions about the use of genetic tests in populations. *Lancet:* 357:702–12.

Wang, Z., P.S. White, M. Petrovic, O.L. Tatum, L.S. Newman, L.A. Maier, and B.L. Marrone. 1999. Differential susceptibilities to chronic beryllium disease contributed by different Glu69 Hla-DPB1 alleles. *Journal of Immunology.* 163:1647–53.

Weinstein, M., M. Widenor, and S. Hecker. 2005. The ethical, legal, and social implications of advances in toxicogenomics on employment practices. *American Association of Occupational Health Nurses Journal* 53:539–33.

CHAPTER 11

Occupational Health and Discrimination Issues Raised by Toxicogenomics in the Workplace

MARK A. ROTHSTEIN

Scientists have long recognized the connection between genetic factors and illnesses caused by workplace exposures. In 1938, geneticist J.B.S. Haldane first suggested the possibility of using genetic screening to exclude workers who were more likely to become ill from occupational exposures. "The majority of potters do not die of bronchitis. It is quite possible that if we understood the causation of this disease, we should find that only a fraction of potters are of a constitution which renders them liable to it. If so, we could eliminate potters' bronchitis by rejecting entrants into the pottery industry who are congenitally disposed to it" (Haldane, 1938, pp. 179–80). Beginning in 1963, a series of scientific articles explored the biochemical genetic basis of predisposition to occupational illness from a variety of sources, including exposure to workers with glucose-6-phosphate dehydrogenase deficiency, glutathione instability, methemoglobin reduction, α_1-antitrypsin deficiency, carbon disulfide sensitivity, reagenic antibodies to allergic chemicals, and sickle cell trait (M.A. Rothstein, 1989, pp. 70–71).

Today, much of the study of the effects of genetic factors and toxic exposures falls under toxicogenomics, the genome-wide study of changes in the structure, expression, and activity of genes and proteins in response to exogenous toxicants (Marchant, 2003). Although scientific advances in toxicogenomics represent an exciting new development, the policy implications of individuals with varying sensitivity to toxic exposures in the workplace have been debated for at least the past twenty-five years (Office of Technology Assessment, 1983). These policy implications include the appropriateness of regulations in the face of scientific uncertainty, weighing the benefits and burdens of regulation, resolving the conflict between autonomy and paternalism in the workplace, and determining the respective rights of employees and employers.

Toxicogenomics raises numerous legal issues in the workplace setting, including workers' compensation claims of individuals with greater sensitivity to toxic substances, product liability actions against manufacturers of toxicants used in the workplace, and actions for discrimination in employment in violation of Title VII of the Civil Rights Act of 1964 (42 U.S.C. §2000e) when adverse employment actions based on toxic exposures have a disparate impact on the basis of race or national origin. This chapter focuses on three other important issues dealing with toxicogenomics: (1) regulation of workplace hazards under the Occupational Safety and Health Act (OSH Act), (2) disability discrimination actions under the Americans with Disabilities Act (ADA), and (3) genetic discrimination actions under state and federal laws.

Regulation under the Occupational Safety and Health Act

The Occupational Safety and Health Act of 1970 (29 U.S.C. §§651–78) is the primary federal law regulating worker safety and health. The OSH Act covers employment in every state and territory—an estimated six million workplaces and ninety million employees (M.A. Rothstein, 2006, p. 8). Unlike many labor and employment laws, there is no minimum number of employees or dollar volume of business needed for coverage. The OSH Act applies to all employers engaged in a business affecting interstate commerce—an easy standard to satisfy.

Among other requirements, each covered employer must comply with two provisions of the statute. First, section 5(a)(1) requires each covered employer to keep its workplace free from recognized hazards that are causing or likely to cause death or serious physical harm to its employees (29 U.S.C. §654(a)(1)). Second, section 5(a)(2) requires each covered employer to comply with occupational safety and health standards promulgated by the Occupational Safety and Health Administration (OSHA) of the U.S. Department of Labor (29 U.S.C. §654(a)(2)). The failure to comply with these requirements may result in the assessment of a range of civil penalties depending on the nature and gravity of the violation as well as on other factors (M.A. Rothstein, 2006, pp. 425–43).

Standard-Setting

Section 6 of the statute provides for the promulgation of standards in three ways. First, under section 6(a), the secretary of labor was authorized from 1971 to 1973 to adopt as OSHA standards, without rule-making procedures, two types of existing standards—national consensus standards (developed by private organizations) and established federal standards (promulgated under other federal laws) (29 U.S.C. §655(a)). This provision was designed to ensure the existence of OSHA standards soon after the effective date of the OSH Act in 1971, by adopting standards with which industry already was familiar. Second, under section 6(b), the secretary may modify, revoke, or issue new standards by complying with detailed rule-making procedures (29 U.S.C. §655(b)). This is the most important standards promulgation provision for new health standards. Third, under section 6(c), the secretary may issue emergency temporary standards in extraordinary circumstances (29 U.S.C. §655(c)), which may remain in effect for up to six months. Because standards promulgated under this provision have been difficult to sustain on judicial review (e.g., *Asbestos Information Association/North America v. OSHA*, 727 F.2d 415 (5th Cir. 1984)), it has rarely been used.

Occupational safety and health standards generally have not been developed with an explicit concern for individual variability in response to toxic substances. Although such standards are designed to provide the maximum protection possible, OSHA has recognized that it may not be possible to protect workers with heightened sensitivity. For example, the preamble to the coke oven emissions standard provides: "Because of the variability of individual response to carcinogens and other factors, the concept of a 'threshold level' may have little applicability on the basis of existing knowledge. Some individuals may be more susceptible than others. Thus, while a 'threshold' exposure level, below which exposure does not cause cancer, may conceivably exist for an individual, susceptible individuals in the working population may have cancer induced by doses so low as to be effectively zero" (29 C.F.R. §1910.1129). New toxicogenomic studies will identify an increasing number of substances for which a particular genotype confers greater risk of illness based on occupational exposures. OSHA will need to decide if, or to what extent, individual variability should be incorporated into the agency's standards promulgation strategy.

As an initial matter, it is necessary to consider OSHA's statutory authority to promulgate health standards and the judicial construction of the exercise of that authority. Section 6(b)(5) of the OSH Act (29 U.S.C. §655(b)(5)), which deals with the promulgation of standards for toxic substances and harmful physical agents, provides in part: "The Secretary of Labor shall set the standard which most adequately assures, to the extent feasible, . . . that no employee will suffer material impairment of health." This seemingly absolute language might be read as requiring OSHA to set standards at a level where even the most sensitive employee could work without ill effects. However, in *Industrial Union Department, AFL-CIO v. American Petroleum Institute* (1980)—also known as the *Benzene* decision—the Supreme Court rejected the notion that the OSH Act requires regulation at the level of zero risk.

The *Benzene* decision involved an industry challenge to OSHA rule making that lowered the permissible exposure limit for benzene from 10 parts per million to 1 part per million. In striking down the benzene standard, the Fifth Circuit held that, based on section 3(5) of the OSH Act (29 U.S.C. §652(5)), the secretary was required to prove that the benefits of the standard bear a reasonable relationship to the costs. The Supreme Court affirmed, but on different grounds. According to the plurality opinion, the secretary must initially demonstrate the need for a new standard by establishing that exposure at current levels poses a "significant risk" of harm (*Industrial Union*, 690). Because the secretary failed to make this finding, the benzene standard was struck down. The Court also cautioned that the duty imposed on employers by the statute was not absolute. "The statute was not designed to require employers to provide absolutely risk-free workplaces whenever it is technologically feasible to do so . . . [but]

was intended to require the elimination, as far as feasible, of significant risks of harm" (*Industrial Union*, 639).

Although the Supreme Court never explicitly stated whether the OSH Act requires employers to set exposure levels that would protect the most sensitive workers, Benzene implicitly holds that it does not. OSHA standards for toxic substances could be set to avoid requiring absolute levels of protection in two main ways: they could be limited to control measures that are economically and technologically feasible, or they could establish permissible exposure levels that would not protect the most sensitive workers. Although these appear to be distinct concepts, as a scientific and practical matter, they are closely related. Figure 11.1 plots a hypothetical linear dose-response curve.

As the dose increases (along the horizontal axis), the percentage of affected workers increases (along the vertical axis), and as the percentage of workers increases, even less sensitive individuals will exhibit the biological response. The lowest feasible level for reducing exposure is in-

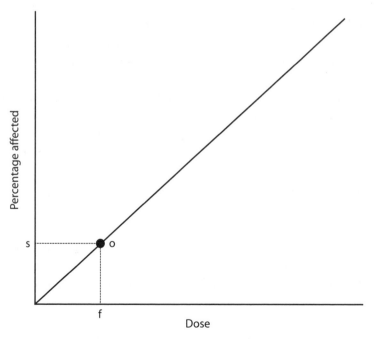

Figure 11.1. The intersection of feasibility and susceptibility in dose-response analysis

dicated by f. The intersection of f with the dose-response line, point 0, results in setting the susceptibility cutoff at s. Consequently, a standard lowering exposures only to the *Benzene* requirement of feasibility will necessarily result in a lack of protection for some of the most susceptible workers.

Genetic Testing

Genetic testing in the workplace setting is a controversial and emotionally charged issue. The scenario of greatest concern involves employers (perhaps even without the individual's knowledge or consent) performing genetic testing and excluding from employment individuals who are genetically predisposed to occupational illness. A related concern is the use of genetic testing or genetic information to exclude individuals at risk of nonoccupational diseases based on employer concerns about absenteeism, turnover, and health care costs. Genetic testing, however, could be performed in other ways and for other purposes: to aid in advising individuals of their increased risk to enable them to make informed decisions about whether to work with potentially harmful exposures, to alert individuals about the possible need to use additional personal protective equipment, and to signal employers and employees of the advisability of additional medical monitoring.

The OSH Act is silent on whether employers are required, permitted, or prohibited from mandating that employees undergo genetic testing before assignment to positions with toxic exposures. OSHA's standard regulating thirteen carcinogens contains the following provision: "Before an employee is assigned to enter a regulated area, a preassignment physical examination by a physician shall be provided. The examination shall include the personal history of the employee, family and occupational background, including genetic and environmental factors" (29 C.F.R. §1910.1003(g)(1)(I)). According to a 1980 clarification by OSHA, the term "genetic factors" does not require genetic testing of any employee or the exclusion of otherwise qualified employees from jobs on the basis of genetic testing (Occupational Safety and Health Administration, 1980).

The issue of genetic testing will arise with increasing frequency as a result of developments in toxicogenomics. The underlying question is whether genetic testing in the workplace setting should ever be considered ethically and legally acceptable. Some commentators have suggested that it would be irresponsible for employers to fail to use genetic tests that might identify individuals at increased risk of developing an occupational disease; moreover, failing to do so could expose the employer to substantial liability (Epstein, 1994; Dichter and Sutor, 1997; Clegg, 2000). Other commentators oppose genetic testing in the workplace because it would violate employee privacy and potentially result in discrimination (Greely, 2001; Gridley, 2001; Kim, 2002; Samuels, 2003).

In my view, overwhelming scientific evidence and extreme caution are needed before using genetic testing in the workplace. Nevertheless, it is inappropriate to adopt an absolute prohibition on genetic testing when there are so many unknown variables, including the absolute and relative risk of the individuals tested, the severity of the relevant conditions, pertinent latency periods, treatment options, and possible risks to the general public. However, in those instances where genetic testing may be warranted to promote occupational health, safeguards are essential. The goals of public policy must be to protect individual autonomy and privacy and to prevent discrimination while allowing the consideration of essential genetic information. I have previously suggested the following guidelines:

1. Employers have a duty to inform applicants and employees of genetic markers of increased risk based on occupational exposures.
2. Individuals should have the option of undergoing genetic testing for these markers at the employer's expense.
3. The testing should be performed by a physician of the individual's choosing.
4. The results should be available only to the individual.
5. The significance of both a positive and a negative test should be explained to the individual.
6. The choice of whether to accept the job should be left to the individual.
7. Only in the rare situations where employment of the individual would constitute a direct, immediate, and severe threat to self or others would the employer be justified in performing its own testing and excluding the individual. (M.A. Rothstein, 2000, pp. 393–95).

Accommodations of High-Risk Workers

If it is unlawful to exclude from employment individuals at a geneti-cally increased risk of occupational illness, does the employer have a duty to provide high-risk workers with additional health protections be-yond those mandated by the applicable OSHA standard? Some examples of these added measures are reassignment, administrative controls (e.g., shift rotation to limit exposure), personal protective equipment (e.g., res-pirators), and medical surveillance.

The issue of additional precautions for high-risk workers has not been resolved under the OSH Act. In *Benzene*, the Supreme Court arguably supported such a possibility when it upheld the principle of "action level" medical testing. According to the Court, testing employees exposed at an action level below the maximum permissible exposure level "could ensure that workers who were unusually susceptible . . . could be re-moved from exposure before they had suffered any permanent damage" (*Industrial Union,* 657 (footnote omitted)). It should also be noted that nothing in the OSH Act prohibits employers from going beyond OSHA standards to provide greater protection for sensitive employees, although special treatment for some workers may raise questions of equity or con-tractual issues under a collective bargaining agreement. The issue of rea-sonable accommodation under the ADA is discussed below.

Warnings

It is not clear whether employers have a duty to provide warnings of the heightened risks to individuals with a certain genotype from expo-sure to toxic substances. OSHA's hazard communication standard re-quires chemical manufacturers and importers to assess the hazards of chemicals they produce or import and requires all employers to provide information to their employees concerning hazardous chemicals by means of hazard communication programs, including labels, material safety data sheets, and access to written records (29 C.F.R. §1910.1200). Additional rule making may be necessary to impose a duty to supply genotype-specific warnings. One concern about overly detailed and com-plicated warnings, however, is that workers will be confused or over-whelmed and therefore will disregard the warnings.

The Americans with Disabilities Act

The Americans with Disabilities Act of 1990 (42 U.S.C. §§12101-13) prohibits discrimination in employment on the basis of physical or mental disability. It also prohibits discrimination in public services and public accommodations. The employment discrimination provisions of the ADA apply to private employers with fifteen or more employees, state and local government employers, and the United States Congress. Federal government employees are covered under section 501 of the Rehabilitation Act (29 U.S.C. §791).

Section 102(a) of the ADA contains the general prohibition on employment discrimination (42 U.S.C. §12112(a)): "No covered entity shall discriminate against a qualified individual with a disability because of the disability of such individual in regard to job application procedures, the hiring, advancement, or discharge of employees, employee compensation, job training and other terms, conditions, and privileges of employment." Under the ADA, the obligations of covered employers go beyond nondiscrimination. Pursuant to section 101(8), employers are required to provide "reasonable accommodations" to the known disabilities of individuals covered by the ADA (42 U.S.C. §12111(8)). As noted below, however, it is unlikely that an individual with a genetic predisposition is a covered "individual with a disability" under the ADA and if not, the employer would have no duty to provide reasonable accommodation.

Coverage under the ADA

Under section 3(2) of the ADA, the term disability means "with respect to an individual—(A) a physical or mental impairment that substantially limits one or more of the major life activities of such individual; (B) a record of such an impairment; or (C) being regarded as having such an impairment" (42 U.S.C. §12102(2)). It is an unresolved question whether the ADA applies to adverse employment actions against asymptomatic individuals who are at a genetically increased risk of illness, including illnesses related to workplace exposures. The statute is silent on the coverage of individuals with a genetic predisposition to illness, and the legislative history is similarly unhelpful (M.A. Rothstein, 1992). In 1995, the Equal Employment Opportunity Commission (EEOC) issued an interpretation of the ADA that when an employer discriminates against an individual on the basis of genetic predisposition, the employer is "regarding" the individual as having a disability, thereby bringing the individual within the third prong of the definition of individual with a disability (Equal Employment Opportunity Commission, 1995).

Although this interpretation has never been challenged in court, a series of Supreme Court cases casts great doubt on whether it would be upheld. In *Sutton v. United Air Lines, Inc.* (1999), twin sisters with correctable vision problems were denied an opportunity to become airline pilots because their uncorrected vision did not meet the airline's medical standards. In the subsequent ADA action, the airline argued that the plaintiffs were not covered by the ADA because in their "mitigated" state (wearing their eyeglasses) they did not have a substantially limiting impairment. The employer's position was that they were too impaired to be hired but not impaired enough to be covered by the ADA. The Supreme Court agreed with the employer and rejected the EEOC's interpretation that impairments should be considered in their unmitigated state. The Court held that in deciding whether an individual is covered under the ADA, the individual should be considered in his or her "mitigated" state (i.e., with medications, eyeglasses, hearing aids). Of particular importance, the Court held that it need not defer to the interpretations of the ADA by the EEOC, because Congress did not authorize the EEOC to issue interpretations of Title I of the ADA. In addition, the Court cited the legislative history and preamble of the ADA to show that the ADA was intended to apply only to a limited number of individuals— the estimated forty-three million Americans with substantially limiting impairments. The "limited coverage" theory of the ADA would undermine attempts to extend coverage to individuals whose "disability" was a genetic predisposition to illness.

In *Toyota Motor Manufacturing, Kentucky, Inc., v. Williams* (2002), the plaintiff alleged that her employer failed to provide reasonable accommodations to her carpal tunnel syndrome. The basis of her alleged disability was a substantial limitation in the major life activity of working. The Supreme Court's decision addressed the issue of when working is a major life activity under the ADA. In adopting a narrow definition, the Court again made reference to the congressional intent of limiting the ADA's coverage to the estimated forty-three million Americans with substantially limiting impairments. Applying this analysis to the coverage of genetic predisposition, it becomes clear that asymptomatic individuals at a genetically increased risk of illness (occupational or otherwise) will not be covered by the ADA under current Supreme Court analysis, simply because virtually every individual is at a genetically increased risk of some disorder.

One other case under the ADA may be relevant. In *Bragdon v. Abbott* (1998), the Supreme Court held that an asymptomatic, HIV-positive woman who was denied dental services in a dentist's office was covered under Title III of the ADA, which prohibits disability discrimination in public accommodations. The Court held that being HIV-positive was a substantial limitation on the plaintiff's major life activity of reproduction. Of particular relevance to toxicogenomics, the Court noted the subclinical effects of HIV in buttressing its argument that an asymptomatic individual had a physical impairment (*Bragdon,* pp. 635–37). Although it could be argued that certain biomarkers or endophenotypes demonstrate comparable physiological manifestations of genetic predisposition, *Bragdon* predates *Sutton.* If presented with such an argument, it is likely that the Court would follow *Sutton* and hold that *Bragdon* is limited to HIV (L.F. Rothstein, 2000).

Direct Threat

Section 103(b) of the ADA (42 U.S.C. §12113(b)) provides that an employee is not qualified for a position if the individual poses a "direct threat to the health or safety of other individuals in the workplace." In *Chevron U.S.A. Inc. v. Echazabal* (2002), an employee who had worked for independent contractors at a Chevron Oil refinery applied for a job with Chevron. On two prior occasions, the employer had withdrawn conditional offers of employment following medical examinations that indicated that Echazabal had asymptomatic hepatitis C. Although he had worked at the Chevron facility for over twenty years without experiencing any health problems, Echazabal was denied employment by Chevron on the ground that exposure to toxic chemicals would damage his liver. He was laid off by his contractor-employer when Chevron requested that he be removed from further exposures. Echazabal then sued under the ADA. The Supreme Court unanimously upheld the validity of an interpretation of section 103(b) of the EEOC that the direct threat defense applies more broadly than the narrow language of the statute to include "self or others." The Court said that section 103(b) uses "threat to others" as a nonexclusive example of a lawful qualification standard.

Reading Sutton and Echazabal together, it is possible that an employer could use predictive genetic information to disqualify an individual from employment on the ground that the individual constituted a direct threat to self, and yet the individual would have no recourse under the ADA because an individual at a genetically increased risk of illness is not covered under the definition of an "individual with a disability." Such a result is contrary to the antidiscrimination principle of the ADA and could encourage the proliferation of inappropriate genetic testing in the workplace.

Genetic Testing and Monitoring

Under the ADA, regulation of medical inquiries and examinations depends on the time at which they are made or performed. The most severe restrictions apply to the preemployment stage. Under section 102(d)(2), an employer may not "conduct a medical examination or make inquiries of a job applicant as to whether such applicant is an individual with a disability or as to the nature or severity of such disability" (42 U.S.C. §12112(d)(2)). The only permissible inquiries are about the ability of the applicant to perform job-related functions. These inquiries, however, must be narrowly tailored.

The most permissive standard for medical examinations and inquiries applies at the preplacement or postoffer stage. Under section 102(d)(3), "[a] covered entity may require a medical examination after an offer of employment has been made to a job applicant and prior to the commencement of the employment duties of such applicant, and may condition an offer of employment on the results of such examination" (42 U.S.C. §12112(d)(3)). These "employment entrance examinations" must satisfy three requirements. First, all entering employees in the same job category, regardless of disability status, must be subject to an examination. The examinations, however, may be of unlimited scope and may include a requirement that the individual sign an authorization to disclose all of the information in the individual's personal medical records to the employer. Second, information obtained at an employment entrance examination must be collected and maintained on separate forms and in separate medical files. The information must be treated as confidential, except that supervisors and managers may be informed regarding necessary restrictions on the work or duties of the employee and necessary accommodations; first aid and safety personnel may be informed, when appropriate, if the disability might require emergency treatment; and government officials investigating compliance with the ADA must be provided with relevant information on request. Third, employers may not use medical criteria to screen out individuals with disabilities unless the medical criteria are job-related. Because there are no limitations placed on medical examinations or inquiries at this stage, employer-mandated genetic testing at the preplacement stage does not violate the ADA.

Pursuant to section 102(d)(4) of the ADA, all medical examinations and inquiries of current employees must be "job-related and consistent with business necessity" (42 U.S.C. §12112(d)(4)). Employers may require medical assessments, including those made by independent examiners, to determine whether an employee remains capable of performing job-related functions safely and efficiently. An employer may offer medical examinations of a non-job-related nature, such as comprehensive medical examinations and wellness programs, but employee participation must be voluntary.

In the context of genetic information, the protections contained in section 102(d) leave several important gaps. First, although medical examinations and inquiries at the preemployment stage are unlawful, some courts hold that a nondisabled individual subjected to illegal medical inquiries is not protected (see, e.g., Conroy v. New York Department of Correctional Services, 2003; Fredenburg v. Contra Costa County Department of Health Services, 1999; and Griffin v. Steeltek, 1998, although better reasoned opinions have held to the contrary (see, e.g., Tice v. Centre Area Transportation Authority, 2001); Armstrong v. Turner Industries, 1998). Thus, inquiring into genetic risk factors might not be unlawful because genetic predisposition is not covered under the ADA.

Second, under section 102(d)(3), if an employer withdraws a conditional offer of employment after a mandatory medical examination, there is no requirement that the employer indicate the reason for the withdrawal. As a result, the individual would not know, unless a lawsuit is later brought, whether the medical examination played a role in the decision or the offer was withdrawn for unrelated economic or human resources reasons.

Third, because there are no limits on the scope of the medical records released pursuant to an authorization signed at the postoffer stage, the results of genetic tests performed in the clinical setting would be disclosed to the employer. Only state laws enacted in California and Minnesota limit employer access at the postoffer stage to job-related medical information (M.A. Rothstein, 1998). Rather than the few cases of documented genetic discrimination in employment, the fact that employers may lawfully gain access to genetic test results is the primary reason many individuals are reluctant to undergo genetic testing.

The ADA does not indicate the types of medical tests that are lawful to perform. The only limitation is that mandatory medical examinations of current employees must be job-related. Whether a test lacking in scientific validity can be considered job-related is an unresolved issue. This is the legal issue raised by the *Burlington Northern* case.

In 2001, the EEOC sued the Burlington Northern Santa Fe Railroad to enjoin the company from conducting genetic tests on employees who submitted claims of work-related carpal tunnel syndrome (*EEOC v. Burlington Northern Santa Fe Railroad Co.,* 2001). The case, which settled in a matter of weeks, generated national attention because it followed closely on the heels of the announcement of the completion of the draft version of the human genome and because it was the first major incident of genetic testing in the workplace. Although the purpose of the railroad's testing program has never been established, most observers assumed that the tests were intended either to help the company develop future medical screening practices or challenge employee claims for carpal tunnel syndrome submitted under the Federal Employers' Liability Act (45 U.S.C. §§51-60), the workers' compensation system for railroad employees.

There is little scientific dispute that the testing performed was totally inappropriate (Schulte & Lomax, 2003). The legal issue, however, is less clear. The EEOC alleged in its complaint that the use of a scientifically unproven test cannot be "job-related" as required by section 102(d)(4). Nevertheless, the statute does not expressly say so, and the test was job-related in the sense that it was designed (albeit poorly) to identify predisposition to the work-related health problem of carpal tunnel syndrome. Therefore, it is not clear that the EEOC would have prevailed at trial, notwithstanding the widespread scientific and public condemnation of the railroad's conduct.

The problem in the *Burlington Northern* case was not so much that the employer was doing genetic testing, even though this is what generated the publicity. It was that the employer was performing medical testing without any informed consent, and it was using a research test unsupported by scientific evidence, inappropriate for the workplace setting, and not designed to benefit the health of the employees. Thus, *Burlington Northern* raises the broader and long-standing concern of physician-patient relations and employer-employee relations in occupational medicine.

Genetic Nondiscrimination Laws

Although there have been few documented instances of employment discrimination or other adverse treatment against individuals based on genetic predisposition, the public is very concerned that genetic information will lead to employment discrimination by employers. One consequence of this widespread concern is a reluctance to undergo genetic testing in the clinical setting (M.A. Rothstein and Hornung, 2003). Consequently, effective employment nondiscrimination and health privacy laws are essential to realizing the promises of modern genomics.

In the absence of effective federal antidiscrimination laws, the states have attempted to fill the gap by enacting laws prohibiting genetic discrimination in employment. About two-thirds of the states have enacted such laws since 1990, and most of the laws are similar. They prohibit employers from requiring or requesting that individuals have a genetic test as a condition of employment, and they make it unlawful for an employer to discriminate in hiring, firing, compensation, benefits, work assignment, or other terms and conditions of employment on the basis of genetic information.

The definition of "genetic information" varies in the states, but all of the state laws apply only to individuals who are asymptomatic (M.A. Rothstein and Anderlik, 2001). Individuals with expressed genetic disorders are considered the same as any other individuals with extant health conditions. There are several other issues reflected in the state laws. In Texas, "genetic information" includes only the results of a DNA-based test. Therefore, refusing to hire an individual because his or her father died of Huntington disease (meaning that the individual would be at a 50% risk) would not be unlawful, because the basis of the decision was not a genetic test of the applicant. Other states vary on whether any genetic test in the workplace (including voluntary medical monitoring) could be considered lawful (National Conference of State Legislatures, 2005).

In 2008, after a thirteen-year battle, Congress finally enacted the Genetic Information Nondiscrimination Act (GINA; Public Law 110–233). GINA prohibits genetic discrimination in health insurance and employment. Employers may not discriminate against an employee (including an applicant) on the basis of genetic information or request, require, or purchase genetic information about an employee or family member. Genetic information includes genetic tests, genetic tests of family members, and family history. A key exception to the prohibition on employer acquisition of genetic information is where the information is used for genetic monitoring of the effects of toxic substances, but only if (1) written notice is provided to the employee; (2) the employee provides voluntary, written authorization or the monitoring is required by law; (3) the employee is informed of individual results; (4) the monitoring is in compliance with applicable regulations; and (5) the employer receives the results only in aggregate form.

The primary goal of GINA is "to fully protect the public from discrimination and allay their concerns about the potential for discrimination, thereby allowing individuals to take advantage of genetic testing, technologies, research, and new therapies" (GINA §2(5)). Although GINA makes it unlawful to request genetic information about an employee, it does not alter the ADA provision permitting employers to require access to all of an individualís health records after a conditional offer of employment. Because it is virtually impossible to distinguish between genetic and nongenetic information in either paper or electronic health records, and despite GINA, most custodians of health records are likely to continue the current practice of sending the entire record in response to employer requests. Without an amendment of the ADA and research and development of new informatics tools to limit disclosures (M.A. Rothstein and Talbott, 2006), GINA and state genetic nondiscrimination laws are not likely to be effective (M.A. Rothstein, 2008).

Conclusion

Most of the focus of commentators and legislators surrounding "genetic discrimination" has been the exclusion of individuals from employment opportunities because they were at a genetically increased risk of ordinary diseases of life, such as various cancers. The issue is whether the law should intervene to prevent employers from taking steps to avoid the likely productivity losses and health care expenditures from employment of individuals at genetically increased risk of disease.

Toxicogenomics raises the separate issue of what, if any, protections and precautions are appropriate to respond to the genetically increased risk of certain individuals based on exposures to toxic substances in the workplace. Scientific developments in toxicogenomics are likely to challenge the existing regulatory paradigm under the OSH Act, under which substantially all individuals are assumed to have comparable risk, and those at higher risk are usually not identifiable in advance of exposure.

Toxicogenomics also challenges the workplace nondiscrimination paradigm, under which asymptomatic individuals are not considered covered under disability discrimination laws because they are not yet sick, and under which genetic-specific laws attempt to prohibit a narrow set of employer practices. As the state of the art in toxicogenomics progresses, the laws on workplace regulation and nondiscrimination will have to keep pace to achieve the dual public policies of promoting occupational safety and health and preventing unfair genetic discrimination.

REFERENCES

Armstrong v. Turner Industries, 141 F.3d 554 (5th Cir. 1998).

Bragdon v. Abbott, 524 U.S. 624 (1998).

Chevron U.S.A. Inc. v. Echazabal, 536 U.S. 73 (2002).

Clegg, R. 2000. Bragdon v. Abbott, asymptomatic genetic conditions, and antidiscrimination law. Journal of Health Care Law & Policy 3:409–29.

Clinton, W.J. 2000. To prohibit discrimination in federal employment based on genetic information. Federal Executive Order No. 13145, 65 Fed. Reg. 6,877 (Feb. 10, 2000).Conroy v. New York Department of Correctional Services, 333 F.3d 99 (2d Cir. 2003).

Dichter, M.A., and S.E. Sutor. 1997. The new genetic age: Do our genes make us disabled individuals under the Americans with Disabilities Act? Villanova Law Review 42:613–33.

EEOC v. Burlington Northern Santa Fe Railroad Co., No. C01-4013 (N.D. Iowa, filed Feb. 9, 2001).

Equal Employment Opportunity Commission compliance manual, vol. 2, EEOC Order 915.002, Definition of the Term "Disability" at 902-45, reprinted in Daily Labor Report, March 16, 1995, E-1, E-23.

Epstein, R.A. 1994. The legal regulation of genetic discrimination: Old responses to new technology. Boston University Law Review 74:1–23.

Fredenburg v. Contra Costa County Department of Health Services, 172 F.3d 1176 (9th Cir. 1999).

Greely, H.T. 2001. Genotype discrimination: The complex case for some legal protection. *University of Pennsylvania Law Review* 149:1483–1505.

Gridley, D. 2001. Genetic testing under the Americans with Disabilities Act: A case for protection from employment discrimination. *Georgetown Law Journal* 89:973–99.

Griffin v. Steeltek, 160 F.3d 591 (10th Cir. 1998), cert. denied, 526 U.S. 1065 (1999).

Haldane, J.B.S. 1938. *Heredity and politics.* London: Allen & Unwin.

Industrial Union Department, AFL-CIO v. American Petroleum Institute. 448 U.S. 607 (1980).

Kim, P.T. 2002. Genetic discrimination, genetic privacy: Rethinking employee protections for a brave new workplace. *Northwestern University Law Review* 96:1497–1551.

Marchant, G.E. 2003. Genomics and toxic substances: Part I—Toxicogenomics. *Environmental Law Reporter* 33:10071–93.

National Conference of State Legislatures. 2005. State genetic discrimination in employment laws. At www.ncsl.org/programs/health/genetics/ndiscrim.htm.

Office of Technology Assessment, United States Congress. 1983. The role of genetic testing in the prevention of occupational disease. Washington, DC: Government Printing Office.

Occupational Safety and Health Administration. 1980. OSHA Instruction STD 1-23.4. Occupational Safety and Health Report Ref. File 21:8212. Washington, DC: U.S. Department of Labor.

Rothstein, L.F. 2000. Genetic discrimination: Why *Bragdon* does not ensure protection. *Journal of Health Care Law & Policy* 3:330–51.

Rothstein, M.A. 1989. *Medical screening and the employee health cost crisis.* Washington, DC: BNA Books.

Rothstein, M.A. 1992. Genetic discrimination in employment and the Americans with Disabilities Act. *Houston Law Review* 29:23–84.

Rothstein, M.A. 1998. Protecting genetic privacy by permitting access only to job-related employee medical information: Analysis of a unique Minnesota law. *American Journal of Law and Medicine* 24:399–417.

Rothstein, M.A. 2000. Genetics and the work force of the next hundred years. *Columbia Business Law Review* 2000:371–402.

Rothstein, M.A. 2005. Genetic exceptionalism and legislative pragmatism. *Hastings Center Report* 35:27–33.

Rothstein, M.A. 2006. *Occupational safety and health law.* St. Paul, MN: Thomson/West.

Rothstein, M.A. 2008. Is GINA worth the wait? *Journal of Law, Medicine, and Ethics* 36:174–78.

Rothstein, M.A., and M.R. Anderlik. 2001. What is genetic discrimination and when and how can it be prevented? *Genetics in Medicine* 3:354–58.

Rothstein, M.A., and C.A. Hornung. 2003. Public attitudes about pharmacogenomics. In *Pharmacogenomics: Social, ethical, and clinical dimensions,* edited by M.A. Rothstein, 17-22 Hoboken, NJ: Wiley-Liss.

Rothstein, M.A. and M.K. Talbott. 2006. Compelled Disclosure of Health Information: Protecting Against the Greatest Potential Threat to Privacy. *Journal of
the American Medical Association* 295:2882–2885.

Samuels, S.W. 2003. Occupational medicine and its discontents. *Journal of Occupational and Environmental Medicine* 45:1226–33.

Schulte, P.A., and G. Lomax. 2003. Assessment of the scientific basis for genetic
testing of railroad workers with carpal tunnel syndrome. *Journal of Occupational and Environmental Medicine* 45:592–600.

Sutton v. United Air Lines, Inc. 527 U.S. 471 (1999).

Tice v. Centre Area Transportation Authority, 247 F.3d 506 (3d Cir. 2001).

Toyota Motor Manufacturing, Kentucky, Inc., v. Williams. 534 U.S. 184 (2002)

CHAPTER 12

Genetic Susceptibility and Radiological Health and Safety

KENNETH L. MOSSMAN

With the publication of the complete human genome in 2001, the door has been pushed wide open to explore fully the genetic basis of human disease. DNA specimens from many individuals can now be examined to identify variants in the 25,000 to 30,000 genes now believed to make up the human genome. Today, DNA chip technology is capable of scanning tens of thousands of genetic variants. Routine genetic screening is just a matter of time. Recognizing and cataloging genetic variants will help to identify specific genes that influence vulnerability to a wide spectrum of human diseases including cancer. Methods of identifying genetic markers for disease, in combination with pathophysiologic studies, will aid in developing diagnostic tests for early detection and individualized therapies. But individuals known to be at risk for specific diseases through genetic screening could be subject to employment, insurance, and social discrimination.

A significant number of genetically based diseases have now been identified that confer heightened cancer risk (Sankaranarayanan and Chakraborty, 2001). This chapter explores individual cancer sensitivity, with a focus on radiation-induced cancer in the workplace environment.

More is known about the cancer-causing effects of ionizing radiation than any other human carcinogen, except perhaps tobacco smoke. There is substantial experience in control of ionizing radiation exposure in the workplace. Management of exposure of the pregnant worker serves as a useful model in developing management strategies for radiosensitive individuals. The developing embryo or fetus is more sensitive to radiation than is the adult. Although pregnancy is a temporary condition, current policies to protect the developing fetus may be of value in developing guidance for protecting workers who are found to be genetically predisposed to cancer.

An individual's sensitivity to ionizing radiation exposure has emerged as an important consideration in protecting workers and members of the public. Identifying radiation-sensitive individuals (through medical screening or disease diagnosis) and providing them with adequate protection raise important policy questions.

Who Is Sensitive to Radiation?

Radiosensitivity (i.e., the response of an individual to a given dose of ionizing radiation) can be defined statistically by the frequency distribution of sensitivities in the population or by the severity of cancer by cancer site. Genetic mutations and polymorphisms have emerged as an important area of research to elucidate the underlying basis of variations in individual cancer sensitivities (National Research Council, 2007). Depending on the underlying genetic mutation, an individual may be at a greater risk than others for lung cancer, breast cancer, colorectal cancer, thyroid cancer, or other cancers from exposure to ionizing radiation. Because cancers have different incidence and mortality rates and present different clinical management challenges (American Cancer Society, 2005), consequences of workplace exposures may be more severe in one person than in another. Having any form of cancer is unfortunate, but certain cancers are more clinically significant than others. Although little evidence is available at this time, sensitivity to radiation may also imply sensitivity to chemical carcinogens, if those sensitivities are determined by common damage and repair pathways.

The proportion of workers and the public who have increased radiogenic cancer risk because of genetic susceptibility is not known but has been estimated to be in the range of 1 to 10 percent. The proportion of

the population that is radiosensitive is difficult to determine directly because of the nonspecificity of radiogenic diseases and because of the small
radiation doses received occupationally and by the general population
(Mossman, 1997; International Commission on Radiological Protection,
1998).

It is assumed that individual sensitivities vary in accordance with a
normal distribution and that radiosensitivity is normally distributed in
the population as are height and other biological characteristics (Figure
12.1). Most people have a radiosensitivity that clusters around a central
estimate (in the figure, the central estimate is 50 relative radiosensitivity
units, assuming radiation sensitivity in the population varies from 1 to
100 relative units). Individuals with sensitivities that deviate significantly
from the central estimate or average are termed to be either radioresis-
tant or radiosensitive. As an illustration, the darkened region in Figure
12.1 represents 10 percent of the area under the curve, and identifies a
radiosensitive subpopulation characterized by individuals with radiation
sensitivities of 70 relative units or more. The actual percentage of indi-

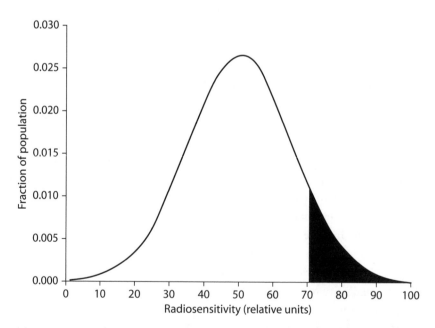

Figure 12.1. Distribution of radiosensitivity plotted as a probability density function.
The darkened portion represents a theoretical radiosensitive subpopulation and is
equal to 10 percent of the total area under the curve.

viduals who are radiosensitive will depend on the variance of the distribution of radiosensitivities in the population (i.e., the spread of the distribution) and the definitional threshold sensitivity level. A definition of radiosensitivity for the purposes of radiation protection has not been established.

Recent studies in molecular genetics suggest that the assumption of a random distribution of radiosensitivity in the population is likely to be overly simplistic. Much of human variation in sensitivity to environmental agents is now thought to result from individual gene variations due to single nucleotide polymorphisms (SNPs)—specific gene codon variations that result in a change of a single amino acid inserted at a specific site in the protein product of the gene. Specific SNP variations are not evenly distributed across the entire human population, but often appear to be heavily concentrated in certain regional or ethnic groups. For example, about one-third of patients with Bloom syndrome (BS), a rare autosomal recessive disease characterized by enhanced cancer risk, are of Ashkenazi Jewish descent (Cleary et al., 2003). Ethnic or regional differences in SNP distributions create serious policy questions regarding protection of specific individuals and population subgroups in the workplace.

Genetic Determinants of the Risk for Cancer

Inherited predisposition for cancer has been shown to be due to specific germ-line mutations in one or more cancer genes (Sankaranarayanan and Chakroborty, 2001). These mutations increase cancer risk because the specific genetic defect compromises cell growth and division or repair of DNA damage. Diseases characterized by increased risk for cancer are either dominant (e.g., familial adenomatous polyposis and neurofibromatosis) or recessive (e.g., xeroderma pigmentosum and ataxia telangiectacsia [AT]).

The accumulation of mutations in cancer genes (i.e., oncogenes and tumor suppressor genes) promotes the development of cancer. DNA repair is a critical cellular response that counteracts the carcinogenic effects of DNA damage. There are several known DNA repair processes, all of which act to remove DNA lesions and prevent mutations, thereby restoring and maintaining genetic integrity. The importance of DNA repair pathways is illustrated by a number of hereditary diseases, in which individuals with defects in DNA repair genes are highly susceptible to cancer. Reduced activity of various DNA repair mechanisms predisposes individuals to lung cancer. Smokers with reduced DNA repair activity have a greater than one hundred-fold higher risk for lung cancer compared to smokers with normal DNA repair capacity (Paz-Elizur et al., 2003).

The only known human genetic diseases characterized by increased radiosensitivity to ionizing radiation and increased cancer risk are AT and Nijmegen breakage syndrome (NBS; National Research Council, 2005). AT is a rare, recessive genetic disorder of childhood that occurs in about one in one hundred thousand persons worldwide. The disease is characterized by neurological complications, recurrent serious sinus and respiratory infections, and dilated blood vessels in the eyes and on the surface of the skin. People have who have the disease usually have immune system abnormalities and are very sensitive to ionizing radiation exposure. They are at high risk of developing and dying of cancer, particularly leukemia and lymphoma. NBS is also a rare autosomal recessive disease that is closely related to, but clinically distinguishable from, AT. The disease affects fewer than one in one hundred thousand persons. NBS is characterized by microcephaly, growth retardation, immunodeficiency, predisposition to cancer, and increased sensitivity to ionizing radiation. BS and Fanconi anemia (FA) are also autosomal recessive disorders associated with increased risk of cancer, but it is uncertain whether increased radiosensitivity is an important clinical feature of these diseases. Affected individuals with AT, NBS, BS, or FA usually do not survive beyond adolescence or early adulthood due to susceptibility to infections and high cancer risks (Table 12.1).

In theory, heterozygote carriers of these recessive genetic conditions may have cancer risks that are lower than affected (i.e., homozygous) individuals, but still higher than normal. For example, Gruber and colleagues have reported increased colon cancer risk in BS heterozygotes (Gruber et al., 2002), but their results could not be duplicated in a Canadian study (Cleary et al., 2003).

The issue of heterozygote sensitivity sparked controversy in the early 1990s over the question of whether mammography should be recommended for women with a genetic predisposition for breast cancer (including AT heterozygotes) in the same manner it is recommended for other women of a certain age and risk profile. Concern focused on whether mammography might cause more breast cancers because of heightened

TABLE 12.1
Selected Autosomal Recessive Disorders with Increased Cancer Risk

Disease	Prevalence (per live births)	Genetic defect	Cancer
Ataxia telangiectasia	1/100,000	DNA repair; induction of p53	Leukemia, lymphoma
Bloom syndrome	1/100 in Ashkenazi Jews	Loss of DNA helicase activity	Colon?
Fanconi anemia	1/300,000	DNA cross-link repair	Leukemia
Nijmegen breakage syndrome	<1/100,000	DNA double strand break repair	Lymphoma

Sources: Sankaranarayanan and Chakraborty, 2001; National Research Council, 2005.

radiation risks in AT heterozygotes. It has been estimated that 1 percent of the U.S. population, or 2.5 million people, are carriers for AT (Sankara-narayanan and Chakraborty, 2001). Swift and colleagues argued that women heterozygous for AT should avoid mammography because of their enhanced radiogenic risk (Swift et al., 1987, 1991). On the basis of two small, related studies, they estimated that irradiation of the breast could result in a five- to sixfold excess risk of breast cancer in blood relatives of AT patients. But breast cancer following diagnostic x-ray exposure in AT heterozygotes has not been confirmed (Boice and Miller, 1992; Hall, Geard, and Brenner, 1992; Kuller and Modan, 1992; Land, 1992; Swift et al., 1992; Wagner, 1992).

There is little evidence demonstrating a link between low-dose diagnostic x-ray and an elevated breast cancer risk in AT heterozygotes. Until such a link is established, and the radiogenic risk is understood in the context of other breast cancer risk factors, it would be unwise for such women to forgo mammography for early detection of breast cancer. Nevertheless, this mammography debate foreshadowed future controversies about how and whether individuals with a genetic sensitivity to radiation should be treated differently because of their potential increased risk.

Prioritizing Risk

Individual cancer risk is governed by a complex combination of genetic, host, and environmental factors. For example, tobacco smoke is the

major cause of lung cancer, but an individual smoker's risk of lung cancer appears to depend on that person's capacity to repair DNA damage
(Paz-Elizur et al., 2003). The combination of genetic and environmental
factors may explain why some smokers get lung cancer and others do
not. Genetic predisposition is an important risk factor for some cancers,
but host factors (such as age and gender) and environmental factors are
the primary determinants of cancer risk. In Doll and Peto's seminal 1981
report on the contributions of various environmental factors to cancer
causation (including ionizing radiation), factors such as diet and cigarette smoking are considered to be significantly more important than genetic causes (Figure 12.2). Together, cigarette smoking and diet account

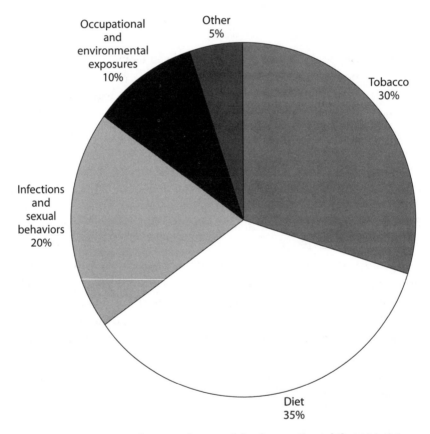

Figure 12.2. Environmental causes of cancer. It has been estimated that 80 to 90
percent of cancers are due to exposures to one or more environmental agents.
Tobacco and diet account for more than 60 percent of all cancer deaths.
Source: Doll and Peto, 1981

for approximately two-thirds of all cancer-related deaths in the United States (Doll and Peto, 1981).

Radiation, included under occupational and environmental exposures, is a relatively weak carcinogen. Ionizing radiation, including exposures from various natural background radiation sources, accounts for only about 2 percent of the total cancer burden in the United States. Although the relevant literature has grown enormously since Doll and Peto's 1981 report (including the emergence of cancers as a result of human immunodeficiency virus infection), the current epidemiological evidence on environmental causes of cancer has not given cause to change the Doll and Peto estimates appreciably (Willett, 1995).

The influence of age, gender, and, to a lesser extent, race as host factors varies considerably with cancer type. Age is a particularly important factor for lung, prostate, and colon cancer. Except for cancers of the breast and prostate, gender and racial differences in cancer risk are relatively minor (Mossman, 1997; American Cancer Society, 2007).

Control of environmental factors is the key to cancer risk management. Modification of personal behaviors related to diet, smoking, and infection or sexual activities can significantly impact the cancer mortality burden in the United States (Figure 12.2). In the future, correction of genetic defects related to repair of DNA damage and control of cell division and growth may also reduce risks for cancer. However, risk management in genetically predisposed individuals via genetic engineering is years or perhaps decades away.

Exposure to pesticides and other environmental and occupational carcinogens has a minor impact on the U.S. cancer burden. These agents are responsible for only a few percent of cancer deaths (Doll and Peto, 1981). Nevertheless, exposure to these agents should be controlled, particularly for members of the public and workers at high risk. The public health challenge is to allocate economic resources to manage health risks with the objective of doing the greatest good for the greatest number of people. However, resources also need to be funneled to manage minor risks, if there are sufficient resources and technical capacity to do so.

Policy Issues

From a public health and radiological protection perspective, genetic diseases predisposing individuals to cancer present challenging problems. The major concerns lie with disease carriers, because affected (i.e., homozygous) individuals usually do not live long enough to reach working age. For those few who live to working age, disease conditions are usually so severe that they preclude employment in almost any nuclear-related industry. Although genetic disease carriers appear normal and do not express signs and symptoms, as stated above it is unclear whether the heterozygous state confers increased risk for cancer. Increased radiosensitivity has been clearly identified in AT and NBS patients, but is an uncertain problem for heterozygotes.

Although age, gender, smoking, and diet are the principal determinants of cancer risk, individual radiosensitivity may also be important in some circumstances. Radiosensitive individuals working in radiological environments could be at higher risk for cancer. It may therefore be prudent to identify such individuals and provide additional protective measures. In the workplace, this might mean providing additional engineering controls to reduce exposures, providing additional worker education and training, or assigning job responsibilities that reduce occupational exposure.

Two general risk-management approaches to protecting radiosensitive workers could be taken, each with its own inherent advantages and disadvantages. First, public and occupational dose limits could be further reduced for all workers to account for radiosensitive subpopulations. By doing so, everyone would be treated equally, and there would be no need to identify sensitive workers. Because everyone would be adequately protected, there would also be no need to segregate sensitive workers by job responsibilities.

More restrictive exposure limits to account for radiosensitive subpopulations are unlikely to result in a net public health benefit. Radiogenic cancer risk estimates are population-derived and likely already reflect the responses of the most radiosensitive component of the population. Further, radiogenic cancers are probably not distributed uniformly in the population. Evidence for this is found in the disproportionate numbers of breast cancers in AT heterozygotes. The 1 percent of the population carrying the AT gene is estimated to constitute 9 to 18 percent of all persons with breast cancer in the United States (Swift et al., 1991). Thus, reducing exposure limits for the entire population would be very costly and would benefit relatively few (radiosensitive) individuals.

In the second risk-management approach, sensitive subpopulations could be identified and provided with additional protection beyond what is normally provided to the general worker population. A more limited, targeted approach would allow for greater reductions in dose than is feasible or practicable for workforce-wide reductions in exposure. Protective measures might include more restrictive dose limits applicable only to radiosensitive subpopulations, job responsibilities with reduced probability of exposure, and additional education and training. Assuming relatively few individuals would be candidates for additional protective measures, this approach is more cost-effective, because additional protection is provided only to the individuals who need it. But genetic screening to identify radiosensitive individuals opens up a Pandora's box. Although some laws and regulations to protect workers are in place, employment, insurance, and social discrimination as a result of genetic screening remain a serious concern.

Genetic testing, whether voluntary or involuntary, raises a number of ethical questions. The rapid evolution in DNA technologies will soon make it possible to obtain quite detailed genetic information on individuals. Some people do not want to know if they carry genes that predispose them to a certain disease; others do want to know, so that they can have the opportunity to prevent its future development by avoiding risks and engaging in preventive behaviors such as eating a healthy diet and exercising.

The most significant problem for radiosensitive individuals in the workplace is the potential for employment and medical insurance discrimination (Lapham, Kozma, and Weiss, 1996). Current international radiological protection programs in various nuclear industries protect workers with a large margin of safety. In the United States nuclear workers are not at increased risk for cancer (Cardis et al., 2005). But individuals identified to be radiosensitive could find themselves to be at a decided disadvantage in the workplace. Employers may decide not to hire such workers, because of the potential insurance liabilities that may occur. Individuals with greater risks for certain medical conditions (identified through genetic or other clinical tests) could be classified as uninsurable, or insurable only at substantially higher rates than normal workers.

Existing legal protections for genetically susceptible workers are uncertain. The Americans with Disabilities Act of 1990 (ADA), section 12112(d), puts some limits on the use of genetic testing in the workplace (Americans with Disabilities Act, 1990). ADA forbids any medical inquiry before a conditional offer of employment. Once an offer of employment has been made, however, the employer can request medical examination, including genetic testing, if such examinations are job-related and consistent with business necessity. Enhanced susceptibility to occupational exposures to carcinogens (including exposure to ionizing radiation) may be a justification for preemployment genetic testing under ADA. Although workers who are radiosensitive and predisposed to cancer may be at higher risk for cancer in a radiological work environment, terminating an employee with a predisposition for a particular work-related disease is prohibited under ADA. However the extent of protection under ADA may be limited for workers with defined disabilities. In *Chevron U.S.A. Inc. v. Echazabal* (2002) the Supreme Court held that employers could refuse to hire or could fire a person with a disability if they believe that person's health or safety would be put at risk by performing the job.

ADA also bars employers from discriminating on the basis of disability in the provision of health insurance. But the Equal Employment Opportunity Commission (EEOC) notes that "blanket pre-existing condition clauses that exclude from the coverage of a health insurance plan the treatment of conditions that predate an individual's eligibility for benefits under that plan also are not distinctions based on disability, and do not violate the ADA" (Equal Employment Opportunity Commission, 1993).

Genetic testing of employees can be construed either as worker discrimination or as a prudent practice in the best interests of the employee and the employer. Individuals with positive screening tests (whether true or false) may be subject to employment, insurance, or social discrimination. Should radiosensitivity be considered a legitimate preemployment condition that requires testing? Should genetic testing for radiosensitivity be left up to the individual only, or are there certain employment situations in which such personal information would be legitimately required by the employer?

Pregnancy as a Precedent for a New Approach

Another risk-management approach is available, one that could reconcile the two risk-management approaches discussed above in an acceptable and practicable manner. The current radiation protection framework includes special considerations for pregnant workers. The experience acquired with formulating protection of pregnant workers may be useful in crafting policy for the protection of radiosensitive individuals. As discussed above, pregnant workers are subject to more restrictive radiation dose limits because of increased embryo or fetus radiosensitivity. The embryo and fetus are more sensitive to the effects of carcinogenic agents because of rapid cell proliferation and tissue and organ development. Adverse pregnancy outcomes generally require direct exposure of the embryo or fetus, which can occur when the mother inhales, ingests, or injects radionuclides or as a result of maternal external exposure to penetrating radiation such as x-rays or gamma radiation. Under existing approaches, a female worker is entitled to "declare" pregnancy and obtain additional protection (U.S. Nuclear Regulatory Commission [NRC], 1992).

Genetic testing for the purposes of identifying radiosensitive individuals should not be a conditional requirement of hiring or continued employment. Genetic testing should be entirely voluntary, and enhanced radiosensitivity should be declarable by the employee in the same way that pregnancy is "declared" (NRC, 1992). Under a declaration provision, the employer would not be obligated to provide additional protections or enforce more restrictive dose limits unless the employee declares a condition involving increased radiosensitivity. The employer's responsibility to provide additional protection is triggered only by the employee's declaration, even if the employer has independent evidence of the employee's condition. The employee would also have the option to "undeclare" a health condition involving increased radiosensitivity. This might occur if the employee was dissatisfied with a job reassignment. Declaration withdrawal would relieve the employer of responsibilities for protection beyond what is provided to other employees. The findings of the U.S. Supreme Court in *Automobile Workers v. Johnson Controls, Inc.* (1991), although addressing discrimination against pregnant workers, may be instructive regarding genetic and other medical conditions: In that decision, the Supreme Court rejected the employer's attempt to prohibit women of child-bearing age from working in the facility because of the potential for lead exposure; rather, the decision of whether to work in such conditions was left to the individual choice of each employee. The decision about the health and welfare of a worker with a genetic predisposition to cancer or other occupationally related disease should be left to the individual.

Orientation programs for all employees in workplaces with potential for radiation exposure should include information about radiosensitivity and the impact of enhanced radiosensitivity on radiogenic risk. Employees who have declared radiosensitivities should be provided with additional information regarding job-specific strategies to reduce dose. Where possible, employers should provide optional job responsibilities to such workers involving reduced radiation exposures. "Declared" employees should not be subjected to different terms and conditions of employment.

Information on an individual's radiosensitivity can also be a relevant factor in the medical arena. For example, there is considerable interest in identifying sensitive individuals who are candidates for cancer therapy. Screening cancer patients for radiation and chemotherapeutic drug sensitivity could be useful in identifying optimal treatments. For example, if a patient with prostate cancer has the option of surgery or radiotherapy treatment, information about radiation sensitivity would be important in the treatment decision. Identification of gene variants may lead to the recognition of patients who may benefit from certain classes of drugs or more important may be inappropriate candidates for certain therapies because of genetic sensitivities.

Studies of molecular epidemiology may prove to be particularly helpful in developing appropriate screening tests, for both workers and patients. Such studies could lead to the development of simple screening tests to identify individuals who are inherently more sensitive to radiation effects. Individual sensitivity has potential implications for radiation protection and use of radiation in medicine (radiotherapy for cancer and high-dose diagnostic procedures such as cardiac angiography).

Conclusion

Individuals who are genetically predisposed to cancer have emerged as an important consideration in radiological protection. Reducing dose limits for all workers to account for radiosensitive subgroups is not a cost-effective solution. Radiosensitivity is a minor contributing factor to carcinogenesis compared with host and environmental factors, but additional protections should be made available to individuals predisposed to cancer, particularly in work environments where occupational risks may be significant. Safeguards must be put in place to protect workers from employment, insurance, and social discrimination as a result of genetic screening. Workers should be given the option to "declare" radiosensitivity in much the same way that female workers "declare" pregnancy. Workers with "declared" radiosensitivity should be informed of the additional health risks associated with radiation exposure, particularly cancer, and should be provided reasonable additional protection including, but not limited to, reassignment to lower health risk work environments.

REFERENCES

American Cancer Society. 2007. *Cancer Facts and Figures, 2007.* Atlanta: American Cancer Society.

Americans with Disabilities Act (ADA). 42 U.S.C. 12112 (d). 1990

Automobile Workers v. Johnson Controls, Inc. 499 U.S. 187. 1991.

Boice, J.D., and R.W. Miller. 1992. Risk of breast cancer in ataxia telangiectasia. *New England Journal of Medicine* 326:1357–58.

Cardis, E., M. Vrijheid, M. Blettner, et al. 2005. Risk of cancer after low doses of ionising radiation: Retrospective cohort study in 15 countries. *British Medical Journal* 331: 77–82.

Chevron U.S. v. Echazabal 536 U.S. 73. 2002.

Cleary, S.P., W. Zhang, N. Di Nicola, et al. 2003. Heterozygosity for the BLM$_{Ash}$ mutation and cancer risk. *Cancer Research* 63:1769–71.

Doll, R., and R. Peto. 1981. The causes of cancer: Quantitative estimates of avoidable risks of cancer in the United States today. *Journal of the National Cancer Institute* 66:1191–1308.

Equal Employment Opportunity Commission. 1993. *Interim Guidance on Application of ADA to Health Insurance Plans. EEOC Compliance Manual.* Washington, DC: Bureau of National Affairs.

Gruber, S.B., N.A. Ellis, G. Rennert, and K. Offit, et al. (2002). BLM heterozygosity and the risk of colorectal cancer. *Science* 297:2013.

Hall, E.J., C.R. Geard, and D.J. Brenner. 1992. Risk of breast cancer in ataxia telangiectasia. *New England Journal of Medicine* 326:1358–59.

International Commission on Radiological Protection (ICRP). 1998. *Genetic Susceptibility to Cancer,* ICRP Publication 79. Oxford: Pergamon Press.

Kuller, L.H., and B. Modan. 1992. Risk of breast cancer in ataxia telangiectasia. *New England Journal of Medicine* 326:1357.

Land, C.E. 1992. Risk of breast cancer in ataxia telangiectasia. *New England Journal of Medicine* 326:1359–60.

Lapham, E.V., C. Kozma, and J. Weiss. 1996. Genetic discrimination: Perspectives of consumers. *Science* 274:621–24.

Mossman, K.L. 1997. Radiation protection of radiosensitive populations. *Health Physics* 72:519–23.

National Research Council. 2005. *Health risks from exposure to low levels of ionizing radiation,* Biological Effects of Ionizing Radiation VII Report. Washington, DC: National Academies Press.

Paz-Elizur, T., M. Krupsky, S. Blumenstein, D. Elinger, E. Schechtman, and Z Livneh. 2003. DNA repair activity for oxidative damage and risk of lung cancer. *Journal of the National Cancer Institute* 95:1312–19.

Sankaranarayanan, K., and R. Chakraborty. 2001. Impact of cancer predisposition and radiosensitivity on the population risk of radiation-induced cancer. *Radiation Research* 156:648–56.

Swift, M., D. Morrell, R.B. Massey and C.L. Chase. 1991. Incidence of cancer in 161 families affected by ataxia-telangiectasia. *New England Journal of Medicine* 325:1831–36.

Swift, M., D. Morrell, R.B. Massey and C.L. Chase. 1992. Risk of breast cancer in ataxia-telangiectasia. *New England Journal of Medicine* 326:1360.

Swift, M., P.J. Reitnauer, T.D. Morrell, and C.L. Chase. 1987. Breast and other cancers in families with ataxia-telangiectasia. *New England Journal of Medicine* 316:1289–94.

U.S. Nuclear Regulatory Commission. 1992. *Code of Federal Regulations,* 10 CFR Part 20. Washington, D.C.: U.S. Government Printing Office.

Wagner, L.K. 1992. Risk of breast cancer in ataxia telangiectasia. *New England Journal of Medicine* 326:1358.

Willett, W.C. 1995. Who is susceptible to cancers of the breast, colon, and prostate? *Annals of the New York Academy of Sciences* 768:1–11.

PART IV

ETHICAL AND PHILOSOPHICAL PERSPECTIVES

CHAPTER 13

Conceptual and Normative Dimensions of Toxicogenomics

ANDREA O. SMITH AND JASON SCOTT ROBERT

Toxicogenetics and toxicogenomics are widely seen to offer considerable promise for environmental risk assessment and rational, knowledge-based environmental policy. As the proponents of such research clearly understand, "it is only through the development of a profound knowledge base that toxicology and environmental health can rapidly advance" (Waters, Olden, and Tennant, 2003, p. 349). But what will constitute this "profound knowledge base"? For some, it will be comprised of molecular knowledge: knowledge about genetic polymorphisms, the molecular signatures of chemicals, and the chemical interactions between genes and toxicants. This would appear to be the perspective of the U.S. National Institute of Environmental Health Sciences, as evidenced by the Environmental Genome Project, the National Center for Toxicogenomics, and related efforts. But without an appropriate context through which to interpret this molecular knowledge, research in toxicogenetics and toxicogenomics may not be able to make good on its promise. From our perspective, this appropriate context includes knowledge about organismal development, ecology, and politics, among other things.

In part, this is because the molecular level does not force itself on us in risk assessment and environmental protection. Scientists and regulators make choices as to whether and how to use molecular data. These are choices with multiple normative dimensions, opportunity costs, and social and scientific consequences. In this chapter, we explore these issues, beginning with a discussion of the recent history of the use of genomic techniques and data in toxicology. Drawing on the tools of the philosophy of science, particularly regarding the identification of conceptual assumptions and the justification of research methods, we discuss both plainly valid though underdeveloped uses (such as DNA microarrays for detecting toxins in biosamples) and some less plainly valid though more common uses of toxicogenomics.

For the authors of many chapters in this volume, their cup runneth over. Ours, by contrast, will seem half-empty. A caveat: though we are skeptical that toxicogenomics will be able to deliver on all the manifold promises made on its behalf, we offer our skepticism not to be "antigene" or technophobic. Rather, as the information produced by toxicogenomics increases in volume and detail, scientists are wrestling with how to understand the meaning of the data—the data far outstrip our ability to interpret them. Should toxicogenomics proceed without resolving issues of validity and inference, for instance, it will promote a false sense of our understanding of environmentally induced disease, having important normative implications. Our claim is a modest one: critical conceptual analysis—and so the philosophy of science—is important to sound progress in environmental science and policy (Robert and Smith, 2004).

Why Toxicogenomics?

Some of the greatest threats to our health arise from exposure to environmental agents. Epidemiologists and environmental health researchers have tracked incidences of exposure, explored the nature of toxic chemicals and their effects on humans and other organisms, and, in some instances, offered remedies, including regulation of suspect (and guilty) toxins. But with the rise of a molecular worldview in biology since the 1940s, and especially in the past two decades, our understanding of environmental influences on human health has come to be dominated by a focus on genes. At first, environmentally induced mutations were explored, as in the Department of Energy's involvement in establishing the

Human Genome Project (Beatty, 2000; Maienschein, 2003). More recently, attention has turned to environmentally sensitive polymorphisms, as in the Environmental Genome Project at the U.S. National Institute of Environmental Health Sciences (Olden and Wilson, 2000; Christiani et al., 2001; Robert and Smith, 2004).

The integration of genetics, and now of genomics, into toxicology has been encouraged in the pursuit of a more mechanistic toxicology. In the 1990s, the National Toxicology Program endorsed this goal and envisioned a future in which toxicology evolved from a descriptive to a predictive scientific enterprise (Goodman, 1994; Bucher and Portier, 2004). By and large, this has yet to be achieved, as toxicologists still grapple with how best to identify detailed mechanisms of toxicity and assess risk posed by chemical agents.

As it is usually defined, toxicogenetics focuses on the identification of genetic susceptibilities through the detection of genetic polymorphisms in populations; by contrast, toxicogenomics is usually defined in terms of its focus on gene expression data, often at the level of the entire genome (Marchant, 2003a, 2003b). Elsewhere we have explored the normative dimensions of toxicogenetics (Robert and Smith, 2004), so what follows focuses largely on toxicogenomics.

High-throughput microarray technologies—used to analyze gene expression—are foundational to toxicogenomics and are now being used to measure genetic reaction to environmental agents. Microarrays are small, usually glass, slides containing thousands of markers, generally either of single-stranded DNA affixed to the slide or short sequences of synthesized DNA (oligonucleotides) photolithographed onto the slide. The philosopher of science Ken Schaffner (2002, pp. 332–33) explains the process for nonexperts:

> To determine which genes have been expressed in a sample, researchers isolate messenger RNA [mRNA] from the samples, convert it to complementary DNA [cDNA], tag it with fluorescent dye, and run the sample over the chip. Typically, there are two samples per slide, i.e., a test and a reference [or control] sample, dyed 'red' and 'green', respectively. The reference samples may be cells at 'time 1', and the test sample cells at 'time 2'. Each tagged cDNA will stick to a probe or oligo with a matching sequence, lighting up a spot on the wafer [or slide] where the sequence is known. A detector, often an automated laser scanner microscope, then scans the slide

and determines which probes or oligos have bound, and hence which genes were expressed.

These data are then analyzed statistically and presented in the form of a matrix (Schaffner, 2002; see also Lander, 1999; Nuwaysir et al., 1999; Hamadeh et al., 2001; Knight, 2001; Choudhuri, 2004; Irwin et al., 2004; Shioda, 2004).

Microarray technologies may be used in a knowledge-driven way, as when knowledge that a toxin interferes with a given receptor can be used to build a microarray to further clarify the nature of the mechanism, or in a pattern-driven way, as when large and heterogeneous microarrays are constructed to assess the pattern of changes in gene expression of a novel toxin (its "molecular signature") by comparison with patterns of changes in gene expression produced by known toxins (Smith, 2001). The latter approach, especially when coupled with proteomics (Schaffner, 2002; see also Pandey and Mann, 2000; Choudhuri, 2004) and metabolite profiling—metabolomics (e.g., Phelps, Palumbo, and Beliaev, 2002)—promises the ability to predict abnormal physiological functioning on the basis of the molecular signatures of chemicals, such that these molecular signatures may then be useful as evidence of exposure and early indicators of adverse effects.

Whether toxicogenomics is, or will be, useful in environmental regulation is still open for debate. Some commentators trumpet a new era in risk assessment revolutionized by genomics (e.g., Nuwaysir et al., 1999; Bishop, Clarke, and Travis, 2001; Hamadeh et al., 2001; Marchant, 2003a; Waters, Selkirk, and Olden, 2003; see also Shostak, 2003, and citations therein); others are considerably more circumspect, expressing skepticism that the data will be properly interpreted, that the analyses will be properly validated, and that the tools will be properly applied in risk assessment (e.g., Smith, 2001; Henry, 2003; Cohen, 2004; Irwin et al., 2004). Nevertheless, despite acknowledged limitations, toxicogenomics is widely anticipated to be applicable to virtually all aspects of toxicology and risk assessment within medium-term time frames (five to ten years).

A survey of the toxicogenomics literature reveals four main themes or areas of application: hazard identification, development of biomarkers of exposure and effect, identification of mechanisms of toxicity, and risk characterization. While these four areas are not entirely independent of

TABLE 13.1

Potential Applications of Toxicogenomics in Environmental Health Sciences and Environmental Regulation

Area of application	Potential uses of toxicogenomics
Hazard identification	• Provides a rapid mechanism for identifying chemicals' effects • Minimizes and eliminates the need for animal models • Helps prioritize chemicals for hazard assessment • Serves as a tool for rapid screening of environmental samples to detect known toxins
Biomarker of exposure and effect	• Supports the development of molecular signatures as biological markers of exposure • Improves the ability to track exposures in the population • Enables preclinical diagnosis of disease resulting from toxic exposure
Mechanism of toxicity	• Develops molecular signatures to serve as informants regarding pathways of response to toxins (a proxy for the aetiology of environmentally induced disease) • Classifies environmental agents by mode of action • Classifies subpopulations by mode of response to toxic exposure
Risk characterization	• Improves precision in use of uncertainty factors in determining reference doses • Aids in assessment of the effects of chemical mixtures and of low doses • Increases accuracy of inferences drawn from laboratory studies • Helps resolve issues of differential sensitivity across groups • Moves toward more accurate predictions of individuals' risk

each other, we will briefly review the applicability of toxicogenomics to each area in turn (as summarized in Table 13.1).

Hazard Identification

We expect developments in two general areas of hazard identification: screening of chemicals for "characteristically toxic" properties and screening of samples for the presence or absence of particular toxins.

Regarding the first area, there are thousands of chemicals for which we have no or minimal data regarding potential health hazards (Schettler et al., 1999). Moreover, the National Toxicology Program estimates that approximately two thousand new chemicals for everyday use are introduced each year (National Toxicology Program, 2005), with more than eighty thousand chemicals currently registered in the United States for commercial and other use. Accordingly, scientists and regulators are seeking a rapid and reliable mechanism for identifying chemicals' likely effects. Hazard assessment is currently based on extrapolating from studies of model organisms. Such studies are costly, take years to execute, and may not always serve as appropriate sources of inference. By analyzing the expression of the human genome, the use of model organisms may be minimized if not eliminated, thus reducing the number of animals subject to experimentation and reducing the cross-species inferential gap. As molecular signatures are developed, the time required to identify the health effects of chemicals may be drastically reduced. Accordingly, hazard identification will be further streamlined; it is hoped that chemicals will be able to be initially screened for any toxic properties by evaluating gene expression resulting from exposure. This would (a) facilitate the initiation of more specific testing into any possible toxic properties and (b) enable the prioritization of chemicals for further testing.

Microarray technology may also be used for rapidly assessing the presence or absence of known toxins in environmental samples. For instance, rather than relying on time- and labor-intensive microbiological assays to determine whether a toxin is present in a water sample, regulators may instead (assuming that microarray technology becomes increasingly cost-effective) use microarrays for the detection of toxins in the water sample. To date, such efforts apparently suffer from a variety of technical and analytical problems, well described by Zhou and Thompson (2002) and Lemarchand, Masson, and Brousseau (2004), though these problems seem to be resolvable over time.

Biomarkers of Exposure and Effect

A biomarker is a biochemical or molecular signal indicating a state or change of state in a biological sample, such as a tissue or a cell. Traditional biomarkers in toxicology include "levels of environmental agents or their metabolites in a tissue or body fluid, usually blood or urine" (Hattis and Swedis, 2001, p. 186), which are measured to assess exposure to environmental toxins. Proponents of toxicogenomics advocate the use of microarray data-derived molecular signatures (chemical profiles, chemical "fingerprints," molecular "types") as biomarkers for this purpose (e.g., Marchant, 2003a), drawing on the successful use of biomarkers in oncology to facilitate diagnostic and treatment decisions on the basis of the molecular signature of tumors (e.g., Ludwig and Weinstein, 2005). Molecular signatures may also be used to prediagnose individuals who have been exposed to particular environmental agents well before they develop symptoms of negative health effects. Successful inference from such molecular signatures depends greatly on how well characterized and validated the putative signatures actually are, beyond proof of principle. Genomic biomarkers of exposure may lead to changes in the classification and definition of particular diseases, such that disease may be diagnosed and modulated prior to onset (e.g., Collins et al., 2003; but see Miller et al., 2006).

Mechanisms of Toxicity

A main goal of the application of genomics in toxicology is to improve the ability to identify molecular mechanisms of toxicity—that is, the pathways by which toxins have their effects, from changes in gene expression onward. It is widely held that more detailed information on pathways of disease development will facilitate hazard identification, risk assessment, and environmental regulation (Hamadeh et al., 2001; Marchant, 2003a). Researchers place heavy emphasis on the alteration of gene expression as a necessary component (though possibly an indirect effect) of toxicity; that is, wherever there is toxic exposure, there are changes in gene expression in affected cells (e.g., Nuwaysir et al., 1999). Molecular signatures—changes in gene expression characteristic of particular agents—promise insight into the mode of action of particular toxins, which in turn will help create a molecular taxonomy of classes of toxins by mode of action (Newton, Aardema, and Aubrecht, 2004) and potentially of subpopulations by toxic response profile.

Risk Characterization

Proponents of toxicogenomics hold that microarray technology will reduce the uncertainty of regulatory decisions by providing detailed information on hazard identification and facilitating the measurement of exposure needed for risk assessment and policy. Some are also hopeful that toxicogenomics will lead to more precise predictions of an individual's risk (Smith, 2001; but see Cohen, 2004). Through the use of molecular signatures of toxicity, toxicogenomics may help to evaluate the effects of exposure to chemical mixtures and the effects of low doses, as well as providing a handle for assessing causation even in the presence of a temporal lag between exposure and phenotypic manifestation— issues that have largely confounded toxicologists to date (Marchant, 2003a; Monosson, 2005). Many observers also hope that microarray technologies will improve the ability to extrapolate from laboratory studies of animal models to human populations "in the wild," while also reducing the sheer numbers of animals required for toxicological assessment. Finally, microarray technology may help to resolve issues of differential sensitivity between populations, such as between adults and children.

Why Not?

Despite the enormous benefits of the potential applications of toxicogenomics in these domains, important challenges remain. This is to be expected: revolutions are, after all, generally bloody affairs.

Some of the challenges facing toxicogenomics are empirical, technical, or logistical. They include developing standardized platforms for microarray analysis (especially to reduce interlaboratory variability), developing and refining statistical techniques for data reduction and conventions for data representation, and enhancing communication among industry, academia, and government in a highly charged (and highly intellectually proprietary) environment (see, for instance, Hamadeh et al., 2001; Schaffner, 2002; Marchant, 2003a; Hackl et al., 2004; Hardiman, 2004; Irwin et al., 2004; Newton, Aardema, and Aubrecht, 2004; Olden, 2004; Pettit, 2004; Shoida, 2004; Grant and Zhang, 2005). But even as these problems may be resolved technically, there may not be enough conceptual ground underfoot of toxicogenomics for the field to deliver on the promises summarized in Table 13.1.

As is evident from the previous section, developing molecular signatures and biomarkers of exposure and effect is at the heart of the potential applications of toxicogenomics. Although toxicogenomics may contribute to a more precise understanding of mechanisms of toxicity at a molecular level, important questions remain regarding the accuracy and validity of the molecular signatures. Orphanides (2003, p. 147) observes that "the increase in the rate at which gene expression data can be generated has not been accompanied by corresponding advances in our ability to interpret them as biologically meaningful information." Similarly, a number of scientists (Smith, 2001; Marchant, 2003a; Olden, 2004) have raised concerns about the need to assess the validity of measures of toxicity based on observations of genetic response, or else their use will be premature. As Schulte (2005) well underscored, establishing the validity of biomarkers is resource-intensive, comprising both a laboratory and a population component, and successful validation will require dynamic interplay between laboratory and population studies.

A cautionary tale from stem cell biology may help to clarify the issue. Attempts to identify the molecular signature of stem cells—the fingerprint of "stemness," or that feature of stem cells that creates their pluripotency and capacity for self-renewal—have to date proven relatively fruitless (see Robert, 2004a). Two studies published in the same issue of *Science* in 2002 proclaimed to have uncovered stemness (Ivanova et al., 2002; Ramalho-Santos et al., 2002). But when the results were compared with each other, and with the results of yet another study attempting to uncover stemness, only one gene was found to be common to all three gene expression profiles (Fortunel et al., 2003)! A number of explanations were proffered, including both technical issues (differences in gene chip technology) and conceptual issues (differences in functional or phenotypic criteria for characterizing stem cells; Ivanova et al., 2003), though many confounders may have been at play (Robert, 2004a). More recent efforts have proven marginally more successful (Sato et al., 2003; Abeyta et al., 2004; Rao et al., 2004), but as yet there is no validated molecular characterization of stem cells. Rather than unique molecular "types," variability is the norm; as for stem cells, so too for genomes. Thus, despite the "microarray stampede" (Pennisi, 2002, p. 1986), microarray technology may not be a panacea.

Let us imagine that the molecular signatures are perfectly validated, the issues of interlaboratory inconsistency are resolved, and the statistical and analytical techniques are perfected. In such a hypothetical world, although we would be farther along than we are now (which may be, but is not necessarily, better than nothing), we would still not have a global picture of toxicity or of the gene-environment interactions that putatively comprise environmentally induced disease. Rather, we would have part of the story of the correlation between changes in gene expression and the presence of environmental agents. But even if these gene expression changes are characteristic (in fact, even if they are demonstrably causally related to exposure), we cannot forget that differential gene expression is only one component of development, disordered or otherwise (Robert, 2003, 2004b). After all, genes do not themselves interact with exogenous environments—bodies do. Bodies are material, dynamic, historical, organic, phenomenal, and are not easily reduced to dots on a slide (cf. Krieger, 2005).

Nancy Krieger articulated the construct and process of embodiment and argued that it is essential to epidemiological inquiry. We extend her insight to toxicology in the era of genetics and genomics. Her starting point is that "our living bodies tell stories about our lives."

> Consider only: food insecurity and fast food profiteering; inadequate sanitation and lack of potable water; economic and social deprivation and discrimination; physical and sexual abuse; ergonomic strain and toxic exposures; and inadequate health care—all leave their marks on the body. As do their converse: the security of a living wage, pensions for old age, and societal support for childcare; universal sanitation and sustainable development; safe workplaces and healthy cities; universal health care and immunizations; and the protection and promotion of human rights— economic, social, political, civil, and cultural. (Krieger, 2005, p. 350)

The notion of embodiment offers hope for making good on at least some of the promises of toxicogenomics. For toxicogenomics to be as scientifically rigorous and as useful for regulatory purposes as it can be, it must be fully embodied, ensconced within organic development and evolution, social and political ecology, person and culture. A molecular signature, to be true to the metaphor, will be a unique manifestation, reflecting different subtleties of the exposed individual's lived experience. These should not be abstracted away in favor of bright lights and beautiful numbers, for that is to miss the forest for the matrices.

Some Conceptual Dimensions of Toxicogenomics

Filling in the gaps in the pathway from exposure to disease development (whether clinical or subclinical) may be interesting from the perspective that it assists us in understanding the mechanisms of toxicity and the precursors to disease development. But, as this evidence is at the molecular level, inferences will still have to be made from particular instances of subcellular activity to other cells to the organism as a whole. The validation of any particular molecular signature requires an examination of many inferential relationships: between exposure and absorbed exposure, absorbed exposure and gene expression, gene expression and physiological changes, and physiological changes and disease. Thus, the development of molecular signatures not only will require extensive efforts in toxicogenomics but also will depend on the expertise of epidemiologists and physiologists (among others), as well as the quality of data contained in a wide variety of biobanks. Hence lies the complexity (both with respect to resources and analysis) of the task of validating molecular signatures. All this for an endeavor that from the perspective of philosophy of science is possibly logically unfeasible, due to untenable assumptions about the nature of genomes, exposures, and gene-environment interactions. We will evaluate each in turn.

Assumptions about the Genome

The attempt to build a molecular taxonomy of environmentally induced human disease relies on the assumption that there is homogeneity of genomic responses to an exposure to a particular chemical. There are good philosophical and scientific grounds for suspecting that this is an inaccurate assumption. First, gene expression is tissue-specific—changes in gene expression in one cell or sample of cells may not be representative of changes in other cells or cell types. We thus cannot make inferences to all cells from changes in gene expression in sampled cells (typically, easily accessible cells such as skin or blood cells). Also, gene expression is exquisitely sensitive to a wide variety of factors, including temperature, diet, menstrual cycle, hydration, infection, and injury (see Shoida, 2004, p. 24, figure 2), such that identifying meaningful changes may prove difficult. Some commentators assume that this is a matter of separating the "noise" from "biologically significant cellular responses to toxic exposures" (Marchant, 2003a, p. 10090). But to take embodiment seriously, this assumption must be called into question. In addition, researchers conducting even well-controlled microarray experiments will have difficulty separating generic from toxin-specific changes in gene expression (Marchant, 2003a).

Second, evidence is accumulating that genetic material can be altered as a result of environmental exposures. Prenatal exposure to polycyclic aromatic hydrocarbons has been found to increase the likelihood of chromosomal damage in newborns (Bocskay et al., 2005; see also Perera et al., 2004). Other research suggests that air pollution has the potential for producing heritable genetic mutations (Somers et al., 2002, 2004). These data suggest that the assumption of the uniformity of the genome and of genomic responses throughout an individual's life is not well founded. Rather than being ahistorical, abstract, immutable "blueprints for development," genomes are themselves historically and context dependent (Robert, 2004b).

Assumptions about Exposure

How representative of human exposure is the introduction of a chemical in a microarray experiment? Exposure measurement is one of the most unexplored facets of environmental health research but certainly not due to its importance. A growing number of scientists (Potter, 2003; Vineis, 2004) acknowledge that it is imperative that measures that accurately capture human exposure be developed. Some of the challenges in accurately measuring exposure arise from the nature of exposure itself; that is, the multiple dimensions of exposure add complexity—such as temporal issues (latency between exposure and disease, differences in exposure over the life course), multiple exposures and chemical mixtures, low-level and chronic exposures, not to mention the pathway of exposure. Thus, the measurement of exposure itself involves normative decisions—health researchers must consciously select which aspects of exposure are relevant for a particular investigation. While toxicogenomics promises to help resolve these challenges through the development of more precise molecular measures, this may be wishful thinking. What is just as likely is that toxicogenomics will develop precise molecular measures of exposures of a specific type (laboratory) and thus not capture the variation that is characteristic of humans and human exposures to toxins.

Moreover, because we health researchers are so bad at measuring exposure (in individuals and populations), any variation that is seen may be inferred as genetic in etiology. As Paolo Vineis (2004) argued, there exists an asymmetry in the accuracy of classifying genotype and environmental exposure, meaning that measurement error of exposure assessment is much greater than that of genetic variants. In statistical terms, this means only genetic effects will be significant—one manifestation of the problem of relying solely on statistics and not philosophy for drawing causal conclusions. Indeed, it amounts to a "self-fulfilling prophecy" in gene-environment interaction research (Vineis, 2004, p. 945) where genes are privileged not only statistically but also ontogenetically and ontologically.

Assumptions about Gene-Environment Interactions

The current focus on molecular signatures risks assuming a linear dose-response relationship, which has been the backbone of toxicology from its inception. In principle, the greater the dose, the more severe the response. As incorporated in toxicogenomics, this logic is best expressed by Waters, Selkirk, and Olden (2003, p. 417): "As exposure to the stressor or agent is increased in time or dose, toxicity or cellular injury will become progressively obvious and various adaptive functions will be expressed. The use of microarrays should thus provide the opportunity to search for signal pathways of toxic injury." Although the assumption of a linear dose-response relationship has often been appropriate in toxicology, there are exceptions to the rule. Most notable among these exceptions is the class of chemicals that acts to disrupt the endocrine system. The effects of these endocrine disruptors can be observed across a range of doses, but large effects may be associated with small doses during particular developmental windows, while large doses during other developmental periods may have negligible effects on ontogeny (Schettler et al., 1999; Melnick et al., 2002; Welshons et al., 2003).

In addition, gene-environment interactions remain sorely undertheorized (as argued, for instance, by Robert, 2000, and as evidenced in Shostak, 2003). While it seems that toxicogenomics researchers acknowledge the complex interplay of multiple factors in disease etiology, to assume that gene-environment interactions are either linear or additive is to ignore the complex, nuanced, systemic, and dynamic nature of development (Levins and Lopez, 1999; Robert, 2004b) and embodiment (Krieger, 2005).

These conceptual assumptions are scientifically interesting and important. But they also have interesting and important social and ethical di-

mensions. To make a conceptual assumption is to make a choice, however unconscious. And choices—in science as elsewhere—demand normative scrutiny.

Some Normative Dimensions of Toxicogenomics

The emphasis on molecular signatures is both a strength and a limitation of toxicogenomics. If molecular signatures are well validated and
appropriately used, they may indeed prove helpful in hazard identification and risk assessment. But that's a big "if." And as long as we understand hazard identification and risk assessment as themselves having
normative and not only technical aspects, what to do with even well-
validated molecular signatures is not entirely straightforward. Recall that
genomic analysis of toxins and their effects is a choice. And not only is
it not forced on us by nature, it is also a moral choice.

Costs and Opportunity Costs

The normative dimensions of toxicogenomics include the assessment
of the cost and the opportunity costs of toxicogenomics, especially in relation to promised health outcomes, and the evaluation of strategies for
conceiving of (and altering) social arrangements in relation to biological
realities. Opportunity costs are often understood retrospectively: money
spent on one thing (say, health care) is money that, *ceteris paribus* (all
else being equal), might otherwise have been spent on something else
(say, education). The *ceteris paribus* clause bears a lot of weight here, for
all else is virtually never equal, and so critics of such retrospective opportunity costs arguments will object that *not* spending money on health
care does not imply that the money saved would have been spent on education. So be it. But let us introduce two twists.

First, opportunity costs may carry on into the future; they may thus be
understood prospectively. This means that spending money on one thing
may in fact rule out spending money on something else in future possibly
because there won't be any money left, or because the initial commitment
of funds channeled attention in one direction rather than other (e.g., investment in high-tech diagnostic equipment might funnel attention toward
acute care rather than prevention; investment in gene sequencers might
funnel attention toward genomes rather than higher levels of organization

and analysis). Second, opportunity costs need not be understood as economic costs; opportunity costs may be practical or epistemic, for instance. Practically: building a city around cars severely undermines alternative forms of transportation—being a pedestrian, riding a bicycle, and building a mass transit system each become considerably more difficult under the regime of road traffic, even if driving a car is less efficient than the alternatives (e.g., Illich, 1978). Epistemically: characterizing a disease as a genetic disease may result in, as a prospective opportunity cost, the delegitimization of alternative characterizations of the disease, alternative etiologies, and even alternative modes of treatment—even if the disease is clearly multifactorial or has nongenetic forms.

Toxicogenomics may have opportunity costs of all sorts. For instance, microarrays are expensive, at least at present. So, at least in the short term, money spent on microarrays (on the challenge of validating biomarkers, for example) is money that is not being spent on more conventional means of monitoring and surveillance. Toxicogenomics may eventually delegitimize the more conventional methods, even if the challenge of validation is not adequately met, such that conventional methods, with all their limitations, are replaced by the techniques of toxicogenomics, with all their limitations. Whether this is a good trade-off is simply not clear. Further, toxicogenomics reduces complex relationships between human bodies and our habitats to interactions between genes and environments. This not only ignores the many facets of human embodiment that constitute us as biological and social creatures and that comprise our prospects for health and illness, it may also prohibit or interfere with attempts to understand and intervene at higher levels of analysis. So, for instance, characterizing some instance of toxicity as an interaction between a toxin and exposure to some specific genotypes may result in ignoring aspects of that toxin's toxicity that are independent of genetic variation and perhaps dependent on other dimensions of exposure. Accordingly, we may choose to regulate the toxin on the basis of its biomarker in relation to a particular population without regard to its actual health effects more broadly or over time. These are all choices with normative dimensions.

Toxicogenomics and Human Health

Beyond the question of opportunity costs, whether toxicogenomics actually will improve human health depends both on how well the risk factors for human disease and disability are tracked by genomics data and on what sorts of social and political responses the data inform.

By focusing on the gene-environment interactions implicated in disease development, toxicogenomics risks ignoring the population-level factors that account for why some people get sick and others do not. Generally speaking, the incorporation of genetic factors into an analysis of etiology is associated with the locating of causes within individuals (Lewontin, Rose, and Kamin, 1985; Hubbard, 1995). While this is very useful in an endeavor such as hazard identification, it is less helpful in risk assessment more generally, as it ignores the interindividual variation of the hazard–exposure–disease relationship. At the very least then, toxicogenomics must be integrated with toxicogenetics.

But it is not clear that the genetic level is the most appropriate level at which to understand the relationships between humans and environmental toxins (Robert and Smith, 2004). And although data about gene expression, and even about gene-environment interactions, may help to identify those subpopulations at greatest genetic risk, there is more to risk than genetic risk. For genetic vulnerability means nothing in the absence of the toxins to which we exhibit vulnerability. And measurement of slightly (or even moderately) elevated genetic vulnerability in the presence of chemicals that are harmful as such, even to those at normal risk, is foolhardy at best.

Given these limitations of toxicogenomic data, we might be faced with odd political choices, including the prospect of regulating on the basis of precision in the absence of accuracy (if the molecular signatures are not properly validated) or in the absence of other relevant data (such as data about the nature of toxic exposure, incidence of disease, prevalence of toxins, or prevalence of exposure). Let us imagine, however, that we have the luxury of both precision and accuracy, and the further luxury of all the quantitative data we could ever want about the geographic distribution of toxins: who is exposed, how they are exposed, and how often; how the exposure manifests phenotypically; and how the phenotypic manifestation significantly impedes social progress. Even with all those data at hand—none of which we have at present and few of which are widely held to be within the domain of toxicogenomics and toxicogenetics—the tasks of risk assessment and risk management would not be any more tractable than they are at present. We cannot pretend that more data are what we need. This is because the tasks of risk assessment and risk management are not strictly empirical tasks but are also political ones.

So in addition to generating a wealth of data, we will need to cultivate the social will to improve health outcomes; science alone won't do the trick, though it should help. Of course, this consideration is not unique to toxicogenomics, but that it is relevant across the board suggests the need to attend to it. Toxicogenomics, like all "-omics" sciences, is presented as a solution to life's many woes. Such presentations of science more generally are familiar, from Vannevar Bush's *Science: The Endless Frontier* onward (see Bush, 1945; and also the excellent discussion in Sarewitz, 2000). Science, we are told, will lead to technological control of nature to benefit all humankind, and we are encouraged to imagine a linear process from scientific research to social return. But there is no such "pipeline" (Branscomb and Florida, 1998)—the relationship between scientific research and beneficial social outcomes is anything but linear. The power of toxicogenomics will be limited by social and political factors far beyond the reach of science; to pretend otherwise is a mistake, however common it may be.

Conclusion

While "everybody knows" that there is more to biology, and so more to development, than the contributions of genes, this apparently common knowledge is bracketed or set aside, typically for heuristic reasons, in the pursuit of genetic explanations (Robert, 2003, 2004b). While perhaps occasionally justified (Schaffner, 1998), the bracketing of development has resulted in inappropriate inferences about causality on the basis of statistical correlations (the *locus classicus* of this critique is Lewontin, 1974), which in turn has led to the use of gene maps to plot out an often nongenic terrain (Lippman, 1992, offers such a criticism; see also Pollack, 2002). We have thus wandered off on a fantastical journey, blinkered and beset by genetic myopia (whether itself genetically caused is unclear!), in search of gene-based explanations, tools, techniques, and interventions for every aspect of organismal life. Sometimes we find them, and more power to us. Too often, however, our never-ending quest yields little along the way, and in fact distracts us from more appropriate, more important, more productive journeys beyond the edges and beneath the surface of what gene maps plot out for us.

Our story here is not antigene. Genes (however construed) are clearly useful in tracking evolutionary and coevolutionary history, transmitting developmental resources from generation to generation, and fashioning bodies and brains anew in each generation. But genes are not supremely powerful, whether methodologically or ontogenetically, and focusing only or primarily on genes comes at a price; in the case of environmental health research, this price may be negotiable with respect to human health—a price perhaps not worth paying (Robert and Smith, 2004).

Accordingly, and against the backdrop of the considerable optimism evidenced throughout this collection, we set off a warning flare. We worry that toxicogenomics offers false hope that technology can resolve the problems of toxicology and environmental health, and that it takes as its starting point the misrepresentation of the problems facing environmental health research as being merely technical. As we've shown, toxicogenomics is unable to account for contextual dimensions of hazard–exposure–disease relationships, a context that is crucial for the accurate identification of risk. Should toxicogenomics take seriously the conceptual challenges elucidated here, in addition to the numerous technical challenges it faces, we believe that it may provide interesting and useful observations of gene-environment interactions. But even then, what is done with these observations is a normative and political matter—not a technical one. Toxic identification and toxic regulation are deeply moral issues, grounded not only in good science but also in the social negotiation of acceptable and unacceptable levels of risk and the political determination of how to achieve improvements in health at both individual and population levels.

ACKNOWLEDGMENTS

We are grateful to Gary Marchant and Sandy Askland for the invitation to present some of this research at a workshop at the Arizona State University College of Law in January 2005 and to Rich Sharp and Paul Schulte for critical discussion of our project. We also thank the Novel Tech Ethics Research Team (www.noveltechethics.ca) for intellectual stimulation and support. Initial research assistance for this work was provided through a Bioethics Grant-in-Aid to JSR from Associated Medical Services, Inc., in 2001; more recently, our work has been supported through grants to JSR from the Canadian Institutes of Health Research (CIHR). The writing and revision of this chapter were financially supported by the School of Life Sciences and the Center for Biology and Society at Arizona State University, and the CIHR Institute of Population and Public Health.

REFERENCES

Abeyta, M.J., A.T Clark, R.T. Rodriguez, M.S. Bodnar, R.A. Pera, and M.T. Firpo. 2004. Unique gene expression signatures of independently-derived human embryonic stem cell lines. *Human Molecular Genetics* 13:601–8.

Beatty, J. 2000. Origins of the U.S. Human Genome Project: Changing relationships between genetics and national security. In *Controlling our destinies: The Human Genome Project from historical, philosophical, social and ethical perspectives,* edited by P.R. Sloan, 131–53. Notre Dame: University of Notre Dame Press.

Bishop, W.E., D.P. Clarke, and C.C. Travis. 2001. Genomics in risk assessment. *Risk Analysis* 21:983–87.

Bocskay, K.A., D. Tang, M.A. Orjuela, X. Liu, D.P. Warburton, and F.P. Perera. 2005. Chromosomal aberrations in cord blood are associated with prenatal exposure to carcinogenic polycyclic aromatic hydrocarbons. *Cancer Epidemiology, Biomarkers and Prevention* 14:506–11.

Branscomb, L.M., and R. Florida. 1998. Challenges to technology policy in a changing world economy. In *Investing in Innovation,* edited by L.M. Branscomb and J.H. Keller, 3–39. Cambridge, MA: MIT Press.

Bucher, J.R., and C. Portier. 2004. Human carcinogenic risk evaluation, Part V: The National Toxicology Program vision for assessing the human carcinogenic hazard of chemicals. *Toxicological Science* 82:363–36.

Bush, V. 1945. *Science: The endless frontier.* Washington, DC: U.S. Government Printing Office.

Choudhuri, S. 2004. Microarrays in biology and medicine. *Journal of Biochemistry and Molecular Toxicology* 18:171–79.

Christiani, D.C., R.R. Sharp, G.W. Collman, and W.A. Suk. 2001. Applying genomic technologies in environmental health research: Challenges and opportunities. *Journal of Occupational and Environmental Medicine* 43:526–33.

Cohen, S.M. 2004. Risk assessment in the genomic era. *Toxicologic Pathology* 32 Supple. 1:3–8.

Collins, F.S., E.D. Green, A.E. Guttmacher, and M.S. Guyer. 2003. A vision for the future of genomics research: A blueprint for the genomic era. *Nature* 422:835–47.

Fortunel, N.O., H.H. Otu, H. Ng, et al. 2003. Comment on "'Stemness': Transcriptional profiling of embryonic and adult stem cells" and "A stem cell molecular signature." *Science* 302:393.

Goodman, J.I. 1994. A rational approach to risk assessment requires the use of biological information: An analysis of the National Toxicology Program (NTP), final report of the Advisory Review by the NTP Board of Scientific Counselors. *Regulatory Toxicology and Pharmacology* 19:51–59.

Grant, T.W., and S. Zhang. 2005. In pursuit of effective toxicogenomics. *Mutation Research* 575:4–16.

Hackl, H., F.S. Cabo, A. Sturn, O. Wolkenhauer, and Z. Trajanoski. 2004. Analysis of DNA microarray data. *Current Topics in Medicinal Chemistry* 4:1357–70.

Hamadeh, H.K., P. Bushel, R. Paules, and C.A. Afshari. 2001. Discovery in toxicology: mediation by gene expression array technology. *Journal of Biochemistry and Molecular Toxicology* 15:231–42.

Hardiman, G. 2004. Microarray platforms—Comparisons and contrasts. *Pharmacogenomics* 5:487–502.

Hattis, D., and S. Swedis. 2001. Uses of biomarkers for genetic susceptibility and exposure in the regulatory context. *Jurimetrics* 41:177–94.

Henry, C.J. 2003. Evolution of toxicology for risk assessment. *International Journal of Toxicology* 22:3–7.

Hubbard, R. 1995. *Profitable promises: Essays on women, science, and health.* Monroe, ME: Common Courage Press.

Illich, I. 1978. *Toward a history of needs.* Berkeley: Heyday.

Irwin, R.D., G.A. Boorman, M.L. Cunningham, A.N. Heinloth, D.E. Malarkey, and R.S. Paules. 2004. Application of toxicogenomics to toxicology: Basic concepts in the analysis of microarray data. *Toxicologic Pathology* 32 Supplement 1:72–83.

Ivanova, N.B., J.T. Dimos, C. Schaniel, et al. 2002. A stem cell molecular signature. *Science* 298:601–4.

Ivanova, N.B., J.T. Dimos, C. Schaniel, et al. 2003. Response to comments on "'Stemness': Transcriptional profiling of embryonic and adult stem cells" and "A stem cell molecular signature." *Science* 302:393.

Knight, J. 2001. When the chips are down. *Nature* 410:860–61.

Krieger, N. 2005. Embodiment: A conceptual glossary for epidemiology. *Journal of Epidemiology and Community Health* 59:350–55.

Lander, E.S. 1999. Array of hope. *Nature Genetics* 21 Supple. 1:3–4.

Lemarchand, K., L. Masson, and R. Brousseau. 2004. Molecular biology and DNA microarray technology for microbial quality monitoring of water. *Critical Reviews in Microbiology* 30:145–72.

Levins, R., and C. Lopez. 1999. Toward an ecosocial view of health. *International Journal of Health Services* 29:261–93.

Lewontin, R.C. 1974. The analysis of variance and the analysis of causes. *American Journal of Human Genetics* 26:400–411.

Lewontin, R.C., S. Rose, and L.J. Kamin. 1985. *Not in our genes: Biology, ideology, and human nature.* New York: Pantheon Books.

Lippman, A. 1992. Led (astray) by genetic maps: The cartography of the human genome and health care. *Social Science and Medicine* 35:1469–76.

Ludwig, J.A., and J.N. Weinstein. 2005. Biomarkers in cancer staging, prognosis and treatment selection. *Nature Reviews Cancer* 5:845–56.

Maienschein, J. 2003. *Whose view of life? Embryos, cloning, and stem cells.* Cambridge, MA: Harvard University Press.

Marchant, G.E. 2003a. Genomics and toxic substances: Part I—Toxicogenomics. *Environmental Law Reporter* 33:10071–93.

Marchant, G.E. 2003b. Genomics and toxic substances: Part II—Toxicogenetics. *Environmental Law Reporter* 33:10641–67.

Melnick, R., G. Lucier, M. Wolfe, et al. 2002. Summary of the National Toxicology Program's report of the endocrine disruptors low-dose peer review. *Environmental Health Perspectives* 110:427–31.

Miller, F.A., M.E. Begbie, M. Giacomini, C. Ahern, and E. Harvey. 2006. Re-defining disease: The nosological implications of molecular genetic knowledge. *Perspectives in Biology and Medicine* 49:99–114.

Monosson, E. 2005. Chemical mixtures: Considering the evolution of toxicology and chemical assessment. *Environmental Health Perspectives* 113:383–90.

National Toxicology Program. 2005. Current directions and evolving strategies, http://ntp.niehs.nih.gov/files/CurrentDirections2005.pdf

Newton, R.K., M. Aardema, and J. Aubrecht. 2004. The utility of DNA microarrays for characterizing genotoxicity. *Environmental Health Perspectives* 112:420–22.

Nuwaysir, E.F., M. Bittner, J. Trent, J.C. Barrett, and C.A. Afshari. 1999. Microarrays and toxicology: The advent of toxicogenomics. *Molecular Carcinogenesis* 24:153–59.

Olden, K. 2004. Genomics in environmental health research: Opportunities and challenges. *Toxicology* 198:19–24.

Olden, K., and S.H. Wilson. 2000. Environmental health and genomics: Visions and implications. *Nature Reviews Genetics* 1:149–53.

Orphanides, G. 2003. Toxicogenomics: Challenges and opportunities. *Toxicological Letters* 140–141:145–48.

Pandey, A., and M. Mann. 2000. Proteomics to study genes and genomes. *Nature* 405:837–46.

Pennisi, E. 2002. Recharged field's rallying cry: Gene chips for all organisms. *Science* 297:1985–87.

Perera, F.P., D. Tang, Y. Tu, L.A. Cruz, M. Borjas, T. Bernert, and R.M. Whyatt. 2004. Biomarkers in maternal and newborn blood indicate heightened fetal susceptibility to procarcinogenic DNA damage. *Environmental Health Perspectives* 112:1133–36.

Pettit, S.D., 2004. Toxicogenomics in risk assessment: Communicating the challenges. *Environmental Health Perspectives* 112:A662.

Phelps, T.J., A.V. Palumbo, and A.S. Beliaev. 2002. Metabolomics and microarrays for improved understanding of phenotypic characteristics controlled by both genomics and environmental constraints. *Current Opinion in Biotechnology* 13:20–24.

Pollack, R. 2002. Gene maps lead medicine down the wrong road. *Perspectives in Biology and Medicine* 45:43–45.

Potter, J.D. 2003. Epidemiology, cancer genetics and microarrays: Making correct inferences, using appropriate designs. *Trends in Genetics* 19:690–95.

Ramalho-Santos, M., S. Yoon, Y. Matsuzaki, R.C. Mulligan, and D.A. Melton. 2002. "Stemness": Transcriptional profiling of embryonic and adult stem cells. *Science* 298:597–600.

Rao, R.R., J.D. Calhoun, X. Qin, R. Reyeka, J.K. Clark, and S.L. Stice. 2004. Comparative transcriptional profiling of two human embryonic stem cell lines. *Biotechnology and Bioengineering* 88:273–86.

Robert, J.S. 2000. Schizophrenia epigenesis? *Theoretical Medicine and Bioethics* 21:191–215.

Robert, J.S. 2003. Constant factors and hedgeless hedges: On heuristics and biases in developmental biology. *Philosophy of Science* 70:975–88.

Robert, J.S. 2004a. Model systems in stem cell Biology. *BioEssays* 26:1005–12.

Robert, J.S. 2004b. *Embryology, epigenesis, and evolution: Taking development seriously.* New York: Cambridge University Press.

Robert, J.S., and A. Smith. 2004. Toxic ethics: Environmental genomics and the health of populations. *Bioethics* 18:493–514.

Sarewitz, D. 2000. Human well-being and federal science—What's the connection? In *Science, technology and democracy,* ed. D.L. Kleinman, 87–102. Albany: SUNY Press.

Sato, N., I.M. Sanjuan, M. Heke, M. Uchida, F. Naef, and A.H. Brivanlou. 2003. Molecular signature of human embryonic stem cells and its comparison with the mouse. *Developmental Biology* 260:404–13.

Schaffner, K.F. 1998. Genes, behavior, and developmental emergentism: One process, indivisible? *Philosophy of Science* 65:209–52.

Schaffner, K.F. 2002. Reductionism, complexity and molecular medicine: Genetic chips and the 'globalization' of the genome. In *Promises and limits of reductionism in the biomedical sciences,* ed. M.H.V. Van Regenmortel, and D.L. Hull, 323–51. New York: Wiley.

Schettler, T., G. Solomon, M. Valenti, and A. Huddle. 1999. *Generations at risk: Reproductive health and the environment.* Cambridge MA: MIT Press.

Schulte, P.A. 2005. The use of biomarkers in surveillance, medical screening, and intervention. *Mutation Research* 592:155–63.

Shoida, T. 2004. Application of DNA microarray to toxicological research. *Journal of Environmental Pathology, Toxicology and Oncology* 23:13–31.

Shostak, S. 2003. Locating gene-environment interaction: At the intersections of genetics and public health. *Social Science and Medicine* 56:2327–42.

Smith, L.L. 2001. Key challenges for toxicologists in the 21st century. *Trends in Pharmacological Sciences* 22:281–85.

Somers, C.M., B.E. McCarry, F. Malek, and J.S. Quinn. 2004. Reduction of particulate air pollution lowers the risk of heritable mutations in mice. *Science* 304:1008–10.

Somers, C.M., C.L. Yauk, P.A. White, C.L.J. Parfett, and J.S. Quinn. 2002. Air pollution induces heritable DNA mutations. *Proceedings of the National Academy of Science USA* 299:15904–7.

Vineis, P. 2004. A Self-fulfilling prophecy: Are we underestimating the role of
the environment in gene-environment interaction research? *International Journal of Epidemiology* 33:945–46.

Waters, M.D., K. Olden, and R.W. Tennant. 2003. Toxicogenomic approaches for
assessing toxicant-related disease. *Mutation Research* 544:415–24.

Waters, M.D., J.K. Selkirk, and K. Olden. 2003. The Impact of New Technologies
on Human Population Studies. *Mutation Research* 544:349–60.

Welshons, W.V., K.A. Thayer, J. Taylor, B.M. Judy, and F.S. von Saal. 2003. Large
effects from small exposures. Part I: Mechanisms for endocrine-disrupting
chemicals with estrogenic activity. *Environmental Health Perspectives*
111:994–1006.

Zhou, J., and D.K. Thompson. 2002. Challenges in applying microarrays to environmental studies. *Current Opinion in Biotechnology* 13:204–7.

CHAPTER 14

Environmental Disease, Biomarkers, and the Precautionary Principle

DAVID B. RESNIK

The commonsense wisdom "an ounce of prevention is worth a pound of cure" provides a basis for a rule for decision making known as the precautionary principle (PP). Scientists, scholars, policy analysts, politicians, and others have invoked the PP as a reason for taking effective action to prevent significant harms from occurring, even when scientific certainty is lacking. The PP has played a role in debates about global warming, environmental regulation, food and drug regulation, genetically modified foods, electric power lines, life extension research, genetic engineering, medicine, and public health (Foster, Vecchia, and Repacholi, 2000; Cranor, 2001; Goklany, 2001; Harris and Holm, 2002; Resnik, 2003, 2004; Engelhardt and Jotterand, 2004; Sandin, 2004; Soule, 2004; Weed, 2004). One of the most influential statements of the PP appeared in the United Nations' Rio Declaration: "To protect the environment, the precautionary principle shall be widely applied by States according to their capabilities. Where there are threats of serious or irreversible damage, lack of full scientific certainty shall not be used as a reason for postponing cost-effective measures to prevent environmental degradation" (United Nations, 1992, p. 10).

Although the PP has a great deal of intuitive appeal, it has generated considerable opposition. Critics have argued that the PP is a vague maxim that is easily manipulated to serve political goals (Bodansky, 1991; Goklany, 2001; Harris and Holm, 2002; Starr, 2003). Critics have also charged that the PP is antiscientific, because people often use the principle to oppose advances in science and technology (Miller, 2001). Proponents of the PP have responded to these objections by carefully defining the principle and showing how it can help guide individual choices and social policies (Foster, Vecchia, and Repacholi, 2000; Cranor, 2001; Resnik, 2003; Sandin, 2004). Proponents have also argued that the PP might support developing advances in science and technology designed to address significant threats to health and safety (Engelhardt and Jotterand, 2004).

This chapter will show how the PP can offer valuable guidance for decisions concerning the use of biomarkers to detect environmentally triggered diseases. To defend this thesis, I first define the PP and then argue that it can be a useful alternative to the risk-assessment paradigm when decision makers do not have enough scientific evidence to conduct sound risk assessments. I then briefly discuss how research in toxicogenetics and toxicogenomics will help scientists develop biomarkers for disease and will apply the PP to using biomarkers to test for environmental diseases.

Defining the Precautionary Principle

The precautionary principle is best understood as a framework for making practical decisions. If the PP is not carefully defined, it can easily become an irrational and risk-aversive doctrine. Three parts of the PP require clarification. The first is epistemological: the PP applies to situations in which one lacks "full scientific certainty." Because science never achieves complete certainty, this phrase should be interpreted as "complete scientific proof or evidence." Scientists prove hypotheses through observation and experimentation. The process of confirmation in science is probabilistic: evidence gathered from observation and experimentation increases or decreases the probability of a hypothesis (Howson and Urbach, 1993). Scientists may decide to accept a hypothesis when its probability increases beyond a specific point, such as .95, or they may decide to reject a hypothesis when its probability falls below a specific point, such as .05. In any case, probability is the coin of the realm in scientific reasoning, and "scientific certainty" is probabilistic knowledge (Haack, 2003).

How should one proceed when one lacks "scientific certainty" (i.e., when one does not have enough evidence to assign a probability to a hypothesis)? Should one respond to every nightmare scenario that one can conceive? Responding to threats that are merely possible would be foolish. It is possible that an alien spaceship will land in my yard and that the aliens will use me in experiments. Even though this threat is possible, I have no evidence that it will happen. Hence, there is no reason for me to respond to this potential threat. One is justified in taking action against a potential threat only when one has some evidence that the threat is plausible or credible (Cranor, 2001; Resnik, 2003). Thus, the PP should address threats that are *plausible.*

How does plausibility differ from probability? A hypothesis is plausible when there is enough evidence in favor of the hypothesis to consider it seriously and subject it to additional testing. A hypothesis is probablistic when there is enough evidence to assign a probability to the hypothesis (Resnik, 2003).[1] Evidence used to demonstrate the plausibility of a hypothesis could come from a variety of sources, such as anecdotes, cases studies, or even causal models. For example, if several people developed heart disease after taking a new drug, the hypothesis that this drug causes heart disease would be plausible. To assign a probability to the hypothesis, additional evidence would be needed from systematic investigations, such as clinical trials, epidemiological studies, or meta-analyses.

The next two parts of the PP that require clarification are practical. A threat should be not only plausible but also *significant.* It would be a waste of time and resources to take precautions against threats that are not significant, even if they are plausible. For example, when I ride my bicycle, a gnat might hit me in the face. But there is no reason to take any precaution against this threat, because it will not cause me serious harm, and the harm that it may cause is reversible. The PP should address only threats that can cause serious or permanent harm to individuals, society, or the environment.

Finally, precautionary measures should be *reasonable:* any response to a plausible and significant threat must balance safety against other values, such as utility, efficiency, convenience, cost-effectiveness, fairness, and freedom. For example, having an accident is a plausible and significant threat every time you drive an automobile. One way of avoiding automobile accidents is never to ride in an automobile. But that response to the threat would be highly inefficient and inconvenient. Unless you live within walking distance of all of your needs and desires, it would be unreasonable never to travel by automobile. For most people, the reasonable response to the threat of an automobile accident is to take measures designed to avoid an accident or reduce its impact, such as wearing a seatbelt, not exceeding a safe speed, not driving while tired or under the influence of alcohol, and so on. The reasonableness provision in the PP brings an important normative dimension to the principle, because acting reasonably always involves making trade-offs among different values (Audi, 2001; Resnik, 2004). As we shall see below, the normativeness inherent in the PP has important implications for making decisions about tests for biomarkers.

With these considerations in mind, we can arrive at a clear and precise version of the PP:

> precautionary principle (def.): Reasonable measures should be taken to avoid or mitigate threats that are plausible and significant.

We shall now see why this principle might be a useful guide to individual choices and public policy in some situations.

Precaution and Risk Management

Precaution plays an important role in many governmental regulations and policies that involve the management of risk. Under the risk-management paradigm for decision making, one attempts to control, minimize, or mitigate risks based on information from risk assessment (Shrader-Frechette, 1991; Cranor, 1993). "Risk" can be understood quantitatively as the products of two measures: the probability that some harm will occur and the severity of that harm. Risk assessment involves two steps, both of which depend heavily on scientific evidence: risk identification and risk estimation (Shrader-Frechette, 1991). In risk identification, the risks (or costs) that may occur are identified. For instance, clinical studies of a new drug, call it drug A, might show that it has the potential to cause liver damage, kidney damage, heart disease, headache, nausea, or dizziness. In risk estimation, the probability of these risks (or costs) occurring under specified conditions is estimated. For example, clinical studies may show that the probability of experiencing a headache while taking drug A is .20, while the probability of sustaining liver damage might be only .01.

Governmental agencies in charge of protecting public health use risk management in regulatory decisions. For example, the U.S. Food and Drug Administration (FDA) attempts to manage risks when deciding whether to approve new drugs (Soule, 2004; Hawthorne, 2005). FDA will approve a new drug only if the benefits of the drug outweigh its risks. To make this decision, FDA reviews evidence pertaining to the assessment of the drug's benefits and risks that is submitted by the pharmaceutical company seeking approval of the drug from its clinical trials and animal studies. FDA might also examine evidence pertaining to the drug from studies that are not sponsored by the company. The U.S. Environmental Protection Agency (EPA) uses risk management to make decisions pertaining to the regulation of pesticides, pollutants, carcinogens, and other toxic compounds that can have an adverse effect on human health or the environment (Grodsky, 2005; Marchant, 2003a, 2003b). EPA will approve the use of a pesticide based on an assessment of the pesticide's risks for causing deleterious effects in human populations at a specified exposure level (or reference dose). EPA will approve the use of a pesticide at a given reference dose if the dose is not likely to have an appreciable risk of a harmful effect on the human population, including sensitive subpopulations. To calculate this dose, EPA obtains evidence for the "no observed adverse effect level" in animals. The agency then divides this dose by three tenfold safety factors to allow for interspecies and intraspecies variation. Thus, the acceptable reference dose for the human population is one onethousandth of the no observed adverse effect level dose in animals.

One might argue that the EPA's pesticide registration process also incorporates parts of the PP, because the interspecies and intraspecies safety factors used by the EPA are not based on a scientific analysis of risk but are precautionary measures that the agency has adopted to protect public health (Grodsky, 2005). Because the potential harms to the public of pesticides are clearly plausible and serious, the justification of these safety factors in environmental regulation would be determined by a careful consideration of the different values at stake, such as protection of the public health, efficacy, and costs. The use of a particular safety factor would be justified, according to the PP, if the protection of the public produced by use of the factor is reasonable in relation to the effectiveness of the factor and the costs of using it.

Even if it is different from the PP, risk management can still be considered a precautionary type of reasoning, because it recommends ways to prevent or minimize risks to human health and the environment. Risk management is also a normative approach to decision making, because normative judgments must be made when deciding how to weigh benefits and risks. However, the risk management applies only when there is enough evidence to make a quantitative assessment of the risk's pertaining to a particular decision. Risk management is a formal and quantitative approach to decision making, whereas the PP is an informal and qualitative approach. Risk management involves the estimation of risks, whereas the PP involves only the identification of risks.

Because we often lack enough evidence to apply the risk-management paradigm, the PP can play an important role in individual and social decisions. For example, consider how society should respond to the threat of asteroids. Clearly, this is a plausible threat because we know that asteroids have hit the earth in the past and that they frequently pass near the earth's orbit. The threat is also serious and irreversible. Although scientists have estimated the probability that the earth will be hit by an asteroid in the next one million years, they have continually revised their estimates as they learn more about asteroids. Until we know much more about the thousands of asteroids that could hit the earth and their potential impact on the human population, we cannot assign a definite probability to this hypothesis, which could be used in risk assessment and risk management. However, until we have more evidence, it would still be wise to take precautionary measures such as identifying and tracking asteroids and designing methods for directing them away from a collision course with the earth. Waiting until the evidence is sufficient to define probability and initiate risk assessment and risk management could have disastrous, possibly apocalyptic, consequences. This is the type of scenario put forth by many proponents of the PP in the environmental field.

Toxicogenomics, Biomarkers, and Precaution

Having defined the PP and having shown how it can apply to individual choices and social policy, I can now consider how it may apply to choices that arise from research in toxicogenetics and toxicogenomics. Toxicogenetics and toxicogenomics study genetic predispositions to toxic reactions to environmental agents such as pesticides, industrial chemicals, pollutants, allergens, or radiation. Toxicogenetics focuses on the relationship between genes and toxicity, whereas toxicogenomics focuses on the relationship between the genome and toxicity (Olden and Guthrie, 2001). A toxicogenetic study seeks to identify genes that predispose people to having toxic reactions to environmental agents and to understand how these genes cause adverse health effects that lead to disease. For example, researchers have identified specific genes that cause people to have an increased risk of adverse reactions to air pollution, such as lung inflammation, injury, and dysfunction (Kleeberger, 2003). Toxicogenomic studies examine gene-activation patterns in response to environmental exposures by using assays that test for thousands of genes at one time, such as DNA microarrays or protein chips (Waters, Olden, and Tennant, 2003). These data can be used to compare gene expression patterns and to study the downstream effects of genes on RNA, proteins, metabolites, cells, and tissues. These studies can allow researchers to identify gene expression patterns that increase susceptibility to diseases related to toxic exposures. Toxicogenetics and toxicogenomics will allow scientists to have a better understanding of the relationship between human heredity and environmentally triggered diseases such as cancer, diabetes, emphysema, multiple chemical sensitivity, and liver or kidney toxicity.

Research in toxicogenomics and toxicogenetics will also help scientists develop tests for biomarkers for environmentally triggered diseases. Biomarkers may include gene polymorphisms, gene expression patterns, proteins, metabolites, and other organic compounds that indicate that an individual is likely to develop a disease. Biomarkers are steps on the causal pathways from toxic exposures to disease (Decaprio, 1997). Many environmental diseases result from changes in genes, protein chemistry, metabolism, cells, or tissues that lead to other events in the body and, eventually, to the clinical manifestations of a disease. For example, elevated blood levels of C-reactive protein have been associated with increased risk of developing hypertension and atherosclerosis (Hackman and Anand, 2003; Sesso et al., 2003). Scientists hypothesize that C-reactive protein is a biomarker for inflammation in the body, which is thought to play a role in the development of hypertension and atherosclerosis.

Biomarkers can be categorized based on their place in the disease process: susceptibility biomarkers are markers of susceptibility to disease, exposure biomarkers indicate that an organism has been exposed to a toxic agent, effect biomarkers indicate that exposure to a toxic agent has had some adverse effect on the organism, and preclinical biomarkers indicate changes in the organisms that immediately precede manifestation of the disease (Decaprio, 1997).

The use of biomarkers is an important medical advance, because it enables physicians to detect, treat, or prevent diseases at an early stage. Tests for biomarkers are precautionary measures, because they can help people prevent, avoid, or mitigate serious harms (i.e., diseases). However, many of the biomarkers that scientists have discovered have not been well validated. To be validated, a biomarker must be biologically relevant, sensitive, and specific (Decaprio, 1997). That is, scientists must have a sound understanding of how the biomarker represents a step on the disease pathway, and the test for the biomarker should be accurate and reliable. In addition, there should be treatments available for patients with the biomarker, because it can do a patient more harm than good to tell him that he is developing a disease, or at elevated risk of developing the disease, but that nothing can be done to stop its progression.

It is worth noting that the use of biomarkers to detect diseases at an early stage raises important questions about the definition of "disease," because diseases are usually equated with clinical signs and symptoms. By using biomarkers to test for effects that precede the clinical manifestation of disease, one can begin medical treatment for a disease long before a person appears to be ill. While there are some obvious advantages to beginning therapy before a disease progresses to the clinical stage, there are also some disadvantages to this strategy, including increased use of medical and economic resources, misdiagnosis, blurring of the lines between health and disease, and the potential for discrimination and bias. I will mention these important issues but not explore them in depth here.[2]

Because many biomarkers have not been thoroughly validated, the scientific community will often lack reliable data on the benefits, risks, and costs of using a particular biomarker in clinical medicine or public health. It is in situations like this, where the risk-management paradigm is not sufficient to determine the proper course of action, that the PP can be useful. For example, scientists and physicians do not now know the benefits, risks, and costs of routine testing patients for C-reactive protein

(Hackman and Anand, 2003). C-reactive protein is a biomarker for car-diovascular diseases, but biomedical researchers do not know whether the benefits of testing people for C-reactive protein outweigh risks and costs, at this point in time. Because we do not have a good understand-ing of the benefits versus risks and costs of C-reactive protein testing, we cannot apply risk-management strategies to decisions concerning the use of this test. To apply the PP to C-reactive protein testing, we can assume that the development of cardiovascular disease as a result of inflamma-tion is a plausible and serious threat. But is the use of the C-reactive pro-tein test a reasonable response to this threat? To answer this question, we must determine whether the test is an effective method of preventing or mitigating cardiovascular disease, how much it costs to use the test, whether use of the test could cause unnecessary stress due to mislead-ing results, and whether the test results could encourage discrimination or other social problems.

Those types of question also arise in the use of biomarkers related to environmental diseases. Let's consider some specific testing scenarios.

Susceptibility Biomarkers

Many biomarkers will indicate that individuals are at increased risk of developing specific diseases in response to environmental toxins. In-dividuals with a mutant allele of the ataxia telangiectasia (AT) gene have an increased risk of developing cancer when exposed to ionizing radia-tion. Approximately .001 percent of the U.S. population has this gene. There is a test of the AT gene, but the reliability of the test in cancer screening is not known (Mossman, 1997). People who work at nuclear power plants face an increased risk of exposure to ionizing radiation in the workplace. Suppose that the company operating a nuclear power plant has taken adequate safety measures to protect its workers from ex-posure to radiation, but that the workers will still face radiation expo-sures in the workplace greater than normal, background radiation levels. Should the company screen its workers for radiosensitivity and use that information to make decisions concerning employment or job assign-ments? Should testing be mandatory or optional? Because the AT test has not been well-validated, the risk-management approach does not offer satisfactory answers to these questions. How would the PP approach these issues? The PP would recommend a testing policy that is a reasonable response to a plausible and significant threat. In this situation, the threat posed by the AT gene is significant and plausible, because there is some evidence that the AT gene increases the risk of cancer, especially breast cancer. Thus, the key question related to testing would involve the reasonableness of a testing policy in this context.

To address the reasonableness of a testing policy, one must balance the different values at stake, including (1) the safety and health of workers, (2) the rights of workers, especially the right to privacy and the right to nondiscriminatory treatment in employment, (3) the cost-effectiveness of the test, (4) the company's financial interests, and (5) justice or fairness. A testing policy would be reasonable, one might argue, only if it (1) protects the health of the workers, (2) is cost-effective, (3) promotes the interests of the companies, (4) does not significantly violate the rights of workers, and (5) is fair. If the test is assumed to be cost-effective and can protect the health of 1 percent of workers, then the key questions in applying the PP to this case would be how the testing policy affects the rights of the workers and the fairness of the policy. Although it is not possible to reach firm decisions concerning any particular testing policy without more data, it is possible to see how the PP would structure such decisions.

Researchers have identified—and will identify—many other genes that increase susceptibility to developing cancer, diabetes, asthma, and environmentally triggered diseases. If and when tests are developed to characterize the increased risk of these genes, should they be used to screen children at birth? Currently, most states have adopted genetic screening programs for a small number of genetic diseases, such as phenylketonuria and sickle cell disease (Newborn Screening and Genetics Resource Center, 2005). In most states, these tests are mandatory; in some they are not. The tests range in cost from $70 to $120, and are included in the hospital bill (Kolata, 2005). An expert panel recommended that all states should test for twenty-nine different diseases (Kolata, 2005). Researchers could one day develop DNA chips to test newborns for thousands of different genes that increase chances of developing disease in response to environmental exposures. These rapid advances in genetic screening technologies will lead to difficult public policy dilemmas (Wilcken, 2003). Should states expand their newborn screening programs as more tests become available?

Because these tests will be new, it is likely that many of them will not have been well-validated, and that we therefore will not have enough evidence to assess their benefits and risks. Hence, the risk-management paradigm probably will not offer useful guidance concerning these tests. Could the PP offer some guidance to help resolve these issues?

In applying the PP, one must first address the question of plausibility: is the threat of a newborn with a particular gene developing a particular disease in response to environmental conditions plausible? Let's assume the answer is "yes" to this question, because the test being considered has been developed on the basis of some evidence. Is the threat significant? Again, the answer is likely to be "yes," because the diseases in question would be harmful and perhaps irreversible. Now the most difficult question must be addressed: what would be a reasonable response to the threat? To answer this question, the different values at stake need to be weighed, such as individual and public health, cost-effectiveness, the psychological well-being of children who are tested, rights to nondiscrimination, and fairness. Even if a test promotes individual and public health at a low cost, one might still oppose use of the test in a screening program if there are currently no methods for treating or preventing the disease that the test predicts will occur, if the test adversely affects the psychological well-being of children that receive it (by causing anxiety about the future, for example), if the test is unfair, or if the test will lead to discrimination and bias against a child that tests positive. Thus, the PP would provide a framework that might favor the adoption of a newborn screening test, or it might not, depending on how conflicting values are balanced in light of the available facts.

Exposure Biomarkers

Biomarkers can also be used to determine whether someone has been exposed to a toxic substance. For example, suppose that workers in a factory are exposed to a toxic substance such as lead during their work. To protect workers from excessive exposure to lead, the employer could institute a program of routine testing of levels of lead in the blood. The employer could use these tests to make changes to the work environment to reduce lead exposure or to make personnel changes to protect employees from exposure. Let's assume that there is not enough information about risks and benefits to apply the risk management paradigm to this decision. How would the PP apply in a situation like this?

The first inquiry would be to evaluate the plausibility of the threat. Because exposure to lead can be harmful to adults and is especially harmful to children, the threat is plausible. Lead exposure can cause mental retardation, learning disabilities, slowed growth, and hearing problems in children, and reproductive problems, high blood pressure, digestive problems, nerve disorders, memory and concentration problems, and muscle and joint pain in adults (U.S. Environmental Protection Agency, 2004). Because these harms are serious and in many cases irreversible, the potential harms posed by the lead threat are significant. The remaining inquiry would focus on the reasonableness of assessing lead exposure in the workplace. The values at stake here would include the health of the employees, the cost-effectiveness of monitoring exposures, the financial interests of the company, the rights of the employees (such as the right to privacy), and fairness. Although it would seem that instituting a lead monitoring program would be a reasonable response to the threat of lead exposure, it might not be a reasonable response if the employees face only a small, negligible chance of being exposed to lead in the workplace. Also, lead monitoring would not be reasonable if it involved testing procedures that did not protect the rights of the employees.

Lead monitoring is a relatively easy case for the PP, because the threat of lead poisoning is plausible and significant, and the tests for lead are inexpensive and accurate. More difficult cases would involve the monitoring of exposures to chemicals where the threats are not as plausible or significant, or the tests are expensive or inaccurate. Here again, however, the PP is useful, even when the variables are more complex, because the PP can structure decision making even when full scientific evidence is not available.

Effect Markers

Biomarkers can also be used to show that exposure to a toxic substance has produced an adverse effect in a person. C-reactive protein, as discussed above, is a biomarker that measures an adverse effect—inflammation—that can cause heart disease. Many different biomarkers can be used to demonstrate adverse effects. For example, damage to cells, tissues, or organs would be adverse effects. Other biomarkers of adverse effects include chromosomal aberrations, enzyme induction, enzyme inhibition, activation of oncogenes, and mutations (Decaprio, 1997). Although effect biomarkers can be useful in predicting the development of disease as a result of toxic exposures, scientists still have not validated many of these biomarkers. Often, the effect produced by a toxic exposure is neutral or adaptive, instead of adverse. That is, the measured effect does not accurately predict disease (Decaprio, 1997).

There are many different situations in which it might be useful to measure effect biomarkers to promote individual or public health. For example, an employer might want to use a test to decide whether employees who have been exposed to toxic agents require medical therapy to prevent or slow the progression of a disease. Thus, an employer might use biomarkers to learn whether employees are susceptible to toxic agents, whether they have been exposed to toxic agents, and whether the agents have produced any adverse effects. The same rationale that applies to testing for exposure biomarkers would also apply to testing for effect biomarkers. If we assume that the threat to employees is plausible and significant, then testing for an effect biomarker will depend on the reasonableness of testing, which will be a function of a careful weighing of the different values at stake. Testing would be justified when it promotes the health of employees without violating their rights and is cost-effective. Testing would not be justified if it was not effective or violated employee rights. This is another case in which the PP provides a useful framework for making decisions when relating to the use of biomarkers when there are not sufficient data to apply the risk-management paradigm.

Conclusion

Because many biomarkers have not been thoroughly validated, it will often be difficult to decide whether to use these tests to prevent, minimize, or mitigate health threats to individual or public health. If we have substantial scientific evidence pertaining to the use of a biomarker in a particular context, then we may able to apply the risk-management paradigm to that decision. When we lack enough evidence to assess benefits and risks, the PP may offer useful guidance. According to the version of the PP described in this chapter, we should use a test for a biomarker to avoid, minimize, or mitigate a threat to individual or public health when the threat is plausible and significant and when using the test would be a reasonable response to the threat, given the circumstances. To determine the reasonableness of a particular test, the different values at stake, such as individual and public health, efficacy, cost-effectiveness, individual rights, business interests, and justice, should be carefully weighed and considered. Although it is difficult to anticipate the form such discussions may take, examples such as those presented above, illustrate how the PP can shed light on debates about the use of biomarkers to detect toxic reactions to environmental exposures.

ACKNOWLEDGMENTS

I would like to thank Ernie Hood, Steve Kleeberger, and Richard Sharp for helpful comments. This research was supported by the intramural program of the National Institute for Environmental Health Sciences, National Institutes of Health. It does not represent the views of the National Institute of Environmental Health Sciences or the National Institutes of Health.

NOTES

1. "Probabilistic" is not identical in meaning to "probable." A hypothesis with a low probability (e.g., .10) would still be probabilistic.

2. For further discussion, see Grodsky (2005).

REFERENCES

Audi, R. 2001. *The architecture of reason.* New York: Oxford University Press.

Bodansky, D. 1991. Scientific uncertainty and the precautionary principle. *Environment* 33:4–5, 43–44.

Cranor, C. 1993. *Regulating toxic substances.* New York: Oxford University Press.

Cranor, C. 2001. Learning from law to address uncertainty in the precautionary principle. *Science and Engineering Ethics* 7:313–26.

Decaprio, A. 1997. Biomarkers: Coming of age for environmental health risk assessment. *Environmental Science and Technology* 31:1837–48.

Engelhardt, H., and F. Jotterand. 2004. The precautionary principle: A dialectical reconsideration. *Journal of Medicine and Philosophy* 29:301–12.

Foster, K., P. Vecchia, and M. Repacholi. 2000. Science and the precautionary principle. *Science* 288:979–81.

Goklany, I. 2001. *The precautionary principle: A critical appraisal of environmental risk assessment.* Washington, DC: Cato Institute.

Grodsky, J. 2005. Genetics and environmental law: Redefining public health. *California Law Review* 93:171–270.

Haack, S. 2003. *Defending science within reason.* New York: Prometheus Books.

Hackman, D., and S. Anand. 2003. Emerging risk factors for atherosclerotic vascular disease: A critical review of the evidence. *Journal of the American Medical Association* 290:932–40.

Harris, J., and S. Holm. 2002. Extending human lifespan and the precautionary paradox. *Journal of Medicine and Philosophy* 27:355–68.

Hawthorne, F. 2005. *Inside the FDA.* New York: Wiley.

Howson, C., and P. Urbach. 1993. *Scientific reasoning: The Bayesian approach,* 2nd ed. New York: Open Court.

Kleeberger, S.R. 2003. Genetic aspects of susceptibility to air pollution. *European Respiration Journal* 40:52s–56s.

Kolata, G. 2005. Panel to advise testing babies for 29 diseases. *New York Times* (Feb. 21).

Marchant, G. 2003a. Genomics and toxic substances: Part I—Toxicogenomics. *Environmental Law Report* 33:10071–93.

Marchant, G. 2003. Genomics and toxic substances: Part II—Toxicogenetics. *Environmental Law Report* 33:10641–67.

Miller, H. 2001. Letter to the Editor: The bogus precautionary principle. *Wall Street Journal* (Mar. 1).

Mossman, K. 1997. Radiation protection of radiosensitive populations. *Health Physics* 72:519–23.

Newborn Screening and Genetics Resource Center. 2005. U.S. National Screening Status Report. At http://genes-r-us.uthscsa.edu/nbsdisorders.pdf.

Olden, K., and J. Guthrie. 2001. Genomics: Implications for toxicology. *Mutation Research* 473:3–10.

Resnik, D. 2003. Is the precautionary principle unscientific? *Studies in the History and Philosophy of Biological and Biomedical Sciences* 34:329–44.

Resnik, D. 2004. The precautionary principle and medical decision making. *Journal of Medicine and Philosophy* 29:281–300.

Sandin, P. 2004. *Better safe than sorry: Applying philosophical methods to the debate on risk and the precautionary principle.* Doctoral thesis, Royal Institute of Technology, Stockholm.

Sesso, H., J. Buring, N. Rifai, G.J. Blake, J.M. Gaziano, and P.M. Ridker. 2003. C-reactive protein and the risk of developing hypertension. *Journal of the American Medical Association* 290:2945–51.

Shrader-Frechette, K. 1991. *Risk and rationality.* Berkeley: University of California Press.

Soule, D. 2004. The precautionary principle and the regulation of U.S. food and drug safety. *Journal of Medicine and Philosophy* 29:333–52.

Starr, C. 2003. The precautionary principle versus risk analysis. *Risk Analysis* 23:1–3.

United Nations. 1992. *Agenda 21: The UN Program of Action from Rio.* New York: United Nations.

U.S. Environmental Protection Agency. 2004. Lead, basic information. At www.epa.gov/lead/leadinfo.htm.

Waters, M., K. Olden, and R. Tennant. 2003. Toxicogenomic approach for assessing toxicant-related disease. *Mutation Research* 544:415–24.

Weed, D. 2004. Precaution, prevention, and public health ethics. *Journal of Medicine and Philosophy* 29:313–32.

Wilcken, B. 2003. Ethical issues in newborn screening and the impact of new technologies. *European Journal of Pediatrics* 162:S62–66.

CHAPTER 15

Rights and the Exceptionally Vulnerable

JAMES W. NICKEL

Let's say that the holder of a legal right is exceptionally vulnerable when that person's condition or circumstances make it unusually difficult and expensive to respect or implement his or her right.[1] For example, people who live in neighborhoods with high levels of crime may be exceptionally vulnerable in regard to their right to safety against crime. Claims about exceptional vulnerability are comparative; they say that exceptionally vulnerable people are far more likely than average people to experience the violation, inadequate implementation, or nonimplementation of some right.

Variation in the costs of respecting and upholding people's rights is large. It may cost the government $5,000 a year, for example, to implement an average person's right to health care while costing hundreds of thousands of dollars a year to provide adequate health care to a person with a severe immune deficiency. The high costs of protecting the exceptionally vulnerable are a general problem, not unique to rights to health care or environmental protection. For example, it is often more difficult and expensive to satisfy the right to a fair trial of someone whom most jurors will despise, such as a person accused of killing or molesting a child. And people whose political beliefs are thought to be subversive are often unusually vulnerable to having their expressive and political liberties violated.

Difficulties in dealing with the exceptionally vulnerable might be taken to be a reason to avoid legal rights, particularly ones that require expensive implementation. When officials with limited budgets of human and financial resources have to satisfy the rights of an exceptionally vulnerable claimant, they can respond either with a justice-though-the-heavens-fall rights fanaticism ("We just have to do whatever it takes to satisfy the rights of such people!") or with a cost-based proposal to disregard or limit the claimant's rights ("There's no way we're going to pay *that* much for this person's health care" or protection or criminal trial or safety!). Because expensive rights confront officials with the dilemma of either adopting a budget-ruining rights fanaticism or arbitrarily imposing cost limits on the exceptionally vulnerable, perhaps we should avoid such rights altogether.[2]

Those attracted by this recommendation should consider whether they are willing to abandon all rights that are expensive to implement. Such rights include rights to safety against crime, rights to fair trial, rights to protection against discrimination, rights to health care, and rights to a safe environment. Perhaps I could live with the idea that we should avoid taking a rights approach to environmental safety, but I am extremely reluctant to abandon legal rights to due process of law. Accordingly, this chapter develops a response to this dilemma that points to a third possibility: a conception of rights that makes them neither fanatically devoted to doing everything necessary for the most vulnerable nor mere fancy packaging for what turns out to be cost-benefit decision making. The key to doing this, I think, is to allow those authoring legal rights to take costs into account in shaping contents or scopes while showing that, once rights are established, they impose transformative constraints on how we deliberate about people's needs and demands in the areas they cover.

Taking Costs into Account in Justifying and Shaping Rights

Respecting and implementing rights is far from cost-free. Rights need budgets for human resources and infrastructure, and the costs associated with a right need to be considered as part of its justification. Containing the costs of legal rights is imperative because (1) there are lots of rights to implement, (2) there are other goods of equal or nearly equal priority (e.g., high levels of education, culture, and scientific knowledge) that must be created and sustained, (3) the country's economy needs to be kept running in a sustainable way in order to pay for these rights and goods, and (4) democratic institutions allow citizens to resist further tax increases to pay for more or better rights.

This point applies to the most basic rights as well as to ones that are less fundamental. For example, having due process when charged with a crime is a very basic right. But this right is expensive to implement and hence is limited in the procedures (hearings, trials, appeals), protections (safety during incarceration), services (free legal help), and time for preparation of a defense that it provides. Similarly, the systems of law, police, courts, and prisons that uphold our fundamental rights to safety of life and property against crime have to compete for budget allocations against expenditures for education, the military, health care, and transportation. A very important right may rightly get larger expenditures for its implementation than those devoted to less important rights, but this does not mean that it can commandeer the entire government budget.

Governments often deal with the costs of rights by providing poor quality implementation that is inequitably distributed. If we viewed those governmental protections as insurance policies we would say that (1) they don't cover all risks or threats, (2) they impose large copays in the form of required self-help, and (3) they make collection difficult—people often have no recourse if a government agency refuses to protect them. Systems of legal rights that provide low-quality, inequitably distributed guarantees are legitimately criticized on grounds of fairness or equal protection.

Adequately implemented rights provide fair and reasonable levels of protection against the most common threats. Henry Shue, in *Basic Rights,* suggests that rights only need to deal with "standard and significant" threats. He does not require that rights protect against every small threat: "I am not suggesting the absurd standard that a right has been fulfilled only if it is impossible for someone to be deprived of it, or that no one is ever deprived of it. The standard can only be some reasonable level of guarantee" (Shue, 1996, p. 17). I will follow Shue in suggesting that legal rights need provide only some reasonable level of guarantee to rightholders, even though this is hard on the exceptionally vulnerable. My purpose here, however, is not to defend a particular view of how tight or loose the limits on the scopes of rights should be but, rather, to defend the principle that such limits are permissible and plausible.

Many universal legal rights are need-based. The benefits a citizen can claim under a right often depend on his or her needs. For example, the right to a trial by jury when charged with a crime is need-based. Citizens who are not facing criminal prosecution are not entitled to a trial just because they would like to be the star of a big public event and gets lots of attention. Further, even among people who need a fair trial because they have been charged with a crime, an adequately implemented right to a fair trial may not provide them with everything that is necessary in their particular case to getting a fair trial. An accused person may have special and expensive needs because the witnesses who could testify that he was not present at the scene of the crime are far away or difficult to locate. The judge may in such cases sometimes rightly refuse to order delays in the trial, additional investigations, or large expenditures for bringing witnesses to court.

The legal philosopher Joel Feinberg proposed a useful distinction between *claims-to* benefits and *claims-against* parties to supply those benefits (Feinberg, 1970, p. 256). Feinberg held that the moral or political justification of a right needs to justify both the claims-to and the claims-against. For example, Feinberg held that to justify a legal right to a fair trial when charged with a crime it was necessary to address both the demand side (the claim-to a fair trial) and the supply side (the claim-against government to provide accused persons with trials). The justification of a right to a benefit is not finished when the claim-to is justified, when it has been shown that the benefit is something that people require in order to enjoy a minimally adequate level of dignity, freedom, or welfare. A complete justification for a right must also justify the claim-against; it must show that it is justifiable to impose the burden of guaranteeing the availability of the benefit on some particular party or agency. And this involves showing, among other things, that the party or agency can actually do the job of providing the benefit while meeting its other responsibilities of equal or higher priority.

To justify the claim-against, it is often necessary to limit the scope of the right. This may be necessary to make the right compatible with other rights—as when we qualify the right to privacy to accommodate the fact that in order to satisfy one person's right to a fair trial other people may be required to testify and thereby reveal things about themselves that they would rather keep hidden. Limiting the scope of a right may also be necessary to make it affordable, to avoid imposing excessive or unsustainable burdens on those to whom the claim-against is assigned.

Consider a person of normal vulnerability (Norm) and an exceptionally vulnerable person (Ev), who both have a justified legal right against their government to some important need-based benefit (B). As equal citizens, both Norm and Ev have equal claims to receive B. Because Ev is exceptionally vulnerable, she needs a lot more of B, or protection of B, than Norm does. Variation in the amount of B needed by rightholders is normal, but suppose that Ev needs a huge and enormously expensive amount.

If we succeed in justifying a legal right to some benefit B by showing that having secure access to B is very important to people's survival, freedom, dignity, or basic welfare, this brings strong considerations of fairness into play. Fairness requires more of legislators and citizens when something extremely important is at stake. To be fair they must be impartially rational. This means that they should care as much about Ev's problems as about Norm's and accordingly try to meet all of her needs in the area covered by the right. But other considerations will push back. There are sure to be lots of justified claims-to for legislators and citizens to consider and they have to try to protect the most important ones in sustainable ways in light of available resources and other obligations.

To deal with this, we may put formal or informal limits on how much B a person like Ev can claim. The guarantees of the availability of B may, like private insurance policies, have limits on how much the guarantor is required to provide in a given time period. These limits may cause no problem to Norm, but they cause big problems for Ev. She gets very inadequate protection given her high level of needs and vulnerability. We have reasons of fairness, welfare, and solidarity to do as much for Ev as we reasonably can. But these reasonable levels of provision in light of available resources may not be sufficient to adequately protect Ev's dignity, freedom, welfare, or survival.

Or course, our assumptions about resources and other obligations may be wrong. Perhaps there are additional resources available in the system that haven't been tapped, or perhaps additional resources are just now becoming available. If so, Ev's prospects for greater assistance ought to improve. But let's suppose that the initial assumptions about resources were correct.

If legislators and citizens have proceeded in the way I described and established these conclusions about resources and the scope of universal rights reasonably, fairly, and in good faith, I believe that Ev has no justified complaint against them (although she has plenty of reason to bewail her bad luck). Legislators and citizens have done everything that morality, fairness, and their recognition of Ev's humanity and equal citizenship requires. They have recognized her personhood and proceeded fairly in evaluating claims and budgeting protection and provision.

Are legislators and citizens required to feel regret about the inadequacy of Ev's protection? Yes and no. They should feel regret in the way that we feel regret about the victims of natural disasters. They should feel regret that their resources and competencies do not allow them to adequately provide for Ev, just as one would feel regret about being unable to swim fast enough to rescue a drowning person. But they should not feel regret for having done something wrong because no bad behavior is present.

Shouldn't Ev have some sort of additional remedy available? Not if we meant it when we concluded that the social resources reasonably available did not allow the government to respond fully to Ev's needs. If we're justifiably certain of that, Ev has to hope for charity, solidarity, and love. Society has made reasonable provision for the rights of all.

In the real world, there will be uncertainty about many of the premises that we use to reach justified hard-heartedness. This should incline us to soften our hard-heartedness, but not so much that we bust the budget, forget other important needs, or kill productivity. Governmental agencies and practices are sure to contain injustice and inefficiency. Resources are wasted through corruption and flawed allocative processes. This should also incline us to soften our hard-heartedness and commit us to political action to remedy those injustices. But it does not justify our pretending that those injustices and inefficiencies do not exist or that we can already spend the savings that will be achieved if they are someday abolished.

If you think my approach does too little for the unusually vulnerable, here is a way to strengthen the rights of the unusually vulnerable without making them fanatical. We can say that being unusually vulnerable in some important area, if that has such a severe impact on one's welfare that it plunges one into the category of the worst off (however we define this category), provides a special but limited reason for protection and assistance. For example, perhaps individuals with medical problems so severe that they fall into the category of worst-off citizens should get some supplement to the scope of their right to health care. This supplement may not be enough to get them everything they need, but it gives them an additional bundle. Such bundles will, of course, increase the costs of implementing the right to health care and will require government do less in other areas. Such limits make the scopes of some people's rights larger, but they do not make those scopes unlimited.

The view of legal rights and their justification that I have presented here certainly avoids the branch of the original dilemma that alleged a fanaticism of rights. It does so by recognizing that legal rights, like private insurance policies, can have limits on their scopes. We now turn to the question of whether the other branch of the dilemma can be avoided. Having allowed budgetary considerations to place limits on the scopes of legal rights, have we abandoned rights for simply deciding on grounds of costs and benefits?

Rights and Cost-Benefit Deliberation

If considerations about costs and resources have been used in justifying, defining, and limiting the scope of a right, does that somehow imply that officials using and applying legal rights are really just making allocations on the basis of costs and benefits? I will argue that it does not.

Let's begin with an analogy. An insurance company offers a dental policy that costs $240 a year and covers up to $1,000 a year in dental expenses. It tells prospective purchasers that if they pay $240 they will have, during the following year, a contractual right to the payment by the insurer of up to $1,000 for dental services, specified on a list, when those services are prescribed and provided by a licensed dentist. Norm buys the policy, betting that his dental costs in the next year will exceed $240. His right to dental care under the policy has a limited scope. If the costs of his dental needs in the next year exceed $1,000, he will have to cover the additional costs himself. In deciding whether to enter into the insurance contract, both the insurer and Norm engaged in cost-benefit calculations. But once the contract is operative, the insurer is not permitted to consider whether Norm's benefits from dental work will be sufficiently great to make it worthwhile for the insurer to pay for them. When Norm makes a claim for $175 for a filling that a licensed dentist prescribed and provided, the only issues are whether dental fillings are on the list and whether they were actually prescribed and provided to Norm by a licensed dentist. If Norm's claim is valid under the contract, the insurance company has to pay. If it doesn't, it will violate Norm's right. There may, of course, be borderline claims that have to be mediated or litigated.

This example gives us a picture of how rights typically work. There is some sort of normative structure (in this case an insurance contract) that gives the holder of the right, Norm, a guarantee of certain benefits. The normative structure also gives at least one party (the duty-bearer) duties or responsibilities to provide such a guarantee. These are specified in the scope or content of the right. It describes what the rightholder may claim and what the duty-bearer must provide.

Rights also have some degree of power or weight as moral or legal considerations. Norm's right to dental care under a valid legal contract is not easily overridden by other considerations. The insurance company cannot escape claims by saying that it has decided to give its employees a yearlong vacation or to invest all of its assets immediately in amusement parks. Unless it wants to be sued by its customers, the company cannot decide that because some of its clients under existing contracts don't benefit very much from dental services it is unilaterally refusing to pay the claims of some of them. No doubt it was permissible for the insurance company to enter into cost-benefit deliberations in deciding whether to offer the contract, but once it was in effect the company had to respect the rights the contract established. Following the duties that correspond to Norm's right is very different from using cost-benefit calculations to decide what to do about Norm's demands. Norm's rights have limited scopes, but within those limits they are legally binding and can be expected to guide behavior. Basing decisions about Norm's claims on costs and benefits may lead to violation of the right.

An objection to the analogy with insurance contracts might suggest that legal rights against government are often poorly defined and hence that shaping the scope of the right is frequently left to judges and administrators as they deal with difficult and contested cases. I agree that legal rights often have undefined or informal limits on their scopes. But this is not always true. In 2005 the state of Florida received approval to set a specific ceiling on spending for each Medicaid recipient (Pear, 2005). Even when a legal right is vague about limits, judges and administrators should not exclusively rely on costs and benefits in deciding on limits. They must also take into account fairness or equal protection of the laws. And they must consider legislative purposes in creating the right and previous decisions by courts and other authoritative decision makers.

Conclusion

How to deal with the exceptionally vulnerable is a significant challenge in designing, justifying, and constructing legal rights. Meeting this challenge often requires limits to the scopes of rights. Many familiar legal rights have such limits formally or informally. Once a legal right is operative the duty-bearers under the right must deliberate in ways that take into account the content of the right and considerations of fairness.

NOTES

1. On the nature of rights, see Wenar, 2005. See also Nickel, 2006, chapters 2 and 3.
2. This formulation of a dilemma emerged from a discussion about the right to a safe environment that I had with my colleague Gary Marchant. See Nickel, 1993.

REFERENCES

Feinberg, J. 1970. The nature and value of rights. *Journal of Value Inquiry* 4:243–257.
Nickel, J. 1993. The human right to a safe environment. *Yale Journal of International Law* 18(1):281–25.
Nickel, J. 2006. *Making sense of human rights,* 2nd ed. Hoboken, NJ: Wiley.
Pear, R. 2005. U.S. gives Florida a sweeping right to curb Medicaid. *New York Times* (Oct. 20).
Shue, H. 1996. *Basic rights,* 2nd ed. Princeton, NJ: Princeton University Press.
Wenar, L. 2005. The nature of rights. *Philosophy and Public Affairs* 33:223–52.

CHAPTER 16

(Almost) Equal Protection for Genetically Susceptible Subpopulations

A Hybrid Regulatory-Compensation Proposal

CARL CRANOR

What would it be like to have legal procedures that exemplify thoroughgoing protection of *all* the public from harm caused by toxic substances? The moral views we use to guide our deliberations about law and regulatory policy can greatly shape the proposals we make. This is not a surprise, because, if our arguments are persuasive, our recommendations follow from the moral premises that support them. I, thus, argue against some quite limited moral theories in the utilitarian tradition. The chapter seeks to exemplify a deeper point, however. Our underlying moral views importantly shape our imagination in conceptualizing possible policies and alternatives to existing practices. Thus, one aim of this chapter is expand our ideas of the extent to which it is possible to protect even quite susceptible persons from harm by suggesting a moral principle by which everyone—even the most susceptible or the most biologically vulnerable—has moral standing to be protected from exposure to toxic substances. I then propose one way in which this principle could be represented in legal structures. I present a hybrid regulatory-compensation proposal to protect susceptible subpopulations from harm that could result from toxic substances. While it is possible that not quite all who will be exposed to toxicants will be protected from harm, the suggestion appears to greatly increase protections compared with current policies and some theoretical alternatives. If the requisite genetic sciences were developed, such legal structures would better protect genetically susceptible subpopulations than do current legal structures.

A Note about Susceptibility

Before turning to moral issues and some institutional devices to protect (almost) all from harm, I want to note a complication with the idea of susceptibility; genetic susceptibility is somewhat subtler than it appears on the surface. For example, people with ataxia telangiectasia, a DNA repair disorder, are highly susceptible to exposure to ionizing radiation (Swift et al., 1991). Persons with xeroderma pigmentosum, another DNA repair disorder, are highly susceptible to ultraviolet radiation (Halpern and Altman, 1999). These appear to be comparatively simple instances of genetic susceptibility. The existence of a genetic tendency makes anyone who has it more susceptible to a particular disease, given a particular exposure, and appears to confer no particular biological advantage.

However, there are genetic susceptibilities that present more varied relationships. For example, people who are "fast acetylators" are less likely than "slow acetylators" to "develop bladder cancer from cigarette smoking and from occupational exposure to bycyclic aromatic amines" (Parkinson, 2001). At the same time, they are at higher risk of cancer from heterocyclic amines (Deitz et al., 2000). Acetylation is a biological process by means of which any chemical substance is transformed in the body to assist in its elimination and excretion. This can be a comparatively quicker or slower process in individuals. Acetylation can facilitate the detoxification of some substances and the activation of the toxicity of others (Deitz et al., 2000). Moreover, the particular features of acetylation appear to vary with population groups: populations of Middle Eastern descent appear to be slow acetylators whereas those of Asian descent tend to be faster acetylators (Deitz et al., 2000). So far, so good.

Here is the complication: the same genetic property in a person, fast acetylation, that increases the toxicity of one substance, decreases the toxicity of another. That is, the property constitutes susceptibility with one exposure and biological strength with another. Is fast acetylation (or slow acetylation, for that matter) a special vulnerability or not? The answer seems to be that often a particular biological state may not by itself always be a special susceptibility. Rather, we should think of at least some susceptibilities as relational properties between the biological state of an organism and the conditions of exposure; for some cases, it appears they cannot be separated. More generally, it is a relation between all the conditions necessary for the induction of a disease—and what one singles out for attention may not be a trivial issue (Rothman, 1986, pp. 19–20).

The larger point that emerges here is that there may be some pure, unequivocal genetic vulnerabilities per se, such as the genetic tendencies to xeroderma pigmentosum and their antecedent susceptibilities. How common they are compared with other kinds of susceptibility awaits further research. Other biological states by themselves are not necessarily susceptible states, but are when a person has one kind of exposure, but not others. My intention is not to make some kind of a priori argument against the idea of susceptibility. Rather, it is to issue a cautionary note that identifying susceptibilities may turn out to be a more complex process than has been appreciated to date, and that this complexity will further complicate the process of treating susceptible subpopulations fairly. For now I will assume the simpler notion of susceptibility for the discussion that follows, but we should remember that susceptibilities might be part of more complex relationships.

Moral Issues

Environmental health regulations may be issued under the authority of several different kinds of statutes with different moral foundations (some of these are discussed below). However, because of other language in the statutes or agency adoption of cost-benefit procedures, or more recently actions by the executive branch (Office of Management and Budget, 2000), in fact many regulations are importantly shaped by cost-benefit analysis, which is a variant of utilitarianism.[1] Despite the widespread use of cost-benefit analysis, it and its moral foundation in utilitarianism or quasi-utilitarianism pose a number of controversial substantive moral issues that are well known to philosophers and can adversely affect regulatory outcomes. Consequently, it is important to explore other possible moral foundations of regulation for protecting susceptible subpopulations.

Utilitarianism and Some Variants

Utilitarianism is a well-known principle for guiding moral deliberations. In the world of regulatory policy, cost-benefit analysis, which
guides actual regulation under many different laws, is a crude species of
utilitarianism. The generic version of the utilitarian principle for distributing social goods is relatively easy to state: in authorizing regulatory
policy, a moral agent (or, in the regulatory world, the administrator of an
agency or the president of the United States) ought to allocate resources
among protecting health, providing for more jobs, increasing social income, and distributing other social goods in such a way as to secure the
overall community good. In technical terms, such decisions should be
made to maximize utility for everyone in the community (Scheffler, 1982).

An important feature of utilitarianism is that it takes into account the
utility of everyone equally. As utilitarians commonly assert, "everyone
counts for one and nobody for more than one." In contrast to a hierar-
chical world, as existed during the Middle Ages, no one has special standing to have his or her "utility"—his or her misery (or the frustration of
desires), on the one hand, or happiness (or the satisfaction of desires),
on the other hand—count more than the utility of others. Thus, one kind
of equality is inherent in utilitarian views.

However, as Annette Baier put it, the normative criterion of right and
wrong action is that utilitarianism "notices or worries about" the wrong-
ness of failing to secure the overall community good or the overall community utility (Baier, 1986). The ultimate consideration of whether a
course of action is right or wrong is whether the overall community good
is realized or not. Putting this somewhat crudely in its optimizing form,
if a policy optimizes overall community good, it is the right course of action to pursue. If it fails to optimize overall good, there must be an alternative policy that would achieve that, and the chosen course of action is
the wrong one. The utilitarian concern with overall community benefits
tends to ignore their distribution (next).

Despite its bedrock of equality, utilitarianism fails in other respects to
give sufficient weight or attention to the distributive effects of policy decisions for individual human beings or particular subpopulations that
might be affected by a decision. It does not attend to particular distributions such as the effects of environmental health policies on particularly

vulnerable individuals or groups, except as a means to the end of promoting the net balance of overall good versus bad consequences that result from a policy decision. Utilitarianism has difficulty with the distribution of benefits and burdens both to particular social groups and to those who might be particularly vulnerable because of genetics or their biology through no fault of their own. Thus, as a matter of logic it will sometimes permit important individual interests to be sacrificed to an efficient production of community utility. It can permit minor benefits to many to outweigh severe harms to a few, if the many who benefit are a large enough group and the few who are harmed are not too many. (In some circumstances, it may also permit inconveniences to many provide some major benefits to a few.) Moreover, it also provides no guarantee of equal or any other particular distribution of health protections; distributions are merely one means to maximizing total utility (Scheffler, 1982). Finally, as Rawls (1971) articulated the point, utilitarianism does not take the separateness of persons seriously. That is, persons live in separate individual bodies and live according to separate individual life plans. Both require certain minimal protections and certain minimal resources and support for persons to flourish. The minimal protections and resources should not be reduced beyond what is required to permit individuals to pursue their own conception of human flourishing in order to secure overall benefits for others.

As a generalization, one might say that, except as it affects overall utility, utilitarianism is in principle indifferent to the sources of utility (e.g., income versus health), the kind of utility produced (e.g., satisfaction of basic human needs or relief of suffering versus nonessential pleasures), or the social group on whom the utility or disutility falls. In addition, utilitarianism tends to undervalue the importance of special relations, such as love, family, or moral relationships (e.g., promises or other commitments). Resources go to the persons or activities that are likely to produce the greatest overall community utility. Consequently, according to a utilitarian view, susceptible subpopulations have no special moral standing except as this affects overall social utility. (Of course, the high marginal losses of especially vulnerable groups could argue for their protection on utilitarian grounds, unless their numbers were too small.)

A policy so conceived may well be, as I have argued previously, "morally numbing" (Cranor, 1997). It might make individuals or vulnerable groups less visible to us and reduce our concern about the effects of policies on them. If it is taken seriously, it may blind us to other possibilities, other ways of thinking about issues. If a utilitarian or cost-benefit analysis produces the optimal amount of social utility among the alternatives that were open to a decision maker in the context, this is the morally right thing to do. There is no moral deficiency in such a decision, because it is morally correct.

Other views would not consider such outcomes as right, even if not everyone could be protected. They would regard policies that did not protect all as possibly morally deficient in some way.

Moral Motivation in Legislation

Despite the frequency of appeals to maximizing social utility in environmental policy and regulation, there are laws that contain more protective language than a utilitarian moral principle or its regulatory counterpart, cost-benefit analysis, would produce. For example, the Clean Air Act (CAA) requires that EPA issue air quality criteria that indicate "the kind and extent of all identifiable effects on public health . . . which may be expected from the presence of [pollutants which may be expected to endanger public health]" (42 U.S.C. 7408 (a)(2)). The legislative history calls attention to effects on elderly people, children, and people with preexisting or special conditions, such as chronic obstructive pulmonary disease, heart disease, or pregnancy (Clean Air Act 1970; Discussion of Provisions, 1990; American Thoracic Society, 1996; *Chevron U.S.A. Inc. v. Natural Resources Defense Council, Inc.,* 1983). While originally the CAA sought to set ambient standards to protect all sensitive groups within the population, because of regulatory paralysis—the regulatory process became so science- and data-intensive in addressing toxicants that it seemed paralyzed—too few toxicants to which people were exposed had been addressed. In turn, this led to greater use of technological controls in an effort to reduce exposures of everyone, with any residual risks affecting susceptible subpopulations left to future ambient exposure controls. This greater emphasis on technological approaches decreased total exposures, but may have attenuated some of the protections of susceptible subpopulations, at least until more protective ambient levels can be set (Grassman, 1996). Technological reductions of air toxicants have now been completed, but reducing residual risks remains in progress. The CAA, with its emphasis on seeking to protect elderly people, children, and those with preexisting conditions, would appear to provide greater protections than cost-benefit analysis would typically authorize, because some of these groups would require greater social resources than cost-benefit analysis would justify.

Sections of the Safe Drinking Water Act direct EPA to determine "maximum contaminant level goals" for each contaminant that may have any adverse effect on the health of persons" (42 U.S.C. Sec. 300g-1(b)(a)(b)). These goals should be "set at a level at which . . . no known or anticipated adverse effects on the health of persons occur and which allow an adequate margin of safety" (Safe Drinking Water Act, 1976, 42 U.S.C. Sec. 300g-1(b)(4)). The language asserting the importance of avoiding "any adverse effect on the health of persons" clearly seems more protective than utilitarian language that would require regulations that maximize the overall social good (or monetary value). However, according to other sections of the law, the health goals must be balanced with economic and technological feasibility considerations to set maximum contaminant levels for regulatory purposes (42 U.S.C. 300g-1(b)(5)). Concessions to feasibility can undermine what are otherwise protective goals expressed in other parts of a statute, but they also recognize concessions to practicality.

The Food Quality Protection Act of 1996, amending the Federal Insecticide, Fungicide and Rodenticide Act, also protects a particular subpopulation, with a special focus on children (Food Quality Protection Act, 1996). It eliminated the Delaney Clause for determining the safety of pesticide residues in processed foods and replaced it with a "reasonable certainty of no harm" standard. The Delaney Clause provided that "no [food additive] shall be deemed to safe if it is found to induce cancer when ingested by man or animal, after tests which are appropriate for the evaluation of the safety of food additives to induce cancer in man or animal" (Office of Technology Assessment, 1987). However, the act authorizes special studies of children's consumption patterns, requires that the "special susceptibilities of children and infants" be taken into account, requires the publication of a "specific determination regarding . . . the safety for infants and children," and requires that "there is a reasonable certainty that no harm will result to infants and children from aggregate exposure to the pesticide chemical residue" (Food Quality Protection Act, 1996; Cranor, 1997). By authorizing special protections for infants and children it is likely to be more protective than typical utilitarian-based language of other statutes.

Other statutes authorizing EPA action, such as the Federal Insecticide, Fungicide, and Rodenticide Act and the Toxic Substances Control Act, require EPA to prevent "unreasonable risks of harm" to people. These do not appear to address sensitive subpopulations and admit of a natural utilitarian reading of the statute. However, even the "unreasonable risk" language would argue for protections for certain susceptible subgroups such as children in various developmental stages or the elderly, if the subgroups include enough people. That is, even the unreasonable risk" language can provide protections for some susceptible subpopulations, provided the numbers are large enough to affect the overall utility of the community.

A few other laws have language that implicitly mandates protection for susceptible subpopulations. For example, the Occupational Safety and Health Act says that "no employee should suffer material impairment of health or functional capacity resulting from a person's working lifetime exposure to toxic substances. However, this law permits the reasonably laudable goals contained in the act to be attenuated by concerns about feasibility or costs. Persons should be protected from harm, to the extent economically and technologically feasible (Occupational Safety and Health Act, 1970).

U.S. legislation suggests that as a society we are morally conflicted in seeking to protect all persons including the most susceptible from toxic substances. That is, some statutes that explicitly or implicitly authorize the protection of susceptible persons in one provision attenuate or modify that protection in other provisions. Nonetheless, the "goal" language of these statutes calls attention to important ideals, possibly forcing recognition of susceptible subpopulations' standing to be protected, even though the goal may be difficult to achieve. How might we do better to realize the goals expressed in some of these statutes? In what follows I will seek to provide the moral outlines of better protections for susceptible subpopulations.

Better Moral Motivation

Moral views that underlie the need to protect sensitive subpopulations from harms associated with exposure to environmental toxicants can be seen in other legal contexts, such as in tort or personal injury law, and their moral genealogy can be found in other moral traditions (Cranor, 2007).

It is interesting to note that the tort or personal injury law contains a principle that provides important insights concerning susceptible persons. This is an area of law that seeks to correct unjust invasions of interest by setting public standards of conduct, which must be privately enforced by the victim. Typically, a defendant is held accountable for unlawful conduct that creates risks of "reasonably foreseeable" harm to others that materializes into harm, or in the case of products that in fact causes harm to others (under strict liability laws). When a victim protected by a negligence law is not within the reasonably foreseeable scope of the risk that a defendant unlawfully created, the defendant is not held liable for the injuries (Keeton et al., 1984).

However, when a victim is within the scope of a risk created by a defendant, the defendant is held accountable for all the harms done to the victim even though it was not foreseeable that the victim was extremely vulnerable.

> It is as if a magic circle were drawn about the person, and one who breaks it, even by so much as a cut on the finger, becomes liable for all resulting harm to the person although it may be death. The defendant is held liable when the defendant's negligence operates upon a concealed physical condition, such as pregnancy, or a latent disease, or susceptibility to disease [psychotic or neurotic predispositions, predisposition to amnesia, ruptured disk, delirium tremens], to produce consequences, which the defendant could not reasonably anticipate. The defendant is held liable for unusual results of personal injuries which are regarded as unforeseeable, such as tuberculosis, paralysis, pneumonia, heart or kidney disease, blood poisoning, cancer or the loss of hair from fright. . . . One of the illustrations which runs through the English cases is that of the plaintiff with the 'eggshell skull,' who suffers death where a normal person would have had only a bump on the head. (Keeton et al., 1984, pp. 291–92)

The defendant is liable, however, "only for the extent to which the defendant's conduct has resulted in an aggravation of the pre-existing condition, and not for the condition as it was" (Keeton et al., 1984, pp. 291–92).

A similar equal protection principle has to some extent been adopted in criminal law. For example, in a case in which an obese, sixty-year-old victim in ill health died from a heart attack caused by stress during a robbery attempt, a California Court articulated a view that is typical in parts of the criminal law:

> So long as a victim's predisposing physical condition, regardless of its cause, is not the *only* substantial factor bringing about his death, that condition and the robber's ignorance of it, in no way destroys the robber's criminal responsibility for the death. So long as life is shortened as a result of the felonious act it does not matter that the victim might have died soon anyway. In this respect, the robber *takes his victim as he finds him.* (Kadish and Schulhofer, 1989, p. 509, emphasis added)

How broadly this principle extends to other aspects of the criminal law is not clear—it might be confined merely to so-called felony-murder rules—but some version of the tort law principle nonetheless appears in the criminal law.

The eggshell skull cases suggest that deeply embedded in our legal system (for more than one hundred years) is a principle that everyone has equal standing to be protected from risk of harm, even though some individuals have eggshell skulls, some are pregnant, some have predispositions to disease, or some even have predispositions to "loss of hair from fright" (*Ominsky v. Chas. Weinhagen & Co.,* 1911), Once persons' interests have been wrongfully invaded, both criminal and tort law seek to protect the healthy and the vulnerable equally—not just the upper 95 percent of the population, not only those whose protection will maximize social utility, but also the most vulnerable, most susceptible, and even those with very rare vulnerabilities (Cranor, 1997).

While tort law seeks to correct unjust invasions of interest that have occurred by requiring defendants to compensate victims and criminal law seeks to correct other unjust acts by punishing the wrongdoer, environmental health law seeks to identify and to prevent some of those invasions from occurring in the first place. Thus, although principles of tort and criminal law do not always transfer easily to the regulatory context (Cranor, 1993), I believe that on the issue of protecting susceptible subpopulations they are both pertinent and revelatory and constitute evidence of long-standing social concerns. Just as there is an "equal protection" from harm principle in tort and parts of the criminal law, it seems that there would be an analogous principle for environmental health protections (Cranor, 1997).

A deeper rationale for this is suggested by the structure of well-known theories such as John Rawls's theory of justice (Rawls, 1971). Rawls proposed a theory in which rational, self-interested agents in an "original position" choose principles of justice (to guide the assessment and design of institutions on grounds of justice) behind what he calls a "veil of ignorance" in which the participants do not know what society they would be in, their particular position in whatever society they would end up in, or even their sex or social role. In these circumstances, he argues, persons would choose two particular principles of justice that he proposes (Rawls, 1971, pp. 60–65, 150–61, 175–81, 302). In short, his view consists of a deliberative position (the original position) from which persons would choose principles of justice, as well as a proposal of the particular principles that he argues would be chosen.

In the original position (OP), each person has equal standing to participate in and have a say in choosing principles of justice that would be used to critique or design legal and other basic institutions of a community. One might say that each has equal standing and "sovereignty" to articulate, propose, and "vote on" principles of justice to guide just institutions. I believe that one can see the remainder of Rawls's theory, in particular his two principles of justice as well as their implications for institutions, as trying to secure the position of citizens affected by his two principles of justice and the practically constrained institutions they authorize as close as possible (and closer than rival principles) to the original equal moral standing that all had in the original position (Rawls, 1971). That is, his two principles of justice would come closer to preserving the initial equal moral standing of those in the original position than would any alternative set of moral principles. This is not the place to argue for that view, but an attraction of it is that in the OP all have equal moral standing—no one is morally superior or inferior to anyone else. The problem for choosing principles, then, is to find those that people in the OP would subscribe to that best preserves their equal moral standing, consistent with any practical constraints that have to be observed in creating institutions and making them function.

I suggest a similar strategy. What principle might be adopted that would preserve as far as is feasibly possible the equal moral standing of all persons in the moral community while protecting them from harms they might incur because of biological features over which they have no control?

If the healthy are entitled to protection from invasion of their interests, others who might be much less healthy and more vulnerable are entitled to the same protections. By contrast, if sensitive subpopulations are not protected, this suggests that they do not have moral standing in the community to warrant protection or moral standing equal to that of others in the community—this is especially true for susceptibilities over which persons have no control, such as genetic susceptibilities and those acquired as a result of involuntary exposure to environmental toxicants.

Such a principle would seem to have greater purchase because of the distributive implications if it were not adopted. If the more susceptible or vulnerable are not provided protections, as a community would we not be authorizing disease or death for some in order to provide noncomparable benefits to others (e.g., reduce the costs of products or business expenses for them)? Such an outcome seems morally unacceptable as well as unfair (Honoré, 1995; Cranor, 1997).

Were we not able to fully protect the susceptible as well as the healthy, we should not see policies as right, or the morally correct outcome, as the utilitarian would. In the interest of a more fine-grained moral view, we should probably not see them as morally justified either. To view the absence of adequate protections for the most susceptible as justified suggests that such policies are not wrong in the circumstances or perhaps (on some accounts) are even right. Instead, if it should turn out that it is not possible to protect some of the most vulnerable among us, we should understand such policies as regrettable or possibly excusable in the circumstances (Morris, 1981).

By approaching the issues concerning susceptible subpopulations in this way, we acknowledge that their claims are not nonexistent or extinguished or eliminated merely because it might be too expensive to protect them (Morris, 1981; Cranor, 1997). If we do not acknowledge the legitimacy of protecting the most susceptible (from diseases that are caused by fellow citizens over which the susceptible have no control), however, we are asserting that they have no standing to be protected and that their claim was nonexistent. This, it seems to me, would be inexcusable on our part. For example, it is difficult, or more likely practically impossible, for the criminal law to ensure that no criminal violates the rights of innocent citizens not to be robbed or raped. Yet we would not want to concede that as a consequence they did not have standing to be protected from these violations.

This too-brief discussion of a more nuanced moral view is in sharp contrast with most utilitarian theories on two counts. It suggests that a better moral view is one that places greater emphasis on the distribution of benefits and harms than utilitarian views do. It also draws on a meta-point that the mere fact that persons cannot be protected does not extinguish their claim to protection. A more detailed discussion would take one into the territory of nonutilitarian views and likely to different theories of moral and legal rights. The remarks above rely on the idea that a person may have standing (or a right or entitlement) to be protected, yet for various reasons, such as costs and other practical considerations; the community may not be able to fully ensure those protections. It does not follow that his entitlement or standing to be protected has disappeared or has not been violated or has not been infringed as a result of this inability to secure adequate protection (Morris, 1976, 1981).

Moreover, one can have duties to compensate others for harm done them even if they do not have a full right in the circumstances. In the law this is exemplified in the idea of an "incomplete privilege" (Morris, 1981). For example, one may be privileged to take a horse to escape an assassin (which the owner would have had a duty to provide were he present), yet still be required to compensate the owner for the death of the horse should it die (Morris, 1981).

These more nuanced moral views are pertinent to environmental regulation. Such views are certainly more subtle than utilitarianism would have it, and it seems to me that they become quite nuanced when one considers a wider range of concepts such as I have sketched above. While I have not presented anything like a full argument for these views, I believe they point in the right direction for an account that would complement the arguments made in this chapter. They also deserve more detailed discussion, but that is beyond this chapter.

In articulating a view for protecting the genetically vulnerable from harm from toxicants, I do not (at least not yet) want to concede that it may not be possible to protect everyone from harms associated with exposure to environmental toxicants; that is a more practical matter. Recall that I seek to address what a legal policy might look like that would protect every citizen, no matter how vulnerable as a result of his or her genetic makeup, from harm resulting from exposure to environmental toxicants.

A Hybrid Regulatory-Compensation Proposal

What legal strategies might there be to more fully protect genetically susceptible subpopulations? Beyond regulations that agencies currently issue to protect the bulk of an average exposed population, they could probably go further. I suggest they should. To begin to protect the most susceptible groups, agencies should set health regulations at the lowest level to protect "average" members of significant susceptible subpopulations, consistent with feasibility. This would recognize the standing that susceptible subpopulations as a group have in the moral-legal community.

This proposal has two elements. Agencies should determine what regulations would be needed to protect an "average" person in significant (by size) susceptible subgroups. This part of the proposal resembles accommodations that must be made under the Americans with Disability Act (ADA)—"reasonable accommodations" for those, in this case, with certain biological "disabilities." Thus, the proposal would be consistent with the legal requirements of the ADA and, for that reason, not unreasonable. Just as the ADA recognizes the equal moral standing of persons with disability in the community to live a life as close to a normal opportunity range as the community can reasonably accommodate (Daniels, 1985), so this suggestion approaches the recognition of the equal moral standing of susceptible groups in the population. Moreover, the ADA analogy suggests that it is possible to extend protections to wider group of susceptible persons (as the ADA does) without bankrupting the community.

However, it is the "average" person of a susceptible subpopulation who should be recognized, not the most vulnerable members of the group. This is a concession to practicality or feasibility—institutional arrangements should acknowledge the practical limits of policies so that they are not dismissed out of hand. At the same time, by creating regulations with concessions to practicality, we should recognize that this is, regrettably, the best that can be accomplished by regulation for the most susceptible. That is, we might be morally forced to regret that they cannot be protected further. Our regret is part of our recognition that, as citizens, they have moral standing for protection from activities in which others are engaged that put susceptible persons at risk, even though we cannot fully achieve those protections consistently without substantially curtailing quite valuable activities or bankrupting ourselves.[2] I am suggesting that in the spirit of providing all citizens (even the most susceptible) with legal protection perhaps more citizens can be reasonably protected as the ADA seems to teach us. If the current state of affairs is the best we can do (consistent with legitimate practical limitations), we should still recognize in other ways the standing of the most susceptible to be protected (next).

For those who are genetically susceptible to harm beyond what can be feasibly protected, is there a way to protect them that continues to recognize their standing to be protected, but will not bankrupt the community or government coffers? I suggest that one way to do so is to provide a legal right for them to receive compensation (1) for actual diseases that have plausibly resulted from a toxic exposure, (2) for conditions that are early warnings of possible future disease (medical monitoring), and (3) for precursors of actual disease (compensation for medical intervention, if that would help).[3]

In legal terms, the idea would be to create an analogue to Vaccine Injury Compensation Program (VICP). This program was created under the National Vaccine Injury Act of 1986 to compensate those who suffer injury or death caused by the administration of certain vaccines (National Childhood Vaccine Injury Act, 1986; Johnson, Drew, and Miletich, 1998, p. 15). Vaccines are expensive to produce, especially those that have to be changed every year or two, but scientists know that vaccines will cause harm to some individuals simply because foreign proteins are being introduced into a person's body. Consequently, in order to have beneficial vaccines available for the vast majority of the population, Congress acted to protect the vaccine manufacturers from liability for harm caused by the vaccines, but preserved the right to compensation for those who were harmed by the vaccines because of their particular vulnerability. Under the program, the federal government assumes liability for compensating vaccine injury victims (Johnson, Drew, and Miletich, 1998). Several aspects of the program are different from traditional torts, but these need not enter the discussion at this point.[4]

For those who contract what one might consider characteristic adverse effects from vaccines, there is a presumption of causation. This applies to well-documented causal relationships between certain vaccines and injuries. These constitute so-called on-Table[5] injuries, making the burden of proving causation virtually nonexistent for petitioners suffering from such characteristic conditions (Johnson, Drew, and Miletich, 1998). These are on-Table injuries because there is actually a table of characteristic adverse effects for such harms. For those who suffer injuries that are not characteristic of vaccine exposure, but for which there is a plausible relationship between exposure and injury, the petitioner must prove cause-in-fact by a preponderance of the evidence "utilizing tort standards of proof" (Johnson, Drew, and Miletich, 1998). These constitute "off-Table" injuries, because they are not characteristic and are not included in the table of such adverse effects.

I suggest that legal institutions similar to the VICP be created to protect susceptible persons from exposures to toxic substances as a result of genetic or other susceptibilities—analogues to the VICP. Under such a program, a list of injuries plausibly associated with toxic exposures would be identified (e.g., acute myelogic leukemia is a typical adverse effect from benzene exposure), and nearly automatic compensation would be authorized. These would be on-Table injuries entitled to compensation. In addition, special courts for off-Table injuries would be established to consider those injuries that are not obviously based on current science, but for which a reasonable scientific argument can be made that they result from the exposure. Moreover, the recovery burdens for the off-Table injuries could be reduced as is done in the vaccine program, for example by creating special masters to review complaints and by having more informal evidentiary rules (Johnson, Drew, and Miletich, 1998). I sketch some issues of compensation below.

The rationales would be largely similar to those for the VICP. For exposures to toxics, I assume that the expenses are too great to use the more elaborate apparatus of the regulatory law to protect literally every single person no matter how susceptible, because there might be individuals who are genetically quite vulnerable. However, because theoretically most people, including the average person in significant susceptible subpopulations, would have been protected by regulation from diseases that result from toxic exposures, those who would not be so protected are not likely to be numerous. Consequently, the costs of recognizing individual rights of compensation suggested above should be considerably lower than trying to protect by regulation every last vulnerable individual. Moreover, because not all who are exposed to a toxicant contract diseases that result from exposure, it is possible that even for susceptible individuals there will be some variation in the manifestation of disease states—that is, even for some susceptible individuals there may not be full penetrance of the adverse effects of exposure.[6] Consequently, the costs of such a compensation program would be substantially lower than regulations that protected the same group of persons with their wide range of susceptibilities.

Moreover, the modest costs of a compensation program instead of an analogous regulatory program are a small price to pay for recognizing that even the most susceptible citizens have moral standing to be protected from harm. Of course, a compensatory program by definition would not protect persons from harm as well as a fully successful regulatory program would, because some would be compensated only after the fact of injury. However, at least by recognizing a right to compensation as a community we would acknowledge that persons have standing to be protected in precisely the same way that eggshell skull victims have a right to compensation in torts. Harming them by exposure to a toxicant is wrong, and they are entitled to be protected from this exposure. Even if they are more vulnerable than the average person, or even the average susceptible person, the most susceptible are entitled to such protections. They have the same standing to be protected from harm as less vulnerable persons—they do not lose this simply because they are more susceptible. In addition, by providing for medical monitoring and medical treatments in the case of precursor conditions, this part of the proposal goes some way toward a more preventive stance than does a program that would merely compensate a person for injuries after harm had occurred.

The proposal has some presuppositions that need further clarification. First, extensive as it seems to be, it would likely not protect every single person harmed by exposure to a toxicant. If it worked perfectly, some would be injured and would only receive compensation after the fact, a morally regrettable issue. As a community, however, we have done the best we could and recognize their moral standing by compensating them for injuries suffered.

Second, the funding for the compensation program could come from one of two leading sources: the community at large, that is, general governmental revenues, or from contributions from the activities that produced typically harmful exposures. I do not argue for one or the other. Using the first source of funding might be based on a principle that the community as a whole recognizes that everyone is entitled to protection from exposures that can harm them and so it provides funding as a matter of recognizing the standing of all to be protected from harm. The second would rest on a narrower principle of fairness, articulated by Honoré among others, that places on every member of the community the burden of bearing the risk that his conduct may turn out to be harmful to others in return for the benefit to himself that will accrue should his conduct turn out beneficially as he plans. The second proposal distributes the costs of harm attributable to human activities that produced it (Honoré, 1995, p. 84).

Third, for the compensation arrangement to work well, the science must be developed further than it is at present. That is, for it to work best there must be some way of identifying who has been exposed to the toxicant in question (i.e., the proposal requires well-understood exposure markers). There would also need to be a way to identify those who are especially susceptible to the exposure (i.e., good susceptibility markers), and those who had suffered adverse effects from the exposures (Resnik, this volume). At present, these are unlikely to have been well developed for most toxic exposures. As genetic technologies advance such markers are more likely to be identified. The more that are identified and the more accurate they become, the easier it would be to implement a compensation regime as suggested above. Short of the genetics' being well developed, there could still be institutions that approximated ideally best structures. For example, if workplace regulations are inadequate to protect all employees from toxic exposures (e.g., as is currently the case with benzene), there could still be compensation programs for those who developed diseases characteristic of those exposures as on-Table injury compensation. For employees who developed different diseases after workplace exposures, injured parties could make a case that they had been injured because of those exposures, but this would more closely resemble a tort proceeding, based on the model of the off-Table injuries of the VICP.

Fourth, similar points would apply to environmental exposures, but here there would more hurdles to overcome. Injured persons would have to show exposure to the toxicants subject to regulation, then contraction of diseases characteristic of the exposure (on-Table proceedings). For diseases not characteristic of the exposure, they would need to demonstrate exposure plus a plausible argument based on analogues to off-Table injuries. Until the genetic sciences are sufficiently improved, this last possibility does not have much to differentiate it from a toxic tort suit, although the proposed procedures might still be easier to satisfy for off-Table injuries than they are in typical tort suits.

Fifth, the special courts suggested for hearing the scientific issues concerning toxic exposures would be better positioned to assess the "off-Table" claims of injury than would general federal or state district courts, which lack any special scientific expertise.

Sixth, as part of the regulatory program to prevent diseases in the first place, agencies could list characteristic injuries from the exposures in question, insofar as they are known, so that this would begin to provide some of the content needed for the companion compensation program.

Conclusion

Acknowledging that persons with genetic susceptibilities are entitled to compensation gives moral recognition to several things. It recognizes that they have a moral right to the protection that, regrettably, administrative law may not be able fully to provide. It also is an acknowledgment that they have been invaded and wronged (even if no one acted wrongly) despite the existence of a law that sought to protect them. Finally, even though it is too costly to protect every genetically susceptible person by administrative regulation, it recognizes that his or her claim to protection is not nonexistent or extinguished or eliminated (Morris, 1981; Cranor, 1997).

In fact, the proposal suggested above that would provide a right to compensation recognizes that the most vulnerable have a right not to be injured in the first place. If they are entitled to medical monitoring when it is established that they have been exposed and are entitled to medical treatment when they have been adversely affected, both entitlements go some way toward recognizing a more preventive entitlement not to be injured at all (as is the case for others of more typical susceptibility). If the science advances so such a legal structure could be reasonably implemented, the community would have taken important steps toward ensuring that everyone has equal standing to be protected from harms resulting from exposures to toxicants.

NOTES

1. A comprehensive account of cost-benefit analysis is offered by the President's Council on Environmental Quality: "Formal cost-benefit analysis is a rigorous, quantitative, and data-intensive procedure. It includes the following steps: identifying all nontrivial effects, categorizing these effects as benefits or costs, making quantitative estimates of the extent of each benefit or cost, translating these benefits and costs into a common metric (such as dollars), discounting future costs and benefits so as to compare them on an equivalent basis, and itemizing the costs and benefits to see which is greater."

2. In proposing the idea of a hybrid regulatory-compensation institutional strategy to implement a robust equal protection principle, the first step, as I have argued elsewhere, is to recognize special susceptibilities in agency risk assessments. Until there is good empirical evidence to provide guidance, agencies should adopt default safety factors or high upper confidence extrapolation models to serve as placeholders for variations in susceptible subpopulations until there is better empirical research. Current tenfold default safety factors to account for variation in human populations may not be large enough; perhaps they should be several hundredfold (Nebert, 1991; Venitt, 1994; Hattis and Barlow, 1996; Hattis, 1997; Perera, 1996). Recently, Hattis, Goble, and Chu (2005) argued that children exposed to a toxicant should be protected with a thirteenfold safety factor instead of the tenfold safety factor indicated under the Food Quality Protection Act. Such safety factors are analogous to presumptions in the law and should be set for factual reasons if the evidence is available and for policy reasons if empirical research has not been done. In doing risk assessment, agencies will have to develop different strategies for both threshold (e.g., noncarcinogens) and nonthreshold (e.g., genotoxic carcinogens) effects for the protection of susceptible individuals.

3. There should be no *res judicata* (no legal barrier to revisiting the issues) on (2) and (3). The idea is that if persons have equal moral standing to be protected from harm as a result of conditions over which they have no control, if they can show that they have conditions that physicians believe likely to lead to disease and resulted from the exposure in question, then they should have access to medical monitoring, so that any more devastating disease effects are detected at as early a time as possible. This is a cause of action that is recognized in torts when persons have been exposed to toxicants that can cause serious injury but is permitted before the disease actually appears. For a case in which the courts have permitted injured parties to revisit events for which some legal remedy has already been provided, but as a result of exposure actual disease later developed, see *Hagerty v. L&L Marine Services, Inc.,* (1986). In effect the court permitted two causes of action: one for the initial invasion by a toxic substance (and the need for medical monitoring) and the second for the development of disease.

For persons who develop precursor conditions, something more than medical monitoring might be justified. I have in mind conditions such as benzene's lowering the white cell count for persons who have been exposed, or ozone's rearranging the structure of the lungs. Neither is yet known for sure to cause disease, so at least medical monitoring would be recommended by the equal protection principle (in order to detect any harm as early as possible and to prevent it if possible). However, there might be some medical treatment of precursor conditions that would prevent development of full-blown disease. If there were such treatment, part of the compensation scheme should go beyond mere monitoring in order to provide treatment that would prevent more serious disease.

4. Because the cases are heard in the Federal Claims Court, the judges in these cases gain their authority from Article I of the Constitution rather than Article III. The judges have jurisdiction to determine both whether petitioners are entitled to compensation and the amount of compensation.

Neither the Federal Rules of Civil Procedure nor the Federal Rules of Evidence legally apply in these cases. Therefore, these hearings are not officially bound by the recent Supreme Court decision in *Daubert v. Merrell-Dow Pharmaceutical, Inc, 509 U.S. 579 (1983).* Finally, procedures in the Claims Court are intended to be less adversarial than in traditional torts (Johnson, Drew, and Miletich, 1998, p. 15).

5. The Vaccine Act included a table of vaccines with known associated injuries. When a petitioner suffers an injury that is recognized as an on-Table injury, the petitioner is entitled to a presumption of causation. However, if the petitioner's injury does not appear on the table or if the injury does not occur within the time periods mentioned on the table, the injury is considered "off-Table" and the petitioner must prove cause-in-fact in order to recover compensation. See Johnson, Drew, and Miletich (1998, p. 13).

6. Penetrance is the "degree or frequency with which a manifests it effect" (American Heritage Dictionary, 1969).

REFERENCES

American Heritage Dictionary. New York: Houghton Mifflin Company, 1969.

American Thoracic Society, Committee of the Environmental and Occupational Health Assembly. 1996. State of the art: Health effects of outdoor air pollution. *American Journal of Respiratory Critical Care Medicine* 153:477–98.

Baier, A. 1986. Poisoning the wells. In *Values at risk* (pp. 49–74), edited by D. MacLean. Totowa, NJ: Rowman & Allenheld.

Clean Air Act. 1970. (amended 1974, 1977, 1990). 42 U.S.C. s/s 7401 et seq. (1970).

Chevron U.S.A. Inc. v. Natural Resources Defense Council, Inc. 467 U.S. 837 (1983).

Cranor, C.F. 1993. *Regulating toxic substances.* New York: Oxford University Press.

Cranor, C.F. 1997. Eggshell skulls and loss of hair from fright: Some moral and legal principles that protect susceptible subpopulations. *Environmental Toxicology and Pharmacology* 4:239–45.

Cranor, C.F. 2007. Toward a Non-consequentialist approach to acceptable risks. In *Risk and philosophy* (pp. 36–53), edited by T. Lewens. London: Routledge.

Daniels, N. 1985. *Just health care.* Cambridge: Cambridge University Press.

Deitz, C.C., W. Zheng, M.A. Leff, M Gross, W.-Q. Wen, M.A. Doll, G.H. Xiao, A.R. Folsom, and D.W. Hein. 2000. N-Acetyltransferase-2 genetic polymorphism, well-done meat intake, and breast cancer risk among postmenopausal women. *Cancer Epidemiology, Biomarkers & Prevention* 9:905–10.

Discussion of Provisions. 1990. Public Law 101-549.

Food Quality Protection Act. 1996. Public Law 104-170.

Grassman, J. 1996. Acquired risk factors and susceptibility to environmental toxicants. *Environmental Toxicology and Pharmacology* 4:195–208.

Hagerty v. L&L Marine Services, Inc., 788 F 2d 315 (1986).

Halpern, A.C., and J.F. Altman. 1999. Genetic predisposition to skin cancer. *Current Opinion in Oncology* 11:132.

Hattis, D. 1997. Variability in susceptibility: How big, how often, for what responses to what agents? *Environmental Toxicology and Environmental Pharmacology* 4:189–94.

Hattis, D., and K. Barlow. 1996. Human interindividual variability in cancer risks: Technical and management challenges. *Health and Ecological Risk Assessment* 2:194–220.

Hattis, D., R. Goble, and M. Chu. 2005. Age-related differences in susceptibility to carcinogenesis. II: Approaches for application and uncertainty analyses for individual genetically acting carcinogens. *Environmental Health Perspectives* 113:509–16.

Honoré, T. 1995. The morality of tort law—Questions and answers. In *Philosophical foundations of tort law,* edited by D. Owen. Oxford: Oxford University Press.

Johnson, M.J., C.E. Drew, and D.P. Miletich. 1998. Use of expert testimony, specialized decision makers, and case-management innovations in the National Vaccine Injury Compensation Program. Washington, DC: Federal Judicial Center.

Kadish, S.H., and S.J. Schulhofer. 1989. *Criminal law and its processes,* 5th ed. New York: Aspen.

Keeton, W.P., D.B. Dobbs, R.E. Keeton, and D.G. Owen. 1984. *Prosser and Keeton on Torts,* 5th ed. St. Paul, MN: West Publishing Co.

Morris, H. 1976. *On guilt and innocence.* Berkeley: University of California Press.

Morris, H. 1981. The status of rights. *Ethics* 92:40–56.

National Childhood Vaccine Injury Act of 1986. 1986. Public Law 99-660, 100 Stat. 3755, codified as amended, 42 U.S.C.A. 300aa-1 *et seq.*

Nebert, D.W. 1991. Role of genetics and drug metabolism in human cancer risk. *Mutation Research* 247:267–81.

Occupational Safety and Health Act. 1970. Public Law 91-596, 84 Stat. 1590 91st Congress, S.2193.

Office of Technology Assessment. 1987. *Identifying and regulating carcinogens.* Washington, DC: U.S. Government Printing Office.

Ominsky v. Chas. Weinhagen & Co. 1911. 129 N.W. Rptr 845-46.

Parkinson, A. 2001. Biotransformation of xenobiotics. In *Casarett and Doull's Toxicology: The basic science of poisons* (pp. 132–224), 6th ed., edited by C.D. Klaassen. New York: McGraw-Hill.

Perera, F. 1996. Molecular epidemiology: Insights into cancer susceptibility, risk assessment, and prevention. *Journal of the National Cancer Institute* 88: 496–509.

Rawls, J. 1971. *A theory of justice.* Cambridge, MA: Harvard University Press.

Rothman, K. 1986. *Modern epidemiology.* Boston: Little, Brown and Company.

Safe Drinking Water Act. 1976. (amended 1987, 1996). 42 U.S.C. 300g-1.

Scheffler, S. 1982. *The rejection of consequentialism.* Oxford: Clarendon Press.

Swift M., D. Morrell, R.B. Massey, and C.L. Chase. 1991. Incidence of cancer in 161 Families affected by ataxia-telangiectasia. *New England Journal of Medicine* 325:1831–36.

U.S. Office of Management and Budget. 2000. *Guidelines to standardize measures of costs and benefits and the format of accounting statements of (Memorandum M-00-08).* Washington, DC: Office of Management and Budget.

Venitt, S. 1994. Mechanisms of carcinogenesis and individual susceptibility to cancer. *Clinical Chemistry* 40:1421–25.

CHAPTER 17

Protecting People in Spite of—or Thanks to—the "Veil of Ignorance"

ADAM M. FINKEL

When society determines that an action to protect public health or the environment is warranted because its benefits exceed its costs, many of us probably conjure up a mental picture of a balance between two discrete quantities, tipping positive. Presumably, all but the most self-contradictory forms of the precautionary principle (discussed by Resnik earlier in this volume) share this mental construct: that is, that the positives that accompany an action outweigh the harms caused by that action or the harms that inaction would perpetuate, even if no attempt is made to gauge costs and benefits in the traditional sense. But these are both abstractions of cost and benefit, and they result from aggregating health, environmental, and economic effects that apply in disparate ways to every individual. When a cost or benefit outweighs its counterpart, it is because a collection of one outweighs that of the other. By looking at only the total bottom line, we can, and often do, luck into sound choices. An individualized assessment, however, can improve collective action in two fundamental and not mutually exclusive ways: (1) it can allow for fine-tuning of the intervention to provide more protection to the individuals most in need or less stringency for those who do not need or prefer not to pay for additional protections; and (2) it can change the level of protection we provide across the board, in light of what we learn about the distribution of costs and benefits.

To see both the whole and the sum of its parts in these situations requires both the will to examine individual costs and benefits and appropriate tools for discerning effects on individuals. *The main thesis of this chapter is that for the past twenty years or more, our technical capacity to individualize estimates of risk and benefit has increased much faster than has our willingness to make use of these new abilities.*

This situation is not simply the result of a lack of vision, as I and others have argued previously (Finkel, 1984; Hattis, 2004). In fact, recent developments suggest that some of the current reticence to exploit our increasing ability to individualize risk stems from legitimate concerns about the side effects of doing so. In this chapter, I attempt to distinguish some of the inevitable downsides of individualized environmental and occupational health protection from other pitfalls that are avoidable. I then sketch out an alternative approach to reconcile the desire to protect individuals according to their unique risks with the reluctance to proceed down such a path: namely, interventions informed by human genetic (and other) variability[1] that are not dependent on identification of the specific individuals motivating society's concern.

This chapter is structured to support the thesis that personal and social decisions that acknowledge variability in risk and cost are more sensible and robust than those that ignore variation or "average it away." In light of the benefits and harms of identifying individuals according to their place on the distribution of risk or cost, I emphasize the concept of "anonymous protection" as a win/win solution to the tension between individualization and identification, or as a worthwhile fallback position that may have unique virtues.

With a debt to John Rawls, who described as the "veil of ignorance" the situation in which individuals know the existence of distributed attributes but not their own personal circumstances (Rawls, 1971), I focus primarily on reasons why this partial "ignorance" may be preferable to complete awareness, despite the connotations of that word. Rawls looks longingly on an unlikely state of ignorance regarding wealth and other obvious attributes, because he sees it as in fact superior to more complete knowledge: "one excludes the knowledge of those contingencies

which sets men at odds and allows them to be guided by their prejudices" (Rawls, 1971, p. 19). In the regulation of environmental and occupational hazards, in contrast, we can choose to place (or to allow) a
"veil of ignorance" over less obvious individual knowledge, and in so
doing we may be able to promote justice at minimal risk to efficiency.

Before sketching out this possible solution, I offer two prefatory sections. In the second section, I place the inattention to individual risk in
the context of similar lapses in several related science-policy arenas. I
summarize the special concerns raised by individual genetic information
relevant to environmental or occupational exposures in the third section.
In the fourth section, I discuss some conceptual objections to calculating
and acting on information about "nonidentifiable variability," and in the
fifth section I present several sets of reasons to explain why such objections may be misguided as well as unduly pessimistic. Finally, I discuss
some policy implications of incorporating nonidentifiable variability into
risk-based decisions about environmental and other issues.

"The Fault Is in Ourselves:" Mishandling Variation May Outlast Our Ignorance of It

It should come as no surprise that our ability to pinpoint environmental risks to individuals has progressed faster than our success in acting
appropriately on such knowledge. There are many analogous situations
where we have had requisite knowledge of interindividual variability at
hand, and yet we have ignored, misinterpreted, or misapplied that knowledge. Such situations can enshrine a self-fulfilling supply-and-demand
problem, as failing to appreciate the benefits of understanding variability in one area can make understanding variability in other areas seem
worthless or even counterproductive. The following examples are meant
to shed light on two different types of failures in responding to available
information about variation. They emphasize how the task becomes even
more difficult in those other cases where we need both to generate and
to incorporate data on interindividual differences.

Ignoring Variability

Sometimes we utterly fail to acknowledge variation that is unambigu-
ously present. Several examples from different contexts are provided below.

Environmental Exposures

Goldstein et al. (1992) analyzed the fatality risks from airplane crashes to persons not on board the plane ("groundlings").[2] They tallied one hundred fifty such deaths in the United States over an eleven-year period (1975–85), divided by the size of the U.S. population in 1980, and converted from an eleven-year window to a seventy-year lifetime, to arrive at an individual lifetime risk of 4.2×10^{-6}. Nowhere in this short paper do the authors even hint at interindividual variability (due primarily to location) in risk: rather, the authors refer to "the risk" as a precisely known quantity[3] and define it as "the likelihood of death due to an airplane crashing on *you* while *you* are on the ground" (emphasis added).

A conclusion drawn from this exercise—that the risk of being hit by a falling airplane is roughly 4.2 times greater than the one-per-million level of risk that sometimes prompts governmental action—later became a central focus of congressional debate (1993–98) over a series of legislative "regulatory reform" proposals to change the way agencies assess and manage risks. John Graham testified on various occasions during this period (Graham, 1993; Graham, 1994) that Congress might rethink the 10^{-6} benchmark, urging members of Congress to consider whether society should strive to reduce risks to a level four times smaller than the implicitly trivial risk each baby born in the United States faces from "being killed while on the ground by a crashing airplane" (Crain, 1995).

Around that time, I suggested (Finkel, 1996) that "these average risks do not reflect the substantial variation in risk that real people undergo; the reason most people probably think the risk of being hit by a falling airplane is remotely low is that for most of us it *is* remotely low." I then offered a "guesstimate" that the 4.2×10^{-6} population average masked a much smaller risk (I guessed 10^{-7}) to perhaps 99 percent of the population living far from any airport flight path, and a much larger risk (I guessed 1.2×10^{-3}) to the remaining 1 percent of Americans living at or near the boundary of airport property.

Five years later, Thompson, Rebouw, and Cooke (2001) analyzed each of the one hundred fifty fatalities and showed that about 3 percent of U.S. residents live less than two miles from an airport runway and face a lifetime "groundling" risk of approximately 1.2×10^{-4}, while for the remaining 97 percent of us, this risk is below 6×10^{-7}. Advancing the original

analysis by one step, from the assumption of no variability to a dichotomous assumption, reveals that for some of us the "groundling" risk is at
least two hundred times larger than it is for others. Qualitatively, of course,
the two subpopulations' risks lie on opposite sides of the 10^{-6} reference
point, suggesting that it may have been particularly misleading to average
a trivial risk to nearly everyone with a large risk to a small minority and
not to disclose or notice the implicit calculation. Note that in this example
proximity to an airport is something observable, without the need for any
sophisticated analysis of an individual's characteristics. This points to the
allure (for the analyst, and perhaps for the recipients of such "risk in perspective") of reducing dichotomies or continuous variation to a single average, even in cases such as these where the variability is so tangible.[4]

Susceptibility to Environmental Disease

Cancer risk-assessment methods depend on many assumptions that
allow us to estimate risks in the face of incomplete data and imperfect
models. Whenever we need to translate information found under the
proverbial lamppost (where we can observe some phenomenon) to a situation of greater interest where no direct observations are available, we
must either assume equivalence or difference, two categories that are mutually exclusive and exhaustive. For example, because we know that mice
and humans breathe different quantities of air during a given time period, we extrapolate across species by trying to quantify that difference.

Extrapolation within a single species, whether this is recognized or
not, similarly challenges us to quantify differences or else to assume that
no meaningful differences exist. Risk assessment for noncarcinogenic
compounds has relied heavily for several decades on quantitative inferences about human interindividual variability. The U.S. Environmental
Protection Agency (EPA) and other agencies routinely decrease allowable
exposures by a factor of ten to account for the possibility that some humans are more susceptible than the typical human, who presumably
would be protected appropriately at the higher level of exposure. A substantial literature suggests that, depending on the compound and assumptions involved, the factor of ten either may be needlessly large (Dourson,
Felter, and Robinson 1996) or that it may be insufficient to protect individuals who are substantially more susceptible than the typical person
(Hattis, Banati, and Goble, 1999). However, the principle of trying to
admit and accommodate intraspecies differences in noncancer risk

assessment will surely survive the ongoing fine-tuning of the precise amount of adjustment.

The situation is completely different with respect to cancer risk assessment, however. EPA and other agencies have, for decades, implicitly treated all humans as identical in susceptibility to the carcinogenic effects of environmental exposures, despite a wealth of information suggesting otherwise. The information that human interindividual variation is substantial began to accumulate before EPA's initial codification of its carcinogenic risk assessment procedures in the late 1970s and is accumulating currently (Finkel, 1995a; Hattis and Barlow, 1996). Nonetheless, whenever cancer risk assessors estimate human risk based on animal bioassay information, they derive a dose-response relationship that is valid for only one hypothetical human being, but they apply the relationship to all persons. In theory, when extrapolating from laboratory animals to humans, it is appropriate to assume that the susceptibility of the test animals (essentially a point estimate because they are inbred for homogeneity) is equivalent to that of the median human (National Research Council [NRC], 1994, p. 210; Hattis and Goble, 2003).

This problem also pervades risk estimation that relies on human epidemiologic data, but here the single, nonvarying dose-response relationship can reflect only the average susceptibility of the human population studied. But this average can differ both at random or systematically from the average susceptibility of the broader population for whom risk is being estimated (Finkel, 1995a), as well as from any individual member of that population. In its 2005 Guidelines for Carcinogen Risk Assessment (p. A-9), EPA does make one passing reference to the "range of human variation" in susceptibility, but only to make the comforting claim that its practice of using a linear (rather than, presumably, a threshold or sublinear) dose-response function "adequately accounts for human variation" (U.S. Environmental Protection Agency [EPA], 2005a). EPA is apparently asserting that the "conservatism" it believes to be inherent in the linear model makes up for concern about individuals of higher-than-average susceptibility—in effect, asserting that it overestimates risk for everyone but just does so less dramatically for some people. This claim is unsupported in that no data exist that suggest that the linear model is in fact conservative[5] or that any upward bias that might occur at this step is sufficient to make up for the downward bias inherent in ignoring the half of the population with above-median susceptibility. Although at least

EPA now admits that humans (unlike laboratory animals bred for genetic homogeneity) have individual dose-response relationships that vary across the population, it does not take this epiphany into account in its cancer risk assessments (with one exception discussed below), as if human variability was a theoretical nicety, rather than a profound challenge to the validity and policy relevance of the agency's cancer risk assessment outputs (NRC, 1994; see especially the committee's recommendation on p. 219).

Medical Decision Making

In contrast to the relationship between the environmental risk manager and the public affected by these risks, the relationship between the clinician and the patient is inherently personal, with the unit of analysis (at least ostensibly) being the individual, rather than the group or population. Physicians are expected to be sensitive to obvious characteristics of the patient that individualize the diagnostic process; for example, the differential diagnosis of hearing loss should not proceed identically in two successive patients, one a teenager and one an octogenarian. To my knowledge, however, no systematic study has ever been carried out to determine the extent to which clinicians successfully (or even attempt to) individualize diagnosis and treatment when such decisions hinge on quantitative variation in risks, even when the underlying variation is obvious. In my experience, supported by many discussions with colleagues who have either given or received medical advice based on quantitative information, physicians often apply population-average values of key probabilities to patients regardless of the extent to which the patient's own probability would seem likely to differ from the average. (See, for example, a book written largely about this subject, Schneider and Lane, 2005.)

As an example, my wife and I faced on several occasions the happy but highly nerve-wracking choice of how many embryos to transfer during in vitro fertilization cycles at several different clinics. In every case, when we expressed concern both about failing to conceive and about the risk of twins and higher-order multiple births, our doctors cited the results of the same recent large trials that had established the average probability (p) of successful implantation per seven-day blastocyst transferred. We became adept at rapidly doing simple binomial expansions to allocate the probabilities of 0 through n births as a function of p and the number of blastocysts we might choose to transfer. Invariably (pun intended), when we asked whether we should make a decision based on the population value of p or on some individualized value that might be higher or lower based on our own characteristics (age, reproductive history, previous attempts, etc.) and on the morphology of the actual blastocysts involved, we were told that the studies had provided all the information available—one value of p for all women in my wife's five-year age category. However, our decision was rather sensitive to small changes in p (Table 17.1). At the population p of 0.5 per blastocyst, we likely would have transferred only one blastocyst to avoid the 25 percent chance of twins with transfer of two. On the other hand, if our individualized p was equal to 0.4 (and we believed that our p was lower than 0.5, due to factors our doctors were well aware of), we would have viewed transferring two as preferable to one, as transferring two would have resulted in a much lower probability of failure with only a 16 percent chance of twins.[6]

My suspicion that clinicians commonly provide quantitative information unmodified by consideration of likely (that is, neither speculative nor difficult-to-discern) factors specific to the patient(s) receiving it is bolstered by a preliminary examination of the medical decision-making literature. Only relatively recently (Winkler and Smith, 2004) have researchers begun to consider methods for communicating uncertainty in one of the most widely used probabilistic analyses—the Bayesian posttest

TABLE 17.1
In Vitro Outcomes as a Function of Transfers and the Probability of Successful Implantation

Number transferred	Number of live births			
	0	1	2	3
1	.6*	.4*	—	—
	.5[†]	.5[†]	—	—
	.4[‡]	.6[‡]	—	—
2	.36*	.48*	.16*	—
	.25[†]	.5[†]	.25[†]	—
	.16[‡]	.48[‡]	.36[‡]	—
3	.216*	.432*	.288*	.064*
	.125[†]	.375[†]	.375[†]	.125[†]
	.06[‡]	.29[‡]	.43[‡]	.22[‡]

Notes: dash = not applicable.
*$p = .4$
[†]$p = .5$
[‡]$p = .6$

probability of disease given a medical test with an assumed sensitivity, specificity, and population prevalence (pretest probability). These articles seem to concentrate on how true uncertainty in one or more of these three parameters affects the patient's posttest probability, rather than the situation where the population parameters can be precisely estimated, but simply differ from patient to patient. One would expect, for instance, the prior disease probability to vary from person to person, based on age, related symptoms, and many other factors.

The tendency to "average away" known or readily ascertainable variability in the clinical setting appears to be writ large in the application of decision theory to public health. Hundreds of analyses of the cost-effectiveness of particular surgical interventions, pharmaceutical therapies, and diagnostic tests have been published over the past twenty-five years, and most of them report either a single value or a small number of subgroup values for the cost-effectiveness result (e.g., a given test may be "cost-effective" for men and not for women, or for women of child-bearing age and not for others). These population cost-effectiveness numbers wield tremendous influence in determining the standard of care for particular conditions, and in determining which interventions will be covered by insurance, and if so, at what frequency. However, any estimate of the cost of a procedure per life-year extended (or a similar metric gauging mortality or morbidity reduction) will vary over the population to whom it applies, in proportion to individual differences in baseline risk, efficacy, valuation, and other factors.[7] Although recent articles in the medical decision-making literature (Zaric, 2003) have begun to explore biases and uncertainties in population cost-effectiveness ratios resulting from ignoring interindividual variability, relatively few sensitivity analyses have been undertaken to explore which decisions might be optimal for populations but suboptimal or flatly incorrect for individuals within them who differ from the group.

Economic Welfare

If risk scientists' progress in acknowledging and quantifying known interindividual variation in risk has been rudimentary, the situation with respect to variation on the cost side of the cost-benefit ledger is even less well-developed. Regulatory economists often define "costs" as the resources that those who must comply with a regulatory or other intervention must expend. A growing literature (see, for example, Goodstein and

Hodges, 1997; Harrington, Morgenstern, and Nelson, 2000) explores the biases, more often than not upward ones, surrounding current estimates of total compliance cost. More recent articles (Pizer and Kopp, 2003) make the point that even an unbiased estimate of total compliance cost is a surrogate for the correct measure, which is social cost—the sum total of economic changes, both negative and positive. These economic changes include compliance costs, but also price changes and benefits and costs to workers and firms that supply the controls or knowledge that the initial compliers must purchase (Porter and van der Linde, 1995; Berck and Hoffman, 2002). But even an accurate estimate of total social cost is itself only a measure that is insensitive to the distribution of individual costs, just as a measure of the number of lives a regulation is expected to "save" is insensitive to the distribution of risk-reducing benefits across individuals. As Pizer and Kopp report, "given the pervasiveness and magnitude of environmental regulation, one would think that comprehensive studies of the cost and benefit distribution of these policies would be bountiful. Ironically, the contrary is true" (p. 33).

As a result, when decision makers compare total benefits with total costs (C), the individual citizen (in a population of size P) has no basis for knowing whether his own share of those total costs will be near zero (or even less than zero), near C, or anywhere in between.[8] The assumption that costs are always borne equally across the population (i.e., that everyone's share is exactly C divided by P) may be useful for some of the population in some cases,[9] but mainstream regulatory economics gives no hint that this may be the rare exception, just as in the "groundlings" example above, where the putative benefits rather than the costs of control are concentrated, but are not acknowledged as such.

Both risks and costs vary across individuals, so the distribution of their ratio or their difference will generally be even broader than the distribution of risk or cost viewed in isolation (Finkel, 1995b). A rejected intervention for which "the (total) costs exceed the benefits," therefore, may mask an underlying reality in which the individual benefit would exceed the individual cost for the majority of affected citizens or vice versa. This is a mathematical property of distributed quantities and does not hinge on the colloquial definition of equity—giving special weight to individuals who are disproportionately affected. Even giving each person identical weight can cause us to conclude that the typical value for individual net benefit may be of a different sign than the value of aggregate net benefit.

These examples show how tempting it often is to regard interindividual variability as an "annoying detail" (Hattis, 2004) that can safely be averaged away, as qualitatively less important than reaching conclusions about group behavior or between-group differences, or even as an impediment to studying those very differences. In risk assessment for environmental health, any impetus to explore and respond to interindividual differences may wane simply because alternatives to expressing risk quantitatively are on the rise. Both the precautionary principle (touted largely from outside the federal regulatory system) and outputs of analysis such as the reference dose or the "margin of exposure" that do not use risk or harm as their currency (developed largely from within the agencies) can drive decision making that is insensitive to risk and hence by definition uninterested in within-population variations in risk.[10]

Mishandling Variability

Even when we acknowledge or emphasize human variation, examples abound of misusing or oversimplifying the information added. I offer six examples of different ways in which disaggregating the population into two or more subgroups can cloud or hinder communication or intervention. These examples are biased toward recent events and commentaries, and for this reason may not be the most apt instances of the phenomena I am trying to categorize. However, they are meant to stimulate thought about the wide array of arenas in which we end up taking initial but unsatisfactory steps toward individualizing risk or benefit.

1. *Splitting the population via a characteristic not causally related to risk, or only partly correlated with it.* The U.S. Food and Drug Administration (FDA, 2004b) published draft guidance that various facilities can use to determine, among other things, which prospective donors of cells and body tissues should be deemed ineligible due to the possibility of HIV transmission to the recipient (during the several-month period in which HIV testing of the donated material may yield a false negative). In particular, the guidance suggests that sperm banks and fertility clinics should reject sperm donors who have had homosexual sex during the preceding five years. However, FDA also recommended that a prospective donor who has had heterosexual sex with a known HIV-positive person more than twelve months before donation be deemed eligible to

donate. Many activists and clinics objected to these recommendations on the grounds that they attach a greater stigma to less risky (monogamous, "safe," possible or documented HIV-negative partner) homosexual practices than they do to riskier (polygamous, unprotected, possible HIV-positive partner or partners) heterosexual practices. FDA acknowledged (FDA, 2004a, pp. 29805–6) that this categorization might incorrectly exclude many prospective donors whose risk of transmitting HIV was lower than other included donors, but noted that one of its advisory committees had determined there were no data that could identify "subsets of men who have had sex with other men . . . [whose risks are] similar to the population at large."[11] Essentially, there are at least two ways to dichotomize a population for such a purpose: via risky behavior or via a different behavior that is imperfectly correlated with risk. FDA has chosen the latter course, putting the onus to improve the sorting mechanism on those who would remedy the new inequities.[12]

2. *Splitting the population via a relevant variable, while ignoring a more powerful one.* Many of the other authors in this volume have referred to the "genetics loads the gun, environment pulls the trigger" model of causation, which holds that few cases of chronic disease arise without some influence from both predisposition and exposure. A possible corollary to this general rule would be that both genetic and environmental variability must be considered when trying to explain the presence or absence of disease in an exposed population. One tidbit of recent anecdotal information may call to mind the frequency of inferences that go astray due to only partial acknowledgment of interindividual variability. A letter to the *New York Times* (Schlack, 2005) notes that "boys account for 80% of all autism cases. Are we to believe that boys received more of the thimerosal vaccine than girls?" Without reaching a conclusion about the existence of a relationship between thimerosal exposure and autism, surely an explanation exists for the gender difference that requires no systematic difference in exposure patterns: boys may simply be more susceptible to the adverse effects of a given exposure to thimerosal than girls are.

3. *Splitting the population via relevant, powerful characteristics that apply to groups rather than (necessarily) to the individuals within them.* The well-known "ecologic fallacy" can yield misleading conclusions about causality or the quantitative strength of a correctly inferred causal relationship, because comparisons of group characteristics may mask con-

flicting or attenuating information about the characteristics and outcomes of individuals. Even in the presence of a correct and precise inference about group behavior, however, policies applied to individuals may be inequitable. One of the "new ideas of 2005" featured in an annual review in the *New York Times Sunday Magazine*—recommending criminals for shorter or longer sentences based on demographic characteristics—may epitomize the dilemma of policies that may be appropriate for groups but not for individuals. Reporter Emily Bazelon (2005) characterized the use of demographic and behavioral risk data by Virginia and other state sentencing commissions as "beginning to make it possible to determine which bad guys really will commit new offenses . . . based on a short list of factors with a proven relationship to future risk."[13] She reported approvingly that when the algorithm was tested on prisoners who had already served their sentences, 12 percent of the felons who would have scored at or below the thirty-five-point cutoff (and therefore would have been recommended for probation or house arrest) committed new crimes, while those who would have scored above thirty-five points had a recidivism rate more than threefold higher (38%). Various critics of this kind of system have focused on the disconnect between most of the attributes in the risk algorithm and "blameworthiness"—some of the variables being immutable (e.g., age) and others (e.g., marital status) reflecting individual opportunities as well as preferences. Bazelon noted that "a woman in her 40's who deals drugs hasn't done anything more to earn trust or deserve a break than a male dealer in his 20's charged with the same offense." But this sort of criticism focuses on the broad relationship between the variables and the outcome, rather than also considering the statistical relationship between the individual and the group "dose-response" functions. The 3:1 relative risk separating those with high and low scores is impressive, but it also implies that 62 percent of those at "high risk" turned out to have been better candidates for mercy than 12 percent of those at "low risk," even though the all of the former offenders would have received harsher sentences. To be sure, the real question here is what the sum of type I and type II errors would be (possibly higher) had the sentencing commissions considered none of the demographic factors and assigned the same sentence to everyone committing a particular crime. This counterfactual gets to the heart of "fairness" in a situation in which we can reduce the misclassification rate by actively tinkering with the intervention or can choose to treat everyone identically. By the former stratagem, some people will receive punishments doubly inappropriate for their true but unknown individual risk of recidivism. The latter approach will probably create more prevalent albeit less severe inequities.

4. *Splitting the population via a relevant explanatory variable, but one for which the within-group variance may exceed the between-group variance.* With the publication of its 2005 "Guidelines for Carcinogen Risk Assessment," EPA took the first small step toward "individualizing" its cancer risk assessments to account for each person's unique susceptibility to carcinogenesis. It divided the human population into three age groups and mandated an additional upward adjustment in some cancer potency factors for two of these groups. For carcinogens thought to have linear dose-response functions in humans, the guidelines incorporate a tenfold upward adjustment for exposures that occur between birth and two years of age and a threefold adjustment for exposures that occur between ages two and fifteen (EPA, 2005b).[14]

According to EPA, therefore, infants as a group are ten times more susceptible than are adults, and exposures during this life stage would need to be one-tenth as high as those allowable for any two-year period in adulthood in order to maintain an acceptably low probability of cancer in either group. The magnitude of this adjustment, however, comes from analysis of many bioassays in which the apparent carcinogenic potency of a given substance in juvenile versus adult animals could be compared (with a "supporting role" given to the one relevant human database, the comparison of cancer incidence in Japanese exposed to atomic bomb radiation as children versus those who were adults in 1945). Because rodents and other test animals are inbred to minimize genetic heterogeneity and are kept in controlled environments that minimize the influence of factors such as disease and concomitant exposures on susceptibility, any observed differences in potency between juvenile and adult animals reflect between-group variations exclusively. However, epidemiologic and biochemical studies of interindividual variability *within* subgroups of the human population (Finkel, 1995a; Hattis and Barlow, 1996), suggest as a first approximation that "typical"[15] adults (and typical children) can differ from each other in their overall susceptibility to carcinogenesis by a factor of twenty-five to fifty or even more, due to differences in metabolism, DNA repair, immune surveillance, and similar factors. An individual adult may therefore need the extra "conservatism" in potency estimation far more than does the average or the "resistant" infant, but only the infants will benefit from EPA's new foray into assessing cancer risk to some individuals.

5. *Splitting the population into any small number of discrete categories when the interindividual variability is continuous.* Even when we recognize that variability is distributed continuously, we often feel compelled to draw "bright lines" that dichotomize the population in order to respond in a workable fashion to the infinite gradations. This practice can, depending on the shape of the function relating susceptibility to risk on either side of the bright line, cause us to focus too little or too much attention on "hypersusceptibles" as defined by a yes/no oversimplification. Hattis (2004) offers an example involving birth weight and infant mortality: he argues that by choosing a 2500-gram cutoff to define low birth weight infants meriting special attention, we fail to intervene to protect babies weighing slightly more than that cutoff, whose individual risks are indeed lower but who collectively account for roughly one-third of all deaths before age one. Similarly, Grodsky (2005) seems to agree with the suggestion Omenn (1982) made over two decades ago: that a bright line of relative risk should govern whether we treat individuals with different genotypes separately from the remainder of the population. If this cutoff was set as high as a 10:1 relative risk (the value Omenn regarded as preferable), people with ninefold-excess susceptibility would be treated as if they were no different from the norm. Such an outcome might reflect a rational balancing of the costs and benefits of providing differential treatment, but such balancing is foreclosed before it can begin when we treat a continuous variable as if it was dichotomous.

6. *Highlighting variability to create a scapegoat.* One additional misuse of information about interindividual variability involves a solid analysis of a relevant source of variation at the individual level, followed by a value-laden adjustment of the result. Arguably, this has taken place with respect to EPA's attempts to estimate the exposure of "the individual most exposed to emissions" as required under the 1990 Clean Air Act Amendments and analogous efforts under other statutes. Beginning in the late 1980s, critics of "conservatism" in risk assessment reserved special derision for EPA's methods for estimating the exposure to the "maximally exposed individual" (MEI); the apotheosis of this effort was probably the argument that only a "porch potato" could be exposed twenty-four hours per day for seventy years (Goldstein, 1989).

EPA may have believed that its procedure to estimate the MEI's exposure yielded a plausible estimate of the extreme tail of the population exposure distribution, perhaps because other assumptions embedded in the calculation, such as breathing rate or environmental concentration, were not in the tails of their respective distributions.[16] Nevertheless, EPA eventually ratcheted back some of the assumptions in the MEI equation and developed constructs such as the "reasonable maximum exposure" and the "high-end exposure estimate," which EPA intended to represent the exposure of an individual between the 90th and 99th percentiles. Most observers, including EPA, have characterized this change as increasing the "realism" of exposure assessment, as if the new type of estimate was simply a more precise (or less fanciful) calculation of the same reference point. But if the reasonable maximum exposure and similar constructs truly represent exposures that between 1 and 10 percent of the population exceed (i.e., perhaps millions of individual U.S. residents), they mark a retreat from the attempt to protect against a true "worst-case" exposure. If so, it appears that focusing on the MEI exposure allowed critics to redefine the "worst case," rather than to confront the benefits and the costs of explicitly rejecting worst-case thinking.

See No Evil: Factors that Opacify the Veil of Ignorance

Although the preceding two sets of examples and discussion are relevant to the subset of human variability that influences risk to environmental and occupational pollutants, the breadth of examples should demonstrate the more general point: that human interindividual variability is often difficult to confront, to depict properly, and to incorporate appropriately into public policy, even when the variation is overt. The challenges only increase when additional research or data-gathering to verify the existence and breadth of variability must precede any analysis and management thereof.

The subset of human variability related to genotype, and the further subset that influences the risk of environmental or occupational disease, carries special baggage that reinforces the general reluctance to begin down the path of individualization. The special hurdles facing genetic susceptibility begin with public discourse about the very possibility of such variation, continue with attempts to quantify its magnitude or to ascribe particular levels of susceptibility to individuals, and ultimately impede attempts to provide information and interventions tailored to individuals according to their susceptibility.

The reluctance to confront these issues is often so strong that the distinction between posing questions and taking irrevocable action based upon the answers has lost much of its meaning. Disquiet over the "tragic choices" we could make with (or without) new knowledge has morphed into revulsion about even seeking the information in the first place. The knowledge that would allow us to consider treating persons differently according to their risk, or to consider treating everyone in a new way because of knowledge about the spectrum of individual risks, is at once both tempting and abhorrent. In recent times, I would argue, abhorrence is carrying the day.

If we continue to see genetic information about environmental susceptibility as a "half-empty" proposition, a negative feedback loop may lock into place. Not wanting our informational capacity to increase could lead to our not advancing the science in ways that could reveal heightened opportunities for public health protection and diminished prospects for mischief. Arguably, this feedback is already occurring, as perhaps seen in Weinstein's chapter in this volume, where he reports that occupational health advocates are generally dismissive of the utility of toxicogenomics in today's regulatory environment.

The prospect of individualizing risk management via genetic information faces a one-two punch from factors one might oversimplify as squeamishness and foreboding. I do not use these terms to imply any unwarranted concerns, only to connote two different phenomena that each may be wholly justified. First, our society has always tiptoed around some manifestations of variation that may be correlated with or caused by immutable characteristics such as race, sex, or age. Even to mention examples where analysis of traits shared by subgroups of the population has revealed apparent associations with other attributes—whether negative or positive—invites both misunderstanding and passion.

To wade briefly into one such controversy, consider the January 2005 speech at the National Bureau of Economic Research by then–Harvard President Lawrence Summers about the underrepresentation of women in tenured faculty positions in science and engineering (Summers, 2005). Summers suggested three possible causative factors, in this "probable order of importance": (1) the possible differential desire of men and women to do "high-powered intense work," exacerbated by the expectations of employers that "the mind is always working on the problems that are in the job, even when the job is not taking place"; (2) the possibility that there are fewer women than men three to four standard deviations above the population mean in mathematical ability (because the variance in mathematical ability among men exceeds that of women, yielding more male mathematical prodigies and more dolts); and (3) the possible influence of the "old boy" network of gender discrimination and "like begets like" hiring practices. I need take no position on the merits or propriety of any of these arguments to observe that at least some of the vitriol that resulted in the unprecedented vote of the Harvard faculty to censure Summers, and that ultimately led to his resignation in 2006, stemmed from his remarks about differential variance in mathematical ability. One professor described those remarks as "reckless and undigested words based in half-baked sociobiological prejudices" (*Harvard Magazine*, 2005, p. 57). Apparently, at least as far back as Darwin's *Descent of Man*, scholars have posited valid reasons why men should and often do exhibit greater genetic variability than do women (Hedges and Nowell, 1995). I suspect, however, that even if Summers had suggested that women have even a higher mean mathematical aptitude but less variability (thus still fewer women at the extreme ends of human mathematical ability), many would still have concluded that one cannot summarize any characteristic of two genetically different groups (in this case, their respective standard deviations) without prejudging (in the pejorative sense) the worth of individuals within them. I suppose that to the extent the characteristic is value-neutral, and to the extent that the genetic difference is wholly uncorrelated with sex, race, or other attributes that define group membership, such observations would be less incendiary. Nevertheless, it seems clear that the very characterization of a group as defined by a genetic commonality makes any further elaboration about that group precarious.

Couple this aversion to genetic information that can open the door to invidious comparisons with a powerful new worry specific to toxicogenomics—foreboding about the deliberate misuse of individual genetic information—and the prospects for personalizing environmental and occupational risk management grow bleaker still. On the one hand, discovering you are at special risk confers potential benefits, such as the ability to protect yourself to a level greater than that enjoyed by those less susceptible or to claim that you deserve such protection in your workplace or community. However, the same discovery can be an unbottled genie that opens you up to a panoply of new harms. In my view, the debate over the peril and promise of toxicogenomics has increasingly accentuated the negative, with some justification (see below). The very term "genetic discrimination" clearly has come to connote something very different from "discriminatory power" in the neutral or positive sense of discerning real differences and intervening appropriately to attenuate or even reward them. Fear of injury, illness, and death has increasingly stepped aside and let other fears play the trump card. Furthermore, in playing one set of rights (for example, the right to die of "natural causes" rather than from involuntary exposures to contaminants in the environment) against the other, I believe we are making little effort to find positive-sum solutions that might extract the benefits of genetic information without accepting the mischief, thereby ensuring that the competing values will remain at odds.[17]

My perspective on these competing rights stems primarily from having worked as a regulatory and enforcement official for the U.S. Occupational Safety and Health Administration (OSHA) and having seen firsthand the repeated failures of our national effort to reduce risks to workers from chronic disease and acute injury to levels that we would consider acceptably low in virtually any other setting. I therefore tend to see a statement such as this one from Silvers and Stein (2002) as an ironic use of the term susceptible: "workers with genetic vulnerabilities to materials found in the workplace . . . seem especially susceptible to rejection on the ground of inability to perform essential functions." The authors clearly intend this as an example of the "dark side" of genetic information and frame "rejection" as the insult—which seems as one-sided as a summary that would say merely that "genetic screening can save the lives of workers who would otherwise face virtual death sentences from exposures that are singularly inappropriate for them," without mentioning the loss of opportunity concomitant with "rejection" (see below).

Given that most OSHA standards (to say nothing of the vast majority of substances for which no OSHA standard exists) allow exposure levels corresponding to lifetime excess risks of 10^{-3} or greater (and as high as roughly 10^{-2} in OSHA's most recent health standard [U.S. Occupational Safety and Health Administration, 2006]), even without accounting for genetic and other variation that may place many workers at even higher individual risk, I find it impossible to view "discrimination" that might lower risks to highly susceptible individuals as solely a detriment to the person or persons involved. Although in environmental policy, typical risk levels (without regard to susceptibility) tend to be two or three orders of magnitude lower than those in the workplace, I still see the potential there to provide highly susceptible individuals with less onerous environmental exposures as a balance that must be struck between competing rights, rather than only as an infringement.[18]

It would be flippant, however, to conclude merely that without life and health, none of the other rights at issue can be enjoyed. Genetic and other information about individual risk potentially impinges on many substantive and cherished rights, raising concerns about

- *Stigmatization.* Identifying persons at high risk of environmental disease because of genetic predisposition raises all of the concerns associated with the original meaning of "stigma"—an indelible mark branding someone as undesirable. This is perhaps the most inchoate but compelling of all the objections to individualized risk assessment, in part because the technology itself is so open-ended. As Silvers and Stein (2002) suggest, acquiescing to a single DNA test, even one where being identified as high-risk confers no stigma, generates personal data that could years later brand you, upon the discovery of a hitherto-unknown genetic marker, as more disadvantaged.[19] The Catch-22 of many of the existing protections against genetic discrimination is that they provide remedies under the Americans with Disabilities Act, thereby making the label "disabled" a price of protection (Silvers and Stein, 2002).
- *Insurability.* Although the federal government (in the 1996 Health Insurance Portability and Accountability Act) and at least forty states have enacted legislation banning some uses of genetic information for denying insurance to otherwise-eligible applicants (Clayton, 2003), concern about insurance companies simply pricing such applicants out of the market remains high. Concern over insurability runs especially high because of an inherent Pandora's box quality of individual genetic information—it can stigmatize or otherwise harm close relatives who were not aware of, or specifically did not consent to have revealed, insights into their own genetic makeup.
- *Job loss.* As several authors in this volume have noted, there currently is no federal law prohibiting private-sector employers from

firing, or refusing to hire, an employee or applicant because of his or her susceptibility to disease. Leaders in the labor movement clearly view employer latitude to screen current and prospective workers for susceptibility as "another form of discrimination against workers" (Sprinker, 2005), rather than as a potential means of selectively reducing the existing discrimination that allows workers as a class to be exposed to risks a thousand to a million times higher than society generally tolerates in the ambient environment (Finkel, 2005). Indeed, the 2002 Supreme Court case *Chevron U.S.A. Inc. v. Echazabal* now explicitly allows employers to deny employment to someone with a medical condition that arguably places him at high risk of disease from exposure to particular substances in that workplace, on the grounds that a basic qualification for employment is the ability to do the job safely, even if the employee's susceptibility places no one else at risk (as would occur in the paradigm scenario of an airline pilot with episodic vertigo).[20]

- *Loss of autonomy.* This concern compasses a variety of harms, beginning with threats to the simple human desire not to know or even to suspect one's susceptibility or disease status—what Diver and Cohen (2001) referred to as the "nocebo effect." [21] This effect might be especially potent when the marker of susceptibility to future exposure implies a grave health problem even in the absence of further exposure.[22] Even if subjects choose to receive the test results, subsequent decisions affecting their autonomy may be beyond their control. The general concern about having to adapt to the environment—keeping one's job but having to wear a respirator, for example—may be as daunting as the prospect of having to leave the environment entirely. Anecdotally, one explanation for the relatively small percentage (about one-quarter) of active OSHA inspectors who, at this writing, have availed themselves of the free blood tests for sensitization to beryllium (Young, 2005) is their concern that a positive test will result in their being assigned to a desk job or prohibited from inspecting those many facilities where beryllium dust could conceivably be present.

- *Debasement.* Some scholars (e.g., Wolf, 1995) believe that the flaws of individualized risk assessment and management do not depend on whether any harms are done to individuals; that a society that embarks on this path debases itself from the outset. Wolf decries

"the eagerness to draw genetic conclusions, the search for suppos-
edly deviant genes, and the conviction that such genes actually deserve disadvantage," and suggests that the "deeper harm" is an
attitude of "geneticism" that derives from repugnant instincts we
should quell. She asserts that seeking and acting upon information
about individual characteristics is offensive "even when based on
accurate rather than exaggerated understanding of the role of genes."
In other words, a test with 100 percent accuracy, used to assess risk
to a single individual without regard to any other characteristics
defining membership in a group (race, sex, age, etc.), dehumanizes
the society that would develop and use it.[23]

Although some of these harms are theoretical, it must be noted that
specific recent uses of information about interindividual variability in
susceptibility tend to validate the concern that the information will be
sought and applied clumsily in practice. Cases such as the blood-testing
policies of Lawrence Berkeley Laboratory, in which African American
employees were reportedly tested repeatedly for sickle cell trait and
syphilis (Silvers and Stein, 2002), and the *Burlington Northern* case referred to throughout this volume, in which the railroad for a time required workers filing claims for carpal tunnel syndrome to submit to
genetic tests for a rare hereditary neuropathy, give credence to a pessimistic stance. These cases and others suggest that fears of misuse, racial
discrimination masquerading as genetic counseling, and blaming the sub-
sidiary cause (the victim) rather than the proximate cause (the environment) are grounded in a sober assessment of economic and social realities.
These concerns are bolstered by examples from the more distant past of
eagerness to distort genetic information (Gould, 1981). The combination
of such specific fears, along with the general reluctance to court social
turmoil, regardless of the case-by-case safeguards that might be built in,
form a potent argument against using many types of scientific information to individualize public health interventions.

I saw these tensions play out as a member of the group that drafted
Executive Order 13145 in 1998–2000 (Clinton, 2000). In developing a
policy that prohibited any federal agency from firing, refusing to hire, or
"classify[ing] employees in any way that would . . . adversely affect that
employee's status" because of information about the employee's genotype (whether gleaned through genetic testing or by information on dis-

ease status of family members), there was essentially no discussion about the potential benefits of such information to heighten protections for individual employees or for the workforce as a whole. Several narrow exemptions were carved out near the end of the process, including a clause (e(1)) that allows OSHA to promulgate future health and safety standards that might allow or require some genetic testing, and a provision (e(3)) that allows the FBI and other agencies to perform genetic testing "to carry out identification purposes," but the order contains no exemptions to protect the health of workers who might face intolerably high excess risks due to genetic susceptibility.

The evolution of subpart (d) of the order, which distinguishes genetic monitoring (the analysis of DNA and other macromolecules to examine mutations acquired during the course of employment) from other genetic testing, indicates how reluctant the other federal agencies in the task force were to "crack open the door" to a perceived genetic technology. When the group hammered out the definition of "genetic test," it was pointed out that "analysis of human DNA . . . to detect disease-related genotypes *or mutations*" (emphasis added) subsumed genetic monitoring, even though that practice cannot reveal information about an individual's or a family member's genotype. By definition, the adducts or point mutations detected are not inborn or shared among relatives, but acquired. The group redefined properly safeguarded "genetic monitoring" as outside the definition of "genetic test," but it nonetheless determined that genetic monitoring would not be permitted in the federal workforce unless the employer "receives results of the monitoring only in aggregate terms that do not disclose the identity of specific employees." The question was left unanswered as to what beneficial use an employer could possibly make of the knowledge that some unknown employee had been overexposed to a workplace contaminant. After all, if the biomonitoring was "nongenetic" in nature, as has been ongoing for many years with respect to measurements of blood lead, urinary cadmium, and other substances in the workplace, we recognize that for the employer to know where engineering controls are inadequate (and to provide paid leave or medical treatment to normalize the excess body burden(s) of the worker(s) affected), she needs to know *whose* test results are abnormal, or at least the work area in which the readings are elevated. Here the concerns over possible misuse of employee-specific (and nongenotypic) information seem to have trumped the intended benefits of a regime with potential for identifying risk-reducing or life-saving interventions—in a microcosm of the direction of the larger debate discussed in this chapter.

Individual genetic information thus repels many thoughtful observers, because it can have far-reaching negative consequences not only for the individuals who submit to testing, but also for their family members, the groups they belong to, and society as a whole. Even when those concerned about the potential for harm acknowledge the possible benefits forgone by restricting the exploration of individual susceptibility, they often damn with faint praise, as in this well-known quote of Francis Collins (Wade, 1998), the director of the Human Genome Project: "This ability to collect very large amounts of [information on] variation on individuals will be quickly upon us. It will empower people to *take advantage of preventive strategies*, but it could also be a nightmare of discriminatory information that could be used against people" (emphasis added).[24]

Rather than a tool to successfully demand an inherently safer workplace or community, individual genetic information is thus portrayed as, at best, information that might force the vigilant individual to work harder to bring about his own health benefit. Similarly, the positive mirror image of susceptibility—"resistance" or immunity—rarely receives attention, yet surely some individuals will benefit (e.g., with lower insurance premiums) from being able to show personal resistance to disease or exposures. Something must explain this overwhelming pessimism, and I offer two observations before proceeding to discuss possible regulatory and public health responses to interindividual variability in susceptibility.

First, perhaps we seek to honor the subset of genetic variation that we need to work hard to detect, as if the genetic code itself hides secrets for a purpose. My sense is that in many of the cases where critics reject differential treatment by genotype, their conclusions would differ if the susceptibility was overt or required no "peeking into the DNA." To oversimplify, I think we would, perhaps reluctantly, agree that albinos (overt variation) should be discouraged from working as lifeguards or hemophiliacs (variation detectable via symptoms or via nongenetic analysis of blood) as meat-cutters—but somehow we conclude that choosing not to know about exposure-specific susceptibilities contained in the genetic code absolves us from confronting such "tragic choices."

Second, perhaps pessimists correctly see individual genetic information as a lose/lose situation, for the following reason: if genetic testing

reveals that individual susceptibility is correlated with group membership, the desire to discriminate against the individual can reinforce or
reawaken the desire to discriminate against the group. But what if—as
seems more biologically plausible in many cases—susceptibility is unrelated to sex, race, age, or ethnicity? Then those identified as high risk become a de facto group, but may be "hung out to dry" because they don't
form a class we otherwise feel poignancy about or because we are reluctant to appear to be discriminating against as a new group.[25] This may
be the most far-reaching concern of all—that individual genetic information can reveal a need to protect, which society can then comfortably
turn its back on, leaving only the stigma behind.

Assuming, therefore, that quantifying susceptibility at the individual
level closes more doors than it opens, the management question remains:
What, if anything, can we do when we know that variation in susceptibility creates a distribution of risks in the environment or workplace, but
when we also believe that learning the identities of those most susceptible carries too high a price?

Does Identifiability Change Everything?

One response to the problem of protecting individuals according to
their susceptibilities would involve lowering the cost of identifying individuals and reducing the likelihood that such identification would be
necessary—in other words, to make identification a last resort when all
other protections have failed and to surround it with additional safeguards. In the occupational setting, executive branch policy or federal or
state legislation could allow for differential treatment of a highly susceptible worker only if several strict conditions were met. Such conditions
might include (1) the diagnosis was reliable and conferred susceptibility
to a specific exposure or exposures in the given workplace; (2) both
relative risk (the degree to which the predisposition elevated the worker's
risk above that of the rest of the workforce) and absolute risk (the probability of harm given exposure) were substantial, so that any "victim-
level controls" such as personal protective equipment or job transfer
would apply only to workers at significant (and significantly elevated)
risk; (3) the information gleaned from any genetic test was the property
of the employee and could not be revealed without consent to any other
party; and (4) differential treatment could not include firing or refusal to

hire, under any circumstances. Most important, the employer seeking to implement a "victim-level" control strategy would have to provide evidence that it was infeasible to further lower ambient exposures, either across-the-board or specific to the susceptible employee or employees. An even more limited role for treating identified hypersusceptible individuals differently might arise in environmental protection; perhaps warnings against excessive consumption of certain contaminated foodstuffs could be targeted primarily at individuals known through genetic testing to be at high relative and absolute risk.

These could be viewed as "stubborn" responses to the tension between rights to health and other rights, with the goal of forcing a balance between them, accepting that some may suffer losses of privacy and autonomy in the name of their own health. *It may be possible, however, to sidestep this tension entirely, by trying to protect populations based on the susceptibilities of unidentified individuals within them.* A "strong form" of such a policy might state that occupational or environmental standards "shall provide acceptably low risk (or 'reasonable certainty of no harm') for X," where X could be defined at a desired level of inclusiveness. Some points along this continuum might include "the entire population including the most susceptible single individual within it," "the population up to and including the average member of the most susceptible subgroup," or "z percent of the population when arrayed in ascending order of susceptibility." A "less strong" form might embrace cost-benefit balancing, but within this framework set monetary values for risk reduction that increase more than linearly as individual risk increases, so that estimates of monetized population risk would not "average away" the disproportionately high risks that susceptible individuals may bear.

Before proceeding any farther to evaluate the merits of either type of policy, one must acknowledge that the very notion that unidentifiable variability could affect public perception or public policy may be illogical or incoherent. Many scholars believe that unidentifiable variability in risk cannot matter, for several reasons. This view generally begins by acknowledging that identifiability clearly makes us much more concerned about high individual risks and those who face them. Jenni and Loewenstein (1997), for example, introduce their paper on the "identifiable victim effect" with a compelling observation made by Thomas Schelling in 1968, attesting to the much higher implicit value we tend to place on human life when we can "rescue" an identified person.[26] If identifiability confers such a premium, it certainly is possible that the converse is true—that absent identifiability, the mere knowledge that someone's risk is intolerably high is of no particular consequence, beyond the proportional effect of those risks on the total risk to the population. More formally, the most powerful argument in favor of the proposition that a distribution of unidentifiable individual risks can and should be reduced to the average probability of harm observes that each individual probability of being susceptible is itself a risk, and asserts that only the expectation of this "second-order probability" should affect the perception of harm.

Consider these hypothetical scenarios, involving two cities, each having one million inhabitants, and a proposal on the table to locate a new source emitting a carcinogenic air pollutant in each city. In city A, the inhabitants all have identical genotypes and environmental histories, such that their additional lifetime risk from the new chemical is 10^{-4}. In city B, ten thousand of the inhabitants are highly (one hundredfold more) susceptible to the carcinogenic effects of the pollutant, such that their excess lifetime risk is 10^{-2}, and the other 990,000 people in city B are immune and face no risk. In both cities, one hundred people are expected to die from their exposures (10^6 people in city A multiplied by a uniform risk of 10^{-4} equals 100; 10^4 susceptibles in city B at a 10^{-2} risk also yields 100).[27] It is thus plausible to argue that any individual, lacking any information on his individual susceptibility, should be indifferent between living in city A or city B; in either case, his expected excess risk with the new pollutant source would be 10^{-4}, or the number of fatalities divided by the population size.

Jenni and Lowenstein (1997) support this view, using a medical hypothetical with slightly different parameters, when they say, "It probably makes no sense to treat a disease that kills 100% of the 10% of the population susceptible to it differently from one that kills 10% of the 100% of the population susceptible to it" (in both cases, the expected individual risk here is 10^{-1}). Adherents to this view presumably allow for departures from risk-neutrality at the societal level. The decision maker concerned about a population of size P may either prefer to accept a distribution of possible numbers of total fatalities whose mean is X to a certainty of accepting exactly X fatalities (risk proneness), or vice versa (risk aversion), but the individual citizen should be indifferent between an uncertain personal risk with mean X ÷ P and a risk known with certainty to

be exactly X ÷ P. Note that in the hypothetical above, the binomial uncertainty in the number of fatalities around X = 100 is small compared
with X and is almost exactly the same in city A versus city B (see below).

If variability in risk has no significance until we can ascribe particular points on the risk distribution to particular persons, then as a practical matter we should feel comfortable censoring information about
interindividual variability that only reveals the breadth of differences
among people. The answer to people who express concern about equity
as well as efficiency would simply be that "people can't be treated inequitably if neither we nor they know who they are."[28] However, it would
be imperative to admit that "the mean is not the message" and perhaps
to control hazards differently based on the distribution of individual risk,
if unidentifiable variability does matter, which I will argue it does.

Is "Someone" Identification Enough?

In contrast to the proposition that only identifiability reifies human
variability, several arguments support the view that the distribution itself may be as compelling as the identities of everyone described by it.

One argument does not even require the individuals themselves to
care about unidentifiable variability. Even if information on the number of fatalities and its uncertainty is sufficient to make risk-management decisions, ignoring interindividual variability in risk can lead to
errors and biases in estimating both the mean and variance of the "body
count." The assessor who focuses on the fatality distribution may not
realize what Feller (1968) referred to as a "striking result": the uncertainty in the number of events from a binomial process is at its *maximum* when the probability of success or failure is identical for each
member of a population.[29] The decision maker in city A above expects
one hundred extra fatalities but should expect a standard deviation of
almost exactly ten around this mean estimate. In city B, however, the
number of fatalities is less uncertain (the standard deviation is approximately 9.95), because in this exaggerated case where the risk is completely concentrated in a subpopulation, there are fewer people who
contribute anything to the "body count." Therefore, a decision maker
who is risk averse (or risk seeking) with respect to the total number of
fatalities in the population may be less (or more) concerned about a
hazard if it applies to a diverse population rather than to a homoge-

neous one. Put another way, ignoring variability known to be present leads to an exaggerated estimate of the actual uncertainty in the number of fatalities or cases of disease, even if the estimate is correct on average—so this may affect the decision even if one is wholly uninterested in the distribution of individual risks.

A different and probably more substantial problem concerns bias, rather than uncertainty, in estimating the expected number of fatalities. The central limit theorem dictates that the observed mean is a useful estimate of the true population mean, but in the presence of unmeasured variability, the errors in that estimate may be much larger and more complicated than elementary statistics suggests. Suppose that the risk of some event was strongly related to income, so we needed to know the average income of the population to estimate risk. In this case, the influence of outliers is strong and asymmetric, such that it is hard to get an accurate estimate of the mean income unless by chance the sample contains the correct proportion of very rich people. Too many billionaires and the estimate of the mean will be much too high; too few, and the opposite will be true. It turns out that for quantities such as income, exposure, and susceptibility, that are nonnegative and distributed approximately normally on a logarithmic scale, the error in sample estimates of the mean is itself lognormally distributed. It is more likely that the observed mean will be slightly below the population mean, but the largest absolute errors will be those less likely instances where the observed mean is much larger than the population mean (Finkel, 1990).[30]

Thus the paradox: even if the average is all that matters, it can be very difficult to find the true average without first exploring the entire distribution which contains it. This is a powerful argument for quantifying variability even when it is nonidentifiable, which would then put us in the position of having to ignore information on variability that we have already accounted for. We can still struggle over how to act on this knowledge, but it seems that treating diverse populations as homogeneous can do violence to efficiency (expected-value decision making) as well as to equity.

Beyond the value of quantifying unidentifiable variability in revealing important characteristics of population risk, various other arguments run counter to the view that individuals should be satisfied with an estimate of their mean risk. Do we really believe that situations where an entire population faces an identical probability of harm are perceptually and ethically equivalent to situations where the mean probability is unchanged but the individual (albeit unidentifiable) probabilities spread farther and farther apart from each other? Is a disease that kills one in ten people at random truly equivalent to one that kills everyone of the 10 percent of the population susceptible to it?

A precondition for answering "no" to these questions is agreeing that individual risks themselves are not merely weights that moderate the ultimate outcome (death, disease, injury, etc.), but have salience of their own.[31] Then, the one in one hundred chance that a resident of city B will face a risk of 10^{-2} is not the same as a certain risk of 10^{-4}; not knowing whether one is at high risk or no risk is simply not the same as knowing for sure that one is at an intermediate level of risk. Put a different way, we often assign a "value of life" estimate to gauge the human cost of imposing an individual risk, the cost to each person being the "value of life" multiplied by the probability of fatality. If the magnitude of that cost has anything but a strictly linear relationship to the size of the risk, then the distribution of risks matters. Only if every risk of magnitude kX is exactly k times as adverse as every risk of X can we reduce the distribution to an average without distorting the conclusion.[32]

I suggest that the very notion of "unacceptable," "intolerable," or "significant" risk says something profound about how we think about individual risk: namely, that as individual risk levels rise, our level of concern may rise faster than dictated by strict proportionality. Guidance on cost-benefit analysis promulgated by the U.S. Office of Management and Budget (2003) cautions that any monetization based on the "value of a statistical life" must be limited to "small changes in fatality risk" (the technique has "no application . . . to very large reductions in individual risks"), reflecting the notion that the total harm done to a million people facing a 10^{-6} risk is qualitatively different from (smaller than) the total harm done to two people, each facing a 50 percent risk, even though one "statistical life" is lost in either case.

Of the various empirical and theoretical arguments that high individual risks matter even before we identify those who face them, the hardest two to decouple relate to fear and fairness. Evidence that people regard the possibility of being highly susceptible (and thus at higher risk) as qualitatively worse than an equivalent certainty of being at lower risk could reflect either what we fear or what we regard as unfair, or both. Either way, widely varying individual risks generally arouse more concern than otherwise identical risks reported as invariant. Lopes (1984) reported that the degree of inequality in a distribution of risks, *ceteris paribus*, is a powerful predictor of the aversion subjects report to the situations. More recently, Ritov and Baron (1990) surveyed whether respondents would vaccinate their own babies against a strain of flu that would kill ten of every ten thousand unvaccinated babies, as they varied the hypothetical probability of death from the side effects of the vaccine itself. On average, respondents would elect not to vaccinate if the side-effect risk exceeded approximately 5.5 per ten thousand. Ritov and Baron concluded that the unwillingness to vaccinate, even when the net risk of doing so was still negative, reflected "omission bias," the special aversion to the chance that an act of commission, rather than one of omission, would result in grave harm. But when respondents were told that 1 percent of babies were highly susceptible to death from side effects of the vaccine (and that the other 99% were immune), the mean risk of side effects at which people were no longer willing to vaccinate dropped significantly (to 4.5 per ten thousand), even though respondents were told that no test could identify which children were susceptible. When respondents were instead told that the susceptible subgroup arose because "the vaccine interacts with a certain chemical naturally produced by the body" in 1 percent of children, the maximum acceptable side-effect risk dropped still farther (to 3.2 per ten thousand). The authors speculated that "the perception of missing information can make people reluctant to act, even when the information is unobtainable," which would explain why the more detailed information about the cause of the susceptibility increased the aversion to vaccination.

An alternative explanation, however, looks to empathy and public perception of fairness. If a risk is found to be confined to 1 percent of the population but has the same mean as reported before, then the individual risk to the susceptibles has been reevaluated at one hundredfold greater than before. Willingness to accept an evenly shared risk of 5.5 per ten thousand, but not a 1 percent chance of a risk of 3.2 per hundred, could suggest that we are repelled to think that some people face risks that large (or that we are afraid that we are among the unlucky or unfortunate). Or perhaps we simply tend to view as more dire those situations where we are not "all in this together." When I first read Cranor's discussion of the "eggshell plaintiff" (Cranor, 1997), I concocted a mental picture of susceptibility as akin to a fanciful situation where a group of a thousand people is confronted with the choice between two "risk rooms." In one room, a rain of gravel will fall from the ceiling, at just the right intensity to kill one of the thousand at random from a hemorrhage in a crucial blood vessel. In the second room, a boulder will drop and crush one of the thousand. In examining why I perceive the second situation as more dreadful, personal fear is not really a satisfactory explanation, because whether I was standing under the boulder or was unlucky enough to be harmed by the gravel, I wouldn't know it until it was too late—it has to be the removal of the shared risk that distinguishes the two rooms. Ex post, someone in the second room turns out to have been facing a crushing risk (literally) all along, while the rest will learn ex post that they were not in fact sharing in this grisly lottery, and this seems to make the one in a thousand chance of facing certain death worse than the certainty of a one in a thousand risk.

Whether fear or fairness (or both) drives this concern, it would be much more useful to be able to gauge *how much* we care about unidentifiable victims in the tail of the risk distribution, beyond the observation that the information may affect us qualitatively. The answer to this estimation problem will doubtless vary across respondents and across situations, but probably the two most important determinants are inversely correlated with each other (for a constant population mean risk, so we can be comparing situations with equal expected fatalities): (1) the proportion of the population at highest risk and (2) how substantially those high risks exceed the typical risks. For example, the population risk in city B would also equal that in "city A" if the susceptible subgroup consisted of 0.1 percent of the population at one thousandfold excess risk, 40 percent of the population at 2.5-fold excess risk, and so on. Qualitatively, I think it possible that at one extreme (the smallest fraction are susceptible and their excess risk is maximal), concern might diminish, on the grounds that those most affected are "too few, too different" (or, regrettably, so frail that protecting them from one risk would only allow them to succumb to one of many other maladies to which they are also hypersusceptible). At the other extreme (very large numbers of individuals at only slightly elevated risk), very minor policy changes, if any, would be needed to account for the variation. This suggests that it is in the intermediate cases where smashing our myths of homogeneity in risk might be most profoundly unsettling to the status quo.

One useful way to summarize and communicate the interplay between the breadth of a risk distribution and the probability that a random person will face greatly elevated risk is to explore the "concentration function," the relationship between the fraction of the population contained within different portions of the distribution and the fractional amount of the total characteristic (in this case, risk) within each portion. Perhaps the most familiar recent use of concentration functions involves various benchmarks of the fraction of total U.S. wealth (or tax burden) associated with different deciles and percentiles of the population (e.g., Johnston [2005], featuring statistics such as "the share of the national income earned by those in this uppermost category [the top 0.1%] has more than doubled since 1980, to 7.4% in 2002").

Figure 17.1 makes use of a simple formula (Finkel, 1990) for the concentration function of a lognormal distribution and shows the fraction of the risk borne by three arbitrary subgroups in a heterogeneous population—those whose susceptibilities place them in the 90 percent of the population at lowest risk, those between the 90th and 99th percentiles, and those above the 99th—as a function of the amount of variability in the population. A vertical line drawn for any degree of variability divides the three groups according to their "mass," or the fraction of the total number of fatalities in the population that will befall each group. For example, at a logarithmic standard deviation of 2.0 (describing a situation where 10 percent of the population faces risks at least thirteen times greater than (or one-thirteenth as great as) the typical person, and 1 percent faces risks at least 105 times greater or smaller), about 39 percent of the fatalities will befall the 9 percent of people in the middle group. That is, if one hundred thousand people face a mean risk of 10^{-3}, thirty-nine of the one hundred expected total deaths would occur among the nine thousand people belonging to this subgroup—and *their* average risk would in fact be thirty-nine in nine thousand, or more than four per thousand.[33]

As the variability increases, the concentration of expected fatalities in the uppermost 1 percent of the population naturally increases as well, but I think it is important to note that the consequences that befall the "reasonably highly susceptible" subgroup (i.e., the height of the dashed arrow in Figure 17.1 in the unshaded portion as it moves across the diagram) is rather insensitive to assumptions about overall variability. For all values of the logarithmic standard deviation between 1.0 and 2.6,

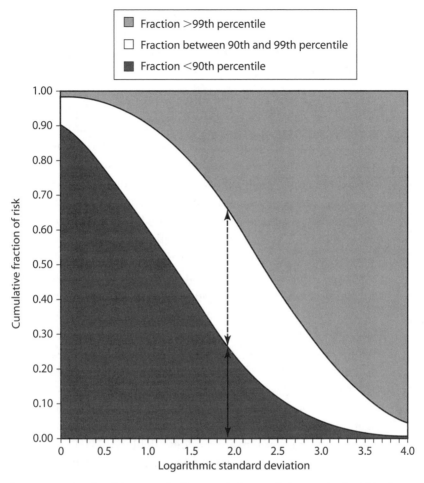

Figure 17.1. Fractional amount of a lognormal characteristic contained within three portions of a heterogeneous population.

roughly one-third of all the risk is concentrated among those more susceptible than most but less susceptible than the "outliers."[34] Perceptions of "how safe is safe enough?" therefore, may be enriched and changed if we consider that perhaps 30 percent of the benefits of more stringent controls (which is to say, 30 percent of the total harm done by stopping short of eliminating the risk) will accrue to those among us who are moderately, but not exceedingly susceptible. Nine percent of the affected U.S. population could comprise upward of 25 million people in the case of a ubiquitous pollutant.

Other, more pragmatic arguments exist in favor of the proposition that knowing the extent of variation in risk may trigger the same perceptual and policy changes as knowing the identities of those at different points on the distribution:

- *Perhaps without realizing it, we already let unidentifiable variability in exposure affect policy.* Although some exposure models allow the analyst to pinpoint the identity of the people whose exposures determine the stringency of a regulatory standard (e.g., sportfishermen who consume a given large amount of their catch), often the models produce an unidentifiable distribution and an unidentifiable reference point. For example, air dispersion models may specify the concentration of a pollutant at the geographic location where an emissions plume exerts its maximal effect but only in terms of the radial distance from the emission source without regard to direction. We learn in such cases how much exposure the MEI receives, but not who the MEI is. Evidently, this circumscribed knowledge is sufficient to drive risk management.[35]
- *Perhaps without realizing it, we also have already let unidentifiable variability in economic burden affect policy.* To the extent that concern over the upper tail of the distribution of compliance costs can cause regulators to relax the stringency of a proposed standard, or abandon a regulatory attempt altogether, often the specific individuals or companies at risk are not identifiable. At OSHA, for example, economists would declare that a proposed exposure limit was infeasible if analysis showed that one or more broad industry classes might have to expend a significant fraction of profits to reduce exposures to that level. The answer to the question "for whom would this standard be economically infeasible?," had anyone ever asked, would have been "someone."
- *Congressional intent motivates attempts to protect identifiable (and probably unidentifiable) subpopulations.* The text of the major environmental statutes, and judicial comment on them, may shed light on what role variability, identifiable or otherwise, can or must play in regulation. Based in large part on Grodsky's (2005) excellent summary, one can conclude that most of EPA's statutes endorse—or even demand—that the agency provide an acceptable level of residual risk for people of heightened susceptibility.

Much of the fine-tuning of regulatory stringency EPA has under-taken (some *sua sponte*, some in response to court rulings) has in-volved the slight ratcheting back of standards that would have protected every conceivable member of the exposed population, suggesting that inclusiveness, rather than protection of the average person, is the default presumption (see, for example, Grodsky's (2005) summary of the D.C. circuit court's instructions that EPA provide a "plausible explanation" why its SO_2 standard would fail to protect all asthmatics undergoing strenuous exercise). The lan-guage from the legislative history of the Clean Air Act of 1970 that the authors cite (protecting "a representative sample of persons com-prising the sensitive group rather than a single person in such group") allows EPA some discretion. This language, though, makes sense only in the context of epidemiology or controlled human ex-perimentation, in which researchers could directly observe expo-sure levels that affect some individuals but do not cause a statistically significant elevation in the health status of the group they belong to. When EPA has to extrapolate from animal toxicol-ogy data to set a standard, there is no "statistically related sample" of humans to study directly, which puts EPA back in the position of having to account for human variability through risk assessment and having to articulate explicitly what fraction of the population its standards are designed to protect.

The more important question for legal interpretation is whether Congress has ever forbidden EPA from protecting subpopulations whose risk can be estimated but whose members cannot or will not be identified. To be sure, references to "identifiable subgroups" per-vade environmental statutes and interpretations, as befits their draft-ing at a time when susceptibility was oversimplified as all-or-none and associated with other salient characteristics such as age and race. However, there appears to be no legal or policy barrier to con-struing these references to include *subgroups defined completely by their susceptibility*, as in "people with α-1-antitrypsin defi-ciency," or even "people whose 'area under the curve' (molecules of a toxic metabolite produced in a target tissue) puts them at the 95th percentile of the distribution of this quantity." I assume that even the more specific language in the Safe Drinking Water Act Amendments of 1996 ("infants, children, . . . or other subpopulations that can be identified and characterized") is perfectly compatible with "identification" in the population sense—estimating the relative size of a subgroup defined by a particular predisposition and estimating the potency of that predisposition to increase disease risk—rather than in the sense of "identifying" the specific individuals at heightened risk.[36]

- *At least one well-known federal regulation is already based on the risk to the unidentifiable individuals at the "reasonably high" end of the distribution of biological variation in susceptibility.* OSHA's regulation of methylene chloride (U.S. Occupational Safety and Health Administration, 1997) demonstrates that quantitative information about interindividual variability in susceptibility can be amassed, analyzed, and used to set a risk-based exposure limit. In the proposed version of the methylene chloride standard, OSHA had generated a point estimate of excess cancer risk to exposed workers using positive mouse tumor data coupled with OSHA's standard assumption that doses could be extrapolated from mice to humans via the relative body weights of the two species. In revising the risk assessment during 1995-97, OSHA decided that various teams of researchers had adequately demonstrated that a physiologically based pharmacokinetic model of methylene chloride metabolism in mice and humans better explained the interspecies differences.

  Data existed, however, pointing to significant interindividual variability in enzyme kinetics and other biochemical parameters within the human population. OSHA staff and contractors used a Bayesian method to integrate published information about the uncertainty in approximately thirty pharmacokinetic parameters in mice and humans with individual data on human variability, taking special care to estimate and account for correlations between relevant pairs of parameters.

  Although my OSHA colleagues and I were unable, due to limitations in the data, to completely decouple uncertainty and variability (and did not attempt to quantify uncertainty or variability in the function relating tumor response to delivered dose), we did develop a probability density function for delivered dose that described the excess risk at a given workplace concentration of methylene chloride for individuals with different pharmacokinetic behavior (U.S. Occupational Safety and Health Administration, 1997). We asserted that it was a reasonable interpretation of the 1980 *Benzene* decision to consider the risk to the (unidentifiable) individual at the 95th percentile of this distribution. The risk at this reference point was approximately tenfold higher than the risk at the median of the new distribution, and approximately threefold higher than the mean risk, because the distribution was right-skewed.[37]

The stakes associated with the OSHA methylene chloride standard may not have been as high as in many of EPA's rule makings. However, the fact that this part of an overall controversial analysis was not challenged during congressional oversight hearings or in ultimately successful negotiations among government, industry, and labor to avoid litigation over the rule, suggests that protecting unidentifiable individuals at the tail of a risk distribution can win acceptance as sound science and as sound science policy.

Conclusion: Toward Embedded Precaution in Risk-Based Policy

Three observations have led me to identify an impasse and to suggest a particular solution to it:

1. Individual risks do matter, and reducing risks to acceptably low levels for as many individuals as possible, consistent with feasibility or other cost-benefit thinking, is the core mission of environmental and occupational health;
2. Knowing the identities of those at highest risk would ensure that we would try to protect them assiduously, but knowing merely that they exist imposes similar, if not identical, ethical duties; and
3. Even if identifiability would cement in place policies that otherwise might be "hard sells," we cannot wait for identification that may never come, because it is held back by legitimate concerns over the use and misuse of individual information related to susceptibility to disease.

In the light of these factors, I prefer a "strong form" (see above) of a science-policy response to unidentifiable variability: we should learn as much as we can about the population parameters of interindividual vari-

ation, and ratchet up our environmental/occupational health goals to acknowledge and protect those—identifiable or not—who would otherwise
be left behind. The foundation of such a policy would be the assertion
that above some individual probability of grave harm (Congress' various
instructions to EPA setting this "bright line" at 10^{-6} may strain the limits of feasibility, while OSHA's clinging to the Supreme Court's uppermost benchmark of 10^{-3} arguably errs in the other direction), involuntary
risks are presumptively unacceptable if they can be reduced further. To
the extent we can do so for all citizens, regardless of their susceptibility
to the effects of a particular substance or stressor, we will recognize, as
Cranor suggests (this volume), that "their claim to protection is not nonexistent or extinguished" because of their genetic makeup or prior exposure history. I therefore endorse the suggestion of Hattis and Anderson
(1999) that agencies should try to extend the mantle of protection to a
relatively high proportion of the entire population, defined either by
choosing a reference point such as the 99th percentile of a continuous
distribution of sensitivities or a related reference point such as "the average member of the most susceptible significant subpopulation" (Cranor, this volume).[38]

The raw material to drive such policies must come from the examination and testing of individual human beings, coupled with sophisticated
biostatistical techniques (Bois, 2001) to separate uncertainty in the measurement of biological parameters from the variability revealed in multiple measurements. Therefore, Congress should consider, as a higher
priority than the recent contentious and long-delayed proposals to regulate genetic information in employment, funding an array of such studies, after establishing a set of strict protections to safeguard the rights of
the smaller number of subjects needed to amass information about population variability. For example, genetic and biochemical information
should be gleaned from volunteers who agree to be studied for this purpose, it should be encrypted, and it should be divulged only to the individual involved (who assents to receive the information) and to no
other party for any reason, in any form that can be traced back to the specific individual tested.[39]

With each new finding of a genetic or other source of human variation that is likely to affect susceptibility to environmental disease, we
need to move quickly to gauge the prevalence of this factor in the human population and the extent to which it heightens susceptibility. The

regulatory agencies need to keep abreast of this information—if any new micromanagement of risk assessment needs to emanate from the Office of Management and Budget or Congress, it is here—for the critical purpose of determining whether existing controls adequately reduce risks to an acceptably large fraction of the population.

I can also easily imagine two "less strong" forms of this policy that might be useful. First, if it is crucial to gauge the monetary benefit of providing acceptable risk to a large fraction of the population, we could accommodate susceptible individuals into a cost-benefit framework, simply by abandoning the fiction that benefit is strictly proportional to the reduction in the average probability of harm. The benefits of eliminating emissions in city B exceed those in city A by an amount we could estimate in light of econometric research, because the benefit to each person freed from a 10^{-2} risk exceeds the benefit to one hundred people freed from a 10^{-4} risk. Second, in many situations we might be able to provide equivalent protection at reduced costs by controlling risks at the "victim level," but in a way very different from the discriminatory methods (e.g., job reassignment) that critics of genetic screening focus on. Rather than identifying hypersusceptible individuals and, for example, providing them bottled water as an alternative to cleaning the groundwater they drink from, we could encourage such "victim-level" controls across-the-board, even if they are necessary for only a small fraction of those who receive them, with the consent of the affected population. This would merely substitute one infringement for another, of course, but here we would be inconveniencing (or worse, I acknowledge) a majority in order not to identify the minority.

A policy goal of protecting unidentifiable individuals may ultimately be an accommodation to the concerns about discrimination, without surrendering to Kierkegaard's concern (see fn 23) that we "heap [people] in a mass and defraud them." Such an approach may be the wave of the future, not only in the environmental and occupational health arena. I see a close analogy between the topic of this volume and the observations Cook (2005) made about medical care and insurance: "It is precisely this danger [genetic discrimination], however, that may lead to a great breakthrough: the inevitable movement to universal health care. . . . Only [thus] will we be able to pool risk for the entire country and share what nature has dealt us; only then will there be no motivation for anyone or any organization to ferret out an individual's confidential, genetic makeup."

Sullivan (2000) said the same thing more pointedly: "In the long run, only the government will be dumb enough or enlightened enough to mandate a national insurance pool that works." Substitute "mandate a system of environmental and occupational health standards that protects people without punishing them for their genes," and you have one prediction about the direction the toxicogenomics revolution may take us.

In either health care or environmental protection, the most serious looming threat to such an evolution seems to be the possible backlash from citizens who realize, as they should, that protecting the tail of risk distributions is tantamount to "overprotecting" the majority. Robert and Smith (2004, p. 511) allude to this, in the context of victim-level controls that remove susceptibles from exposure, by stating "we may witness pressure to increase the tolerable level of toxins in the environment," but that same concern has always applied to across-the-board controls that might increase economic costs to many in the name of protecting the few.

In trying to predict whether such a backlash will occur, I am partly comforted by the track record of overestimation of regulatory costs (Goodstein and Hodges, 1997), which suggests that the price of "overprotection" may not be nearly as high as agencies and the regulated community initially portray. But fairness and fear, especially if they reinforce each other, may be even more important than cost in determining the overall tenor of environmental protection in the age of toxicogenomics. On fairness, echoes of support for protecting unidentifiable individuals can be found in an ancient source: Maimonides's "eight degrees of charity" (Sacks, 2005). Other than giving someone a job so they no longer need charity (the highest degree), the highest form of charity, according to Maimonides, occurs when neither the giver nor the recipient know each other's identities. The practical downsides of identifying those most in need of protection thus encourage us to embrace a system in which we all, depending on the hazard, can participate in this rarefied form of altruism.

In our field of endeavor, with the new knowledge that "genetics loads the gun" for each one of us as we live in a sea of environmental stressors, the line between fairness and self-interest has begun to blur more and more. Many observers of risk assessment and management, notably Justice Breyer (1993), have interpreted the following passage of John Donne (1624/1839) as an appeal to altruism: "Any man's death diminishes me, because I am involved in mankind; and therefore never send to know for whom the bell tolls; it tolls for thee." But in light of genetic and environmental variability, I have always read this passage as an appeal to self-interest as well and have found that the original title of Donne's "Meditation 17," from which this passage is drawn, supports that reading. That title, "Nunc Lento Sonitu Dicunt, Morieris," means "now this bell, tolling for another, says to me 'thou must die.'" So "the bell tolls for thee" not only because humanity is morally interconnected, but also because our risks and our vulnerabilities are shared. Later in this meditation, Donne provides the ultimate argument for the "strong form" of reducing unidentifiable risks: "by this consideration of another's danger, I take mine own into contemplation, and so secure my self."

ACKNOWLEDGMENTS

I gratefully acknowledge helpful suggestions from L.A. (Tony) Cox, David Hassenzahl, Gary Marchant, Richard Sharp, and Troy Tucker.

NOTES

1. The examples used in this chapter reflect many different types of human interindividual variability: differences in exposure, susceptibility, economic burden, preferences, and so on. Most of the prescriptive discussion will deal with variability in susceptibility, defined here as a predisposition—due to genotype or other factors such as health status, nutrition, concomitant exposures, and the like—to disease caused by specific exposures in the workplace or the general environment. Occasionally, I will further distinguish "genetic susceptibility" from susceptibility governed by those other factors.

2. All of the analysis and discussion of this issue raised in this article occurred before the events of September 2001, which have forever changed the way we think about "groundlings," so this example must be viewed wholly apart from that tragedy. The cited articles did not specify "unintentional" airplane crashes, although the data therein still apply to fatalities caused by factors other than terrorist acts.

3. Although at one point Goldstein et al. say that the risk was "shown to be in the range of 10^{-5} to 10^{-6} lifetime," in context this clearly seems to be an attempt to calibrate the risk with reference to the subset of risks at this rough order of magnitude, not a statement about the uncertainty or variability in the risk. The authors refer to this range as "a range in which our society seems to have achieved a consensus that governmental action to protect public health is appro-

priate in environmental matters, yet well below the range of usual everyday risks to which we react on a personal level."

4. Although the "groundlings" example involves exposure to safety hazards, the literature on exposure to environmental hazards is replete with similar population-based thinking. For example, Mossman (1997) concludes that "radio-sensitivity is a minor host factor in carcinogenesis," on the grounds that "cigarette smoking and diet each account for 15-18 times as many cancer deaths as ionizing radiation." But to an individual person who does not smoke but who is exposed to appreciable levels of radiation in the workplace or the home, the national "body count" matters not at all—from his vantage point, radiation may be far more important.

5. In fact, earlier versions of the guidelines attempted to justify the decision not to adjust individual or population risk estimates to account for human variation in susceptibility by citing studies (Allen, Crump, and Shipp, 1988; Goodman and Wilson, 1991; Hoel and Portier, 1994) showing that linear extrapolation using animal data tended on average neither to overestimate nor underestimate expected cancer death rates for the same substances as verified by epidemiologic data. A process that accurately estimates the population risk cannot, of course, overestimate risk for all or nearly all members of that population; it must underestimate risk to many. EPA may have realized that the conclusion and the explanation contradict each other: in the final version of the guidelines, only the conclusion remains, as if the explanation was a Cheshire cat.

6. We transferred two blastocysts and were blessed with one healthy daughter.

7. Aversion to one possible outcome over another is, of course, another factor that varies dramatically across individuals. Guidelines that assume a single set of preferences for every patient can impel "irrational" decisions. For example, the recommendation that pregnant women undergo amniocentesis when their risk of carrying a fetus with Down syndrome exceeds the risk of a procedure-induced miscarriage implicitly assumes equal aversion to each negative outcome (Harris et al., 2001).

8. Lack of interest in the distribution of costs may also reveal a fundamental illogic in cost-benefit policy. In theory, actions that benefit "winners" in total more than they harm "losers" are "potential Pareto-optimal" because the winners can compensate the losers such that everyone's benefit increases (or does not decrease). Many concerns have been raised about whether the ex post compensation ever occurs in practice (Ackerman and Heinzerling, 2004)—but without taking an interest in the distribution of costs (i.e., identifying those who should provide compensation and those who ought to receive it), voluntary or mandatory compensation can't even be contemplated in theory.

9. In general, the more ubiquitous the product or process whose externalities (pollution) are controlled, the more the costs of control tend to be shared across the entire population. More citizens participate in spreading out the costs of reducing pollution from gasoline combustion than from golf club manufacture, so

the implicit assumption that costs are shared universally and equally is more dubious in the latter case.

10. Perhaps ironically, economists working within the risk analysis system have kept the pressure on for decisions informed by quantitative risk determinations rather than by nonrisk measures such as the reference dose or the "margin of exposure" (Workshop, 2000).

11. Note that this phraseology may also encompass subsets of homosexual men whose risks are even lower than that of the general population, although perhaps it is significant that this category is not specifically acknowledged.

12. A similar example from the environmental and occupational arena can be seen in the debate over whether EPA should be required to use "real data" on the number of years the average resident lives in his home before moving to another location (Hamilton, Vicusi, and Dockins, 1997), rather than assuming exposure for a seventy-year life span. The analogous issue at OSHA contrasts the standard assumption of a forty-five-year working lifetime with data indicating that the average worker changes jobs five or more times during a career (Burmaster, 2000). In either case, advocates for a data-driven approach often seem oblivious that changing homes (or jobs) is not tantamount to changing exposures. If we allow every point source of chemical X to emit seven times more of it because people live near the source for only one-seventh of a lifetime, on average, then only those fortunate enough to move to pristine areas in every subsequent move will not see their risks rise by up to the factor of seven (see NRC, 1994, pp. 217-18, for a recommendation that EPA not succumb to this fallacy). The same problem holds in the workplace, where the relevant variable is years of exposure, not years of employment at any particular establishment or job title.

13. Virginia's algorithm sums nine subscores to generate a total score of between 3 and 76. Factors leading to a higher total score include: larceny as the precipitating offense; offender being male, younger than thirty, not regularly employed, or unmarried; prior arrest within the previous eighteen months; and number of prior incarcerations (especially if both as a juvenile and as an adult). As a result, a twenty-nine-year-old unmarried, unemployed male would start with thirty-six points (above the cutoff), even if he had no prior criminal record.

14. For exposures throughout the life span, the net effect of this three-tiered potency system is to multiply risk by a factor approximately 60 percent above its value under the assumption that susceptibility is not heightened in younger persons. The tenfold factor applies for $2 \div 70$ of the life span, and the threefold factor for an additional $13 \div 70$ of the life span: $10(2 \div 70) + 3(13 \div 70) + 1(55 \div 70) = 114 \div 70$, or 1.63. As the main text suggests, however, a factor of 1.6 may be dwarfed by the actual variation among children or among adults.

15. "Typical" in this context refers to individuals who don't display profound (and often obvious) characteristics, such as Down syndrome, that can inflate susceptibility to cancer even more markedly than can combinations of less profound predispositions.

16. Certainly twenty-four hours is at the 100th percentile of the distribution of hours per day of possible exposure. In many other cases, however, parameters criticized for being "outside the distribution" have (or already had) been found to underestimate the extreme value in the population. Many of EPA's early assumptions about food consumption patterns were later found to underestimate consumption among defined subpopulations. Similarly, OSHA risk assessments continue to use forty-five years as the maximum time that any employee can possibly be exposed to a particular hazardous substance in the workplace, even though the agency routinely receives public comment from workers and their families attesting to longer exposure periods (with the same employer, or in a series of jobs with identical exposures).

17. In a recent presentation of (Finkel, 2007), I argue that the brief history of policy analysis of a similar issue—the emphasis on the possible risk-increasing side effects of interventions to reduce environmental risk—has also been marked by the pitting of one set of problems against another with a bias toward inaction. Inevitable risk-risk trade-offs may strongly argue against trying to control a primary risk, but the concern over side effects could instead motivate the search for actions that reduce both the primary and offsetting risks.

18. If, as various analyses suggest, environmental health risk assessments may underestimate risk to highly susceptible individuals by a factor of fifty- or one hundredfold, risk-based standards that reduce average risks to 10^{-5} may mask individual risks in the 10^{-3} range. At that high level, weighing the probability of infringement against the possibility of serious physical harm may cease to be a speculative trade-off.

19. This could still be a danger even if the original sample was destroyed, as the new marker could be so highly correlated with the original one that the former result implies the latter.

20. In this case, Mr. Echazabal had a chronic condition (hepatitis C), and his diagnosis did not rely on any genetic information.

21. A subcurrent in the literature on the harms of testing for genetic (or other) predisposition to disease argues that the uncertainty in the information gleaned from such tests makes them particularly harmful. This argument seems to me analogous to a fallacy in the risk assessment arena: that imprecise statements about uncertainty can possibly be worse than no acknowledgment of uncertainty at all.

22. For example, the test for susceptibility to malignant hyperthermia, a life-threatening reaction to many common surgical anesthetics, also appears to reveal that the susceptible person may well develop one of several other rare neuromuscular disorders, whether or not he is ever exposed to the anesthetics (Mathews and Moore, 2004).

23. This current of thought strikes me as a very pessimistic outlook on human interindividual differences. In addition to the potential for providing life-saving information, individual genetic testing could conceivably elevate rather than debase society. Kierkegaard (1849/1941, p. 160), in *The Sickness unto Death,* sug-

decreases (which is what happens as the size of the sample whose mean is estimated increases).

31. A strong contrary view can be found in Adler (2005), who argues that we should ignore all estimates of individual risk, because until risk finds its fruition in harm, no harm has been done. He constructs an example in which "P" is asleep in his bed while an intruder creeps to his bedside, spins the chamber of a revolver loaded with one bullet, and pulls the trigger to find that an empty chamber was in position. According to Adler, "no pair of possible worlds differing merely in P's level of frequentist risk are different for P's welfare (and obviously, then, they are not for anyone else's either)." By this logic, it seems to me, we can conclude that a risk was unacceptable all along (at least in the case of fatality risks) only after the victim has died.

32. In general (unless all relevant relationships are linear), the expected value of a function is not equal to the function evaluated at its expected value. So for the function relating risk level to cost (or to "disutility"), if we believe that a risk of one in ten is more than one hundred times worse than a risk of one in one thousand, then a gamble between those two risks is worse than a certain prospect that the risk is at its expected value.

33. Note that the average risk in this subgroup is only four times higher than the overall mean, because for this distribution the mean is itself roughly seven times higher than the median. Also, all of the descriptions in this paragraph could be recast in terms of income or wealth, as in "39 percent of the income in this population accrues to the 9 percent of persons whose income is between 13 and 105 times that of the typical person."

34. To provide some reference points, the logarithmic standard deviation of personal income in the United States is approximately 0.7 (and for personal net wealth it is about 1.0); the logarithmic standard deviation of susceptibility in the methylene chloride example discussed below is approximately 1.5, and independent estimates by Hattis and Barlow (1996) and Finkel (1995a) suggest that the logarithmic standard deviation of susceptibility to a typical carcinogenic substance may be on the order of 2.0. For all of these cases, therefore, roughly 25 to 30 percent of the characteristic (income, wealth, risk) is concentrated within the 9 percent of the population in the lower nine-tenths of the topmost decile.

35. Another way to look at this is to recognize that some important determinants of susceptibility actually affect the extent of exposure to individuals. As the National Academy of Sciences / National Research Council Committee on Risk Assessment of Hazardous Air Pollutants pointed out (National Research Council, 1994, p. 216), "the individual most exposed to emissions" may in fact be someone breathing less of a particular pollutant than the MEI, but whose metabolizing enzymes actually deliver more of the pollutant to target cells.

36. I believe OSHA's congressional mandate is even clearer than is EPA's in this regard, with a highly prescriptive statute that sets a goal of considering 100 percent of the affected population. To those who would argue that OSHA may not be permitted to set standards to protect hypersusceptible employees (Bergeson, Campbell,

gested that failing to admit differences among us may debase us in a differer
way: "And, oh, this misery, that . . . as for the masses of men, that people em
ploy them about everything else, utilize them to generate the power for the the
ater of life, but never remind them of their blessedness; that they heap them in
mass and defraud them, instead of splitting them apart so that they might gaii
the highest thing."

24. When one of the prime developers of a new technology is in the vanguarc
of those cautioning against its use, technological optimists need to take particu
lar notice.

25. Consider, for example, the collection of men and women of all ages, races
and ethnicities who have an otherwise silent point mutation that may make them
particularly prone to developing chronic beryllium disease (McCanlies et al.,
2004).

26. "Let a six-year-old girl with brown hair need thousands of dollars for an
operation that will prolong her life until Christmas, and the post office will be
swamped with nickels and dimes to save her. But let it be reported that without
a sales tax the hospital facilities of Massachusetts will deteriorate and cause a
barely perceptible increase in preventable deaths—not many will drop a tear or
reach for their checkbooks" (Schelling, 1968).

27. Later in this chapter, I will refer to this hypothetical again in the context
of continuous distributions of susceptibility. If the one million inhabitants of city
C had susceptibilities distributed lognormally, with a logarithmic standard deviation of 2 and a median risk of 1.35×10^{-5}, the average individual risk (10^{-4})
and the expected number of fatalities (one hundred) would also align with those
in the other two cities.

28. I deliberately phrased this summary to emphasize the "tree falling in a forest
with no one to hear it" quality of this argument. Not being able to identify the people facing inequities doesn't erase the disparate result—it simply obscures it. However, because so much of risk management is wrapped up in how we perceive reality,
what we discern is also important. I believe that the "inequality we can't pinpoint
can't matter" argument is plausible but perhaps somewhat self-fulfilling.

29. For example, flipping one thousand fair coins should yield approximately
five hundred heads, but the standard deviation of that number will be approximately 16 (the square root of npq, where $n = 1000$ and p (probability of heads on
each flip) and q (probability of tails) both equal $\frac{1}{2}$—so it is very possible that
more than 516 or fewer than 484 heads will appear. But if you have one thousand unfair coins whose mean probability of heads equals $\frac{1}{2}$ (distributed equally
among one hundred different probabilities of heads, ranging from .01 to .99), the
standard deviation of the expected number of heads (which is still five hundred)
will be only about 13 rather than 16—showing the (perhaps) counterintuitive
property that the more different the members of the population are, the less variable the expected number of events in the population will be.

30. This property is consistent with the central limit theorem, as lognormal
distributions asymptotically become normal in shape as their standard deviation

and Bozof, 2002), I asked (Finkel, 2003), in effect, "What part of '*no employee* will suffer material impairment of health or functional capacity even if such employee has regular exposure to the hazard dealt with by such standard for the period of his working life' (emphasis added) don't you understand?" Read in the context of the *Benzene* decision's definition of "significant risk" as the probability of harm to an individual (not as the number of cases in the population, which the justices certainly could have chosen as the guide to distinguishing between significant and insignificant threats), it seems obvious that OSHA can reject a standard that eliminates significant risk for every employee if it would be infeasible, but not because of any hint that OSHA should be satisfied with protecting employees of average susceptibility.

37. The permissible exposure limit (PEL) of 25 parts per million (ppm) proposed in 1991 and the final PEL promulgated were identical. In part, this occurred because OSHA's economists had, inexplicably, not analyzed the costs and feasibility of a lower PEL in 1991, even though the risk at 25 ppm estimated in the proposal was 2.3 per 1,000 using body-weight extrapolation. Although the pharmacokinetic analysis indicated a slightly higher risk (3.6 per 1,000) at the 95th percentile reference point we chose, it would have prolonged this long-delayed rule even further to re-propose the standard with an economic analysis for a 10 ppm limit, the level at which estimated excess risk would have approached the 1 per 1,000 ceiling suggested by the *Benzene* court. Any comparison between the old and new risk estimates would be precarious, because both the method and the output (a distribution versus a point estimate of unknown "conservatism") changed so dramatically between the proposed and final versions.

38. My own preference is to concentrate society's effort on risk reduction rather than on ex post compensation, although I see various merits in Cranor's "hybrid proposal." I believe his proposal may have an illogical aspect, though, in that a susceptible person damaged by exposure deserves compensation in his scheme, whereas an average person damaged by exposure does not. If a priori risks are made acceptably low for both people, it seems odd to distinguish between someone unlucky enough to develop disease despite low risk from someone unlucky enough to do so at a somewhat higher underlying probability.

39. One statistical wrinkle needs to be anticipated here: for some small data sets exhibiting very large interindividual variability, very high percentiles of the fitted distribution may exceed the maximum individual measured value. This is not a defect in the estimation procedure, but one of its strengths.

REFERENCES

Ackerman, F., and L. Heinzerling. 2004. *Priceless: On knowing the price of everything and the value of nothing.* New York: New Press.

Adler, M.D. 2005. Against "individual risk": A sympathetic critique of risk assessment. *University of Pennsylvania Law Review* 153:1121–50.

Allen, B.C., K.S. Crump, and A.M. Shipp. 1988. Correlation between carcinogenic potency of chemicals in animals and humans. *Risk Analysis* 8:531–44.

Bazelon, E. 2005. Sentencing by the numbers. *New York Times Sunday Magazine* (Jan. 2).

Berck, P., and S. Hoffmann. 2002. Assessing the employment impacts of environmental and natural resource policy. *Environmental and Resource Economics* 22:133–56.

Bergeson, L.L., L.M. Campbell, and R.P. Bozof. 2002. Toxicogenomics. *The Environmental Forum* 19:28–39.

Bois, F.Y. 2001. Applications of population approaches in toxicology. *Toxicology Letters* 120:385–94.

Breyer, S. 1993. *Breaking the vicious circle: Toward effective risk regulation.* Cambridge, MA: Harvard University Press.

Burmaster, D. 2000. Distributions of total job tenure for men and women in selected industries and occupations in the United States, February 1996. *Risk Analysis* 20:205–24.

Chevron U.S.A. Inc. v. Ezachabal. 2002. 536 U.S. 73.

Clayton, E.W. 2003. Ethical, legal, and social implications of genomic medicine. *New England Journal of Medicine* 349:562–69.

Clinton, W.J. 2000. To prohibit discrimination in federal employment based on genetic information. Federal Executive Order No. 13145, *Federal Register* 65:6877.

Cook, R. 2005. Decoding health insurance. *New York Times* (May 22):13.

Crain, W. 1995. Risks and public policy: An interview with John Graham. *IEEE Power Engineering Review* (December):3–4.

Cranor, C.F. 1997. Eggshell skulls and loss of hair from fright: Some moral and legal principles that protect susceptible subpopulations. *Environmental Toxicology and Pharmacology* 4:239–45.

Diver, C.S., and J.M. Cohen. 2001. Genophobia: What is wrong with genetic discrimination? *University of Pennsylvania Law Review* 149:1439–72.

Donne, J. 1839. The works of John Donne, Vol. III, edited by Henry Alford. London: John W. Parker. (Originally published in 1624)

Dourson, M.J., S.P. Felter, and D. Robinson. 1996. Evolution of science-based uncertainty factors in noncancer risk assessment. *Regulatory Toxicology and Pharmacology* 24:108–20.

Feller, W. 1968. *An introduction to probability theory and its applications,* 3rd ed. New York: Wiley.

Finkel, A.M. 1984. Heterogeneity in human susceptibility to environmental carcinogens: Public health, regulatory, and ethical implications. Discussion Paper #E-84-06, John F. Kennedy School of Governmental Energy and Environmental Policy Center, Cambridge, MA.

Finkel, A.M. 1990. A simple formula for calculating the 'mass density' of a lognormally-distributed characteristic: Applications to risk analysis. *Risk Analysis* 10:291–301.

Finkel, A.M. 1995a. A quantitative estimate of the variations in human susceptibility to cancer and its implications for risk management. In *Low-dose extrapolation of cancer risks: Issues and perspectives*, ed. S. Olin, D.A. Neumann,
J.A. Foran, and G.J. Scarano, 297–328. Washington, DC: International Life Sciences Institute.

Finkel, A.M. 1995b. Toward less misleading comparisons of uncertain risks: The
example of aflatoxin and alar. *Environmental Health Perspectives* 103:376–85.

Finkel, A.M. 1996. Comparing risks thoughtfully. *Risk: Health, Safety & Environment* 7:325–59.

Finkel, A.M. 2003. The other side of toxicogenomics [Letter]. *Environmental Forum* 20(3):4–5.

Finkel, A.M. 2005. "Kilo-disparities": Prevailing concentrations of carcinogenic
air pollutants in U.S. workplaces and the ambient environment. Presentation
to the Society for Risk Analysis Annual Meeting, Orlando, FL, December 5.

Finkel, A.M. 2007. Distinguishing from straw men risk-risk tradeoffs legitimate
Presentation to the Society for Risk Analysis Annual Meeting, San Antonio,
TX, December 11.

Goldstein, B.D. 1989. The maximally exposed individual: An inappropriate basis
for public health decision-making. *Environmental Forum* 6:13–16.

Goldstein, B.D., M. Demak, M. Northridge, and D. Wartenberg. 1992. Risk to
groundlings of death due to airplane accidents: A risk communication tool.
Risk Analysis 12:339–41.

Goodman, G., and R. Wilson. 1991. Predicting the carcinogenicity of chemicals
in humans from rodent bioassay data. *Environmental Health Perspectives*
94:195–218.

Goodstein, E., and H. Hodges. 1997. Polluted data: Overestimating environmental costs. *American Prospect* 35:64–69.

Gould, S.J. 1981. *The mismeasure of man*. New York: Norton.

Graham, J.D. 1993. Testimony before joint hearing of the House Subcommittee on
Health and Environment (Committee on Energy and Commerce) and the Senate Committee on Labor and Human Resources, Sept. 21, 1993

Graham, J.D. 1994. The role of risk analysis in environmental protection. Testimony before the U.S. House Committee on Government Operations, February
1, 1994.

Grodsky, J.A. 2005. Genetics and environmental law: Redefining public health.
California Law Review 93:171–270.

Hamilton, J.T., W.K. Viscusi, and P.C. Dockins. 1997. Conservative versus mean
risk assessments: Implications for Superfund policies. *Journal of Environmental Economics and Management* 34:187–206.

Harrington, W., R.D. Morgenstern, and P. Nelson. 2000. On the accuracy of regulatory cost estimates. *Journal of Policy Analysis and Management* 19:297–322.

Harris, R.A., A.E. Washington, D. Feeny, and M. Kuppermann. 2001. Decision
analysis of prenatal testing for chromosomal disorders: What do the preferences of pregnant women tell us? *Genetic Testing* 5:23–32.

Harvard Magazine. 2005. At odds. May–June, 55–67.

Hattis, D. 2004. The conception of variability in risk analysis: Developments since 1980. In *Risk analysis and society: An interdisciplinary characterization of the field,* ed. T. McDaniels and M.J. Small, 15–45. Cambridge: Cambridge University Press.

Hattis, D., and E.L. Anderson. 1999. What should be the implications of uncertainty, variability, and inherent "biases"/"conservatism" for risk management decision-making? *Risk Analysis* 19:95–107.

Hattis, D., P. Banati, and R. Goble. 1999. Distributions of individual susceptibility among humans for toxic effects: How much protection does the traditional tenfold factor provide for what fraction of which kinds of chemicals and effects? *Annals of the New York Academy of Sciences* 895:286–316.

Hattis, D., and K. Barlow. 1996. Human interindividual variability in cancer risks: Technical and management challenges. *Human and Ecological Risk Assessment* 2:194–220.

Hattis, D., and R. Goble. 2003. The red book, risk assessment, and policy analysis: The road not taken. *Human and Ecological Risk Assessment* 9:1297–1306.

Hedges, L.V., and A. Nowell. 1995. Sex differences in mental test scores, variability, and numbers of high-scoring individuals. *Science* 269:41–45.

Hoel, D.G., and C.J. Portier. 1994. Nonlinearity of dose-response functions for carcinogenicity. *Environmental Health Perspectives* 102 Suppl. 1:109–13.

Jenni, K.E., and G. Loewenstein. 1997. Explaining the "identifiable victim effect." *Journal of Risk and Uncertainty* 14:235–57.

Johnston, D.C. 2005. Richest are leaving even the rich far behind. *New York Times* (June 5).

Kierkegaard, S. 1941. The sickness unto death. In *Fear and trembling and sickness unto death,* translated by Walter Lowrie. Princeton University Press, Princeton, NJ. (Originally published 1849)

Lopes, L.L. 1984. Risk and distributional inequality. *Journal of Experimental Psychology: Human Perception and Performance* 10:465–85.

Mathews, K.D., and S.A. Moore. 2004. Multiminicore myopathy, central core disease, malignant hyperthermia susceptibility, and RYR1 mutations: One disease with many faces? *Archives of Neurology* 61:27–29.

McCanlies, E.C., J.S. Ensey, C.R. Schuler, K. Kreiss, and A. Weston. 2004. The association between HLA-DPB1[Glu69] and chronic beryllium disease and beryllium sensitization. *American Journal of Industrial Medicine* 46:95–103.

Mossman, K.L. 1997. Radiation protection of radiosensitive populations. *Health Physics* 72:519–23.

National Research Council. 1994. *Science and judgment in risk assessment.* Washington, DC: National Academies Press.

Omenn, G.S. 1982. Predictive identification of hypersensitive individuals. *Journal of Occupational Medicine* 24:369–74.

Pizer, W.A., and R. Kopp. 2003. Calculating the cost of environmental regulation. Discussion Paper 03-06, Resources for the Future, Washington, DC.

Porter, M.E., and C. van der Linde. 1995. Toward a new conception of the environment-competitiveness relationship. *Journal of Economic Perspectives* 9:97–118.

Rawls, J. 1971. *A theory of justice.* Cambridge, MA: Harvard University Press.

Ritov, I., and J. Baron. 1990. Reluctance to vaccinate: Omission bias and ambiguity. *Journal of Behavioral Decision Making* 3:263–77.

Robert, J.S., and A. Smith. 2004. Toxic ethics: Environmental genomics and the health of populations. *Bioethics* 18:493–514.

Sacks, J. 2005. Covenant and conversation: Charity as justice. At www.chiefrabbi .org/thoughts/reeh5765.pdf.

Schelling, T.C. 1968. The life you save may be your own. In *Problems in public expenditure analysis,* ed. Samuel Chase. Washington, DC: Brookings Institution.

Schlack, L. 2005. Evidence of harm. *New York Times Sunday Magazine* (May 15):6.

Schneider, S.H., and J. Lane. 2005. *The patient from hell: How I worked with my doctors to get the best of modern medicine and how you can too.* Cambridge, MA: Da Capo Press.

Silvers, A., and M.A. Stein. 2002. An equality paradigm for preventing genetic discrimination. *Vanderbilt Law Review* 55:1341–95.

Sprinker, M. 2005. Genetic testing: How can we protect workers' rights to privacy? Abstract 117682 for the 133rd Annual Meeting of the American Public Health Association, Dec. 12, Philadelphia, Pa; http://apha.confex.com/apha/ 133am/techprogram/paper_117682.htm..

Sullivan, A. 2000. Promotion of the fittest. *New York Times Sunday Magazine* (July 23):16–17.

Summers, L.H. 2005. Remarks at the National Bureau of Economic Research Conference on Diversifying the Science and Engineering Workforce. At www .president.harvard.edu/speeches/2005/nber.html.

Thompson, K.M., R.F. Rabouw, and R.M. Cooke. 2001. The risk of groundling fatalities from unintentional airplane crashes. *Risk Analysis* 21:1025–37.

U.S. Environmental Protection Agency. 2005a. *Guidelines for carcinogen risk assessment.* Washington, DC: Author.

U.S. Environmental Protection Agency. 2005b. *Supplemental guidance for assessing susceptibility from early-life exposure to carcinogens.* Washington, DC: Author.

U.S. Food and Drug Administration. 2004a. Eligibility determination for donors of human cells, tissues, and cellular and tissue-based products. *Federal Register* 69:29786–834.

U.S. Food and Drug Administration. 2004b. Guidance for industry: Eligibility determination for donors of human cells, tissues, and cellular and tissue-based products. *Center for Biologics Evaluation and Research* (May):52.

U.S. Occupational Safety and Health Administration. 1997. Occupational exposure to methylene chloride: Final rule. *Federal Register* 62:1494–1619.

U.S. Occupational Safety and Health Administration. 2006. Occupational exposure to hexavalent chromium. Final rule. *Federal Register* 71:10100–10385.

U.S. Office of Management and Budget. 2003. Circular A-4: Regulatory analysis. At www.whitehouse.gov/omb/circulars/a004/a-4.pdf.

Wade, N. 1998. In the hunt for useful genes, a lot depends on 'snips'. *New York Times* (August 11).

Winkler, R.L., and J.E. Smith. 2004. On uncertainty in medical testing. *Medical Decision Making* 24:654–58.

Wolf, S.M. 1995. Beyond "genetic discrimination": Toward the broader harm of geneticism. *Journal of Law, Medicine and Ethics* 23:345–53.

Workshop on the Convergence of Risk Assessment and Socio-Economic Analysis to Better Inform Chemical Risk Management Decisions. 2000. Proceedings of a workshop sponsored by U.S. EPA, the Government of Canada, the American Chemistry Council, the International Council on Metals and the Environment, the Society for Risk Analysis, Resources for the Future, the Procter & Gamble Company, and the Organization for Economic Co-operation and Development, Arlington, VA, May 1–2. At www.riskworld.com/Nreports/2000/RA-EAWork-shopMay2000.pdf.

Young, J. 2005. Dems press to strengthen standards on inspectors' exposure to beryllium. *The Hill* (June 9).

Zaric, G.S. 2003. The impact of ignoring population heterogeneity when Markov models are used in cost-effectiveness analysis. *Medical Decision Making* 23:379–96.

APPENDIX

Applications of Toxicogenomic Technologies to Predictive Toxicology and Risk Assessment

The Human Genome Project, which set the goal of determining the complete nucleotide sequence of the human genome, was among the most important biologic research projects of all time. First envisioned in the late 1980s and considered by many to be technologically impossible at the time, it was the combination of adequate resources and strong scientific leadership of the project that fostered development of the requisite rapid DNA sequencing technologies. These new technologies were so successful that the genomic sequence of the bacterium *Haemophilus influenzae* was obtained only a few years later in 1995. Since then, the genomes of dozens of organisms have been elucidated and made available to the research community, and most important, the reference human genome sequence was made available by the year 2000, several years ahead of schedule.

To capitalize on the enormous potential of having access to genome-wide sequence information, scientists, clinicians, engineers, and information scientists combined forces to develop a battery of new molecular and bioinformatic tools that now make it possible to obtain and analyze biologic datasets of unprecedented magnitude and detail. Generally referred to as genomic technologies, these approaches permit sequence analysis—as well as gene transcript, protein, and metabolite profiling—on a genome-wide scale. As a result, the Human Genome Project and the technologic innovations and computational tools that it spawned are having profound effects on biologic research and understanding.

The application of these technologies to toxicology has ushered in an era when genotypes and toxicant-induced genome expression, protein, and metabolite patterns can be used to screen compounds for hazard identification, to monitor individuals' exposure to toxicants, to track cellular responses to different doses, to assess mechanisms of action, and to predict individual variability in sensitivity to toxicants.

This potential has prompted a plethora of scientific reviews and commentaries about toxicogenomics written over the past several years that attest to the widely held expectation that toxicogenomics will enhance the ability of scientists to study and estimate the risks different chemicals pose to human health and the environment. However, there are limitations in the data that are currently available, and fully understanding what can be expected from the technologies will require a greater consolidation of useful data, tools, and analyses. Given the inherent complexity in generating, analyzing, and interpreting toxicogenomic data and the fact that toxicogenomics cannot address all aspects of toxicology testing, interested parties need to prepare in advance. This preparation will help them understand how best to use these new types of information for risk assessment and for implementing commensurate changes in regulations and public health, while preparing for the potential economic, ethical, legal, and social consequences.

Committee's Charge

In anticipation of these questions, the National Institute of Environmental Health Sciences (NIEHS) of the U.S. Department of Health and Human Services, asked the National Academies to direct its investigative arm, the National Research Council (NRC), to examine the potential impacts of toxicogenomic technologies on predictive toxicology. NIEHS has invested significant resources in toxicogenomic research through establishment of the National Center for Toxicogenomics, funding of the National Toxicogenomics Research Consortium, development of the Chemical Effects in Biological Systems database for toxicogenomic data, and other collaborative ventures.

In response to the NIEHS request, the NRC assembled a panel of 16 experts with perspectives from academia, industry, environmental advocacy groups, and the legal community. The charge to the committee was to provide a broad overview for the public, government policy makers, and other interested and involved parties of the benefits potentially arising from toxicogenomic technologies; to identify the challenges in achieving them; and to suggest approaches that might be used to address the challenges.

Committee's Response to Its Charge

The committee clarified its task by defining the terms "toxicogenomics" and "predictive toxicology" as follows:

- *Toxicogenomics* is defined as the application of genomic technologies (for example, genetics, genome sequence analysis, gene expression profiling, proteomics, metabolomics, and related approaches) to study the adverse effects of environmental and pharmaceutical chemicals on human health and the environment. Toxicogenomics combines toxicology with information-dense genomic technologies to integrate toxicant-specific alterations in gene, protein, and metabolite expression patterns with phenotypic responses of cells, tissues, and organisms. Toxicogenomics can provide insight into gene-environment interactions and the response of biologic pathways and networks to perturbations. Toxicogenomics may lead to information that is more discriminating, predictive, and sensitive than that currently used to evaluate exposures to toxicants or to predict effects on human health.

- *Predictive toxicology* is used in this report to describe the study of how toxic effects observed in model systems or humans can be used to predict pathogenesis, assess risk, and prevent human disease.

Because of the belief that toxicogenomics has the potential to place toxicology on a more predictive footing, the committee describes the momentum channeling the field in this direction and some of the obstacles in its path. The committee approached its charge by identifying, defining, and describing several proposed applications of toxicogenomics to hazard-identification screening, mechanism-of-action studies, classification of compounds, exposure assessment, defining genetic susceptibility, and reducing the use of animal-based testing. Studies supporting each of these putative applications were then critically evaluated to define limitations, to enumerate remaining challenges, and to propose viable solutions whenever possible. Finally, the committee outlined realistic expectations of how these applications can be validated and how they can be used in risk assessment. The second part of this summary reviews these applications and what is needed for each of them.

In evaluating the putative applications, the committee recognized some overarching themes and steps necessary for the field to move forward.

Overarching Conclusions and Recommendations
Reproducibility, Data Analysis, Standards, and Validation

After evaluating the different applications, the committee concluded that, for the most part, the technologic hurdles that could have limited the reproducibility of data from toxicogenomic technologies have been resolved, representing an important step forward. To consolidate this advance, those who use these tools need to make a unified effort to establish objective standards for assessing quality and quality-control measures. Across the different applications, validation efforts are an important next step: actions should be taken to facilitate the technical and regulatory validation of toxicogenomics.

There is also a need for bioinformatic, statistical, and computational approaches and software to analyze data. Thus, the committee recommends the development of specialized bioinformatic, statistical, and computational tools and approaches to analyze toxicogenomic data.

Use of Toxicogenomics in Risk Assessment

Improving risk assessment is an essential aim of predictive toxicology, and toxicogenomic technologies present new opportunities to enhance it by potentially improving the understanding of dose-response relationships, cross-species extrapolations, exposure quantification, the underlying mechanisms of toxicity, and the basis of individual susceptibilities to particular compounds.

Although the applications of toxicogenomic technologies to risk assessment and the regulatory decision-making process have been exploratory to date, the potential to improve risk assessment has just begun to be tapped. Toxicogenomic technologies clearly have strong potential to affect decision making, but they are not currently ready to replace existing required testing regimes in risk assessment and regulatory toxicology. Toxicogenomic technologies are assuming an increasing role as adjuncts to and extensions of existing technologies for predictive toxicology. Toxicogenomics can provide additional molecular level information and tests that add to the "weight of the evidence" for refining judgments about the risks posed by environmental toxicants and drugs. Ultimately, however, they are envisioned to be more sensitive and informative than existing technologies and may supplant some approaches currently used or at least be a component of batteries that will replace certain tests.

To move forward, the committee recommends that regulatory agencies enhance efforts to incorporate toxicogenomic data into risk assessment. The following actions are needed: (1) substantially enhance agencies' capability to effectively integrate toxicogenomic approaches into risk assessment practice, focusing on the specific applications below; (2) invest in research and personnel within the infrastructure of regulatory agencies; and (3) develop and expand research programs dedicated to integrating toxicogenomics into challenging risk assessment problems, including the development of partnerships between the public and private sectors.

Need for a Human Toxicogenomics Initiative

Several themes emerged throughout evaluation of the different applications discussed below, including the need for more data, the need to broaden data collection, the need for a public database to facilitate sharing and use of the volumes of data, and the need for tools to mine this database to extract biologic knowledge.

Concerted efforts are necessary to address these needs and propel the field forward. Fully integrating toxicogenomic technologies into predictive toxicology will require a coordinated effort approaching the scale of the Human Genome Project. It will require funding and resources significantly greater than what is allocated to existing research programs and will benefit from public-private partnerships to achieve its goals. These types of investments and coordinated scientific leadership will be essential to develop toxicogenomic tools to the point where many of the expected benefits for predicting the toxicity of compounds and related decision making can be realized.

To achieve this goal, NIEHS should cooperate with other stakeholders to explore the feasibility and objectives of a human toxicogenomics initiative (HTGI), as described in Box S-1. The HTGI would support the collection of

---

BOX S-1 Human Toxicogenomics Initiative

NIEHS should cooperate with other stakeholders in exploring the feasibility and objectives of implementing a human toxicogenomics initiative (HTGI) dedicated to advancing toxicogenomics. Elements of the HTGI should include the following:

1. Creation and management of a large, public database for storing and integrating the results of toxicogenomic analyses with conventional toxicity-testing data.
2. Assembly of toxicogenomic and conventional toxicologic data on a large number (hundreds) of compounds into the single database. This includes the generation of new toxicogenomic data from humans and animals for a number of compounds for which other types of data already exist as well as the consolidation of existing data. Every effort should be made to leverage existing research studies and infrastructure (such as those of the National Toxicology Program) to collect samples and data that can be used for toxicogenomic analyses.
3. Creation of a centralized national biorepository for human clinical and epidemiologic samples, building on existing efforts.
4. Further development of bioinformatic tools, such as software, analysis, and statistical tools.
5. Consideration of the ethical, legal, and social implications of collecting and using toxicogenomic data and samples.
6. Coordinated subinitiatives to evaluate the application of toxicogenomic technologies to the assessment of risks associated with chemical exposures.

toxicogenomic data and would coordinate the creation and management of a large-scale database that would use systems biology approaches and tools to integrate the results of toxicogenomic analyses with conventional toxicity testing data.

The information generated from toxicogenomic experiments is on a scale vastly exceeding DNA sequencing efforts like the Human Genome Project. The heft of these outputs, consisting of multidimensional datasets that include genotype, gene expression, metabolite, and protein information; design factors such as dose, time, and species information; and information on toxicologic effects warrant the creation of a public database. This database is needed to compile and analyze the information at a more complex level than the current "one disease is caused by one gene" approach. Curation, storage, and mining of these data will require developing and distributing specialized bioinformatic and computational tools. Current public databases are inadequate to manage the types or volumes of data to be generated by large-scale applications of toxicogenomic technologies and to facilitate the mining and interpretation of the data, which are just as important as their generation and storage.

Although the database and tools are important, the database itself is not sufficient. Data on a large number of compounds are needed so that comparisons can be made and data can be mined to identify important relationships. To collect and generate these toxicogenomic data, it will be important to leverage large publicly funded studies and facilitate the production and sharing of private sector data.

In addition to data, work is needed in the collection of physical samples appropriate for toxicogenomic research. Specifically, a national biorepository for human clinical and epidemiologic samples is needed so that toxicogenomic data can eventually be extracted from them. In addition, when possible and appropriate, the collection of samples and data should be incorporated into major human studies. The collection of human samples and their corresponding data raises a number of ethical, legal, and social issues of the type described below, which need to be addressed.

Because the realization of the goals articulated here will require significantly higher levels of funding, leadership, and commitment than are currently allocated to toxicogenomics, planning and organizing research should begin immediately. Collaborations among government, academia, and the private sector not only will expedite discovery but will ensure optimal use of samples and data; prevent unnecessary duplication or fragmentation of datasets; enhance the ability to address key ethical, legal, and social effects; reduce costs; and promote intellectual synergy.

The resulting publicly accessible HTGI data resource would strengthen the utility of toxicogenomic technologies in toxicity assessment and thus enable more accurate prediction of health risks associated with existing and newly developed compounds and formulations.

Specific Applications of Toxicogenomics

To address the expectation that toxicogenomics will revolutionize predictive toxicology, the committee explored several proposed applications of toxicogenomics, including hazard screening, the study of toxicologic mechanisms of action, exposure assessment, and characterizing variability in susceptibility. These and the other applications can be used in conjunction with risk assessment, although they are also important in predictive toxicology, which is removed from the risk assessment process. In the following sections, the committee reports findings from the evaluation of these topics that were assimilated into the conclusions of the report.

Exposure Assessment

The application of toxicogenomics for defining biomarkers of exposure will require consensus on what constitutes an exposure biomarker. Standardized toxicogenomic platforms that are appropriate for identifying signatures of environmental or drug exposures in target and surrogate tissues and fluids will also be required. Additional technical challenges include the individual variation in response to an environmental exposure and the persistence of a toxicogenomic signature after exposure.

Toxicogenomic technologies should be adapted and applied for the study of exposure assessment by developing signatures of exposure to individual chemicals and perhaps to chemical mixtures. To facilitate the development of exposure-assessment tools based on toxicogenomics, large human population studies should include a collection of samples that can be used for transcriptomic, proteomic, metabolomic, or other toxicogenomic analyses in addition to traditional epidemiologic measures of exposure.

Hazard Screening

Toxicogenomic technologies provide new and potentially useful indicators for use in toxicity screening. Near-term applications include current uses in drug development and the validation of categories of compounds for screening chemicals found in the environment. In contrast to applications in evaluating new drug candidates, screening approaches for environmental chemicals will need to address a broader range of exposure levels and a more comprehensive set of adverse health effects.

Toxicogenomic screening methods should be integrated into relevant current and future chemical regulatory and safety programs upon validation and development of adequate databases. To move toward this goal, it is important to improve the quantity and quality of data available for deriving screening profiles and to develop a database to organize this information. The process of creating such a database could be accelerated by addressing proprietary and legal hurdles so at least some of the toxicogenomic data currently in private databases could be made available, and by integrating toxicogenomic assays into ongoing chemical screening and testing initiatives such as those conducted by the National Toxicology Program. In addition, regulatory agencies should continue to develop and refine guidance documents for their staff on interpreting toxicogenomic data.

Variability in Susceptibility

People vary in their susceptibility to toxic effects of chemical exposures. Toxicogenomic technologies (including the analysis of gene sequences and epigenetic modifications) offer the opportunity to use genetic information in a prospective fashion to identify susceptible subpopulations and assess the distribution of differences in susceptibility in larger populations. Toxicogenomic technologies could also reduce the uncertainty surrounding assumptions used in regulatory processes to address population variability.

Toxicogenomic information should be used to prospectively identify, understand the mechanisms of, and characterize the extent of genetic and epigenetic influences on variations in human susceptibility to the toxic effects of chemicals. Animal models and genome-wide human studies should be used to identify genetic variations that influence sensitivity to chemicals, using existing large human studies when possible to investigate the effect of genetic variations on responses to a wide array of chemical exposures and pharmaceutical therapies. More attention should be focused on modeling effects involving multiple genes and the study of context-dependent genetic effects (that is, gene-gene interactions as well as the impact of developmental age, sex, and life course).

Mechanistic Information

Toxicogenomic studies are improving knowledge of the molecular level events that underlie toxicity and may thus advance the consideration of mechanistic information in risk assessment and decision making. Tools and approaches should continue to be developed to advance the ability of toxicogenomics to provide useful mechanistic information. Developing richer algorithms and models that can integrate complex and various types of toxicogenomic data (for example, metabolomic and proteomic data) may make it possible to shift the focus of mechanistic investigations of single genes to more integrated analyses. These will encompass more of the complexity of biologic systems as a whole as well as the multidimensionality of the dose- and time-related effects of toxicants.

Cross-Species Extrapolation

Toxicogenomic technologies offer the potential to significantly enhance confidence in animal-to-human toxicity extrapolations that constitute the foundation of risk evaluations. Using toxicogenomics to analyze species differences in toxicity will help explain the molecular basis for the differences and improve the translation of animal observations into estimates of potential human risk. In addition, by providing molecular level comparisons between humans and other species, toxicogenomics may assist in identifying those animal species and strains that are most relevant for specific assays.

Toxicogenomics should continue to be used to study differences in toxicant responses between animal models and humans, and genotyped and genetically altered animal model strains should continue to be used as experimental tools to better extrapolate results from animal tests to human health. Algorithms must be developed to facilitate accurate identification of genes and proteins that serve the same function in different organisms and species—called orthologous genes and proteins—used in toxicologic research.

Dose-Response Relationships

Toxicogenomics has the potential to improve the understanding of dose-response relationships, particularly at low doses. Future toxicologic assessment should incorporate dose-response and time-course analyses appropriate to risk assessment. Analyses of toxic compounds that are well characterized could provide an intellectual framework for future studies.

Developmental Exposures

Although recognized to be important in a number of disorders, relatively little is known about the health impacts of fetal and early-life exposures to many chemicals in current use. Because of their sensitivity, toxicogenomic technologies are expected to reveal more than previously was possible about the molecules involved in development and the critical molecular level events that can be perturbed by toxicants. Toxicogenomics may also enable screening for chemicals that cause gene expression changes associated with adverse developmental effects. In short, toxicogenomic technologies should be used to investigate how exposure during early development conveys susceptibility to drug and chemical toxicities.

Mixtures

Although much toxicology focuses on the study of single chemicals, humans are frequently exposed to multiple chemicals. It is difficult to decipher how exposure to many chemicals will influence the effects of each one. It is unlikely that toxicogenomic signatures will be able to decipher all interactions among complex mixtures, but it should be possible to use mechanism-of-action data to design informative toxicogenomic experiments, including screening chemicals for potential points of biologic conversion (overlap) such as shared activation and detoxification pathways, enhancing identification and exploration of potential interactions, and moving beyond empirical experiments. Toxicogenomic approaches should be used to test the validity of methods for the ongoing challenge of estimating potential risks associated with mixtures of environmental chemicals.

Ethical, Legal, and Social Issues

The committee evaluated ethical, legal, and social implications of toxicogenomics. As toxicogenomic data linked to clinical and epidemiologic information are collected, it is critical to ensure adequate protections of the privacy, confidentiality, and security of toxicogenomic information in health records and information used in studies. Safeguarding this information will further advance important individual and societal interests. It will also prevent individuals from being dissuaded from participating in research or undergoing the genetic testing that is the first step in individualized risk assessment and risk reduction.

Toxicogenomics is also likely to play a role in occupational, environmental, and pharmaceutical regulation and litigation. Regulatory agencies and courts should give appropriate weight to the validation, replication, consistency, sensitivity, and specificity of methods when deciding whether to rely on toxicogenomic data.

Ethical, legal, and social issues that affect the use of toxicogenomic data and the collection of data and samples needed for toxicogenomic research should be addressed. This could occur through legislative improvements to enhance individual protection, exploration of how to facilitate large-scale biorepository and database research while protecting individuals, and consideration by courts and regulatory agencies of appropriate factors when deciding how to consider toxicogenomic data. Finally, special efforts should be made to address the impact of toxicogenomic research and findings on vulnerable populations.

Education and Training in Toxicogenomics

Given the complexity of toxicogenomics, the generation, analysis, and interpretation of toxicogenomic information represents a challenge to the scientific community and requires the collaborative cross-disciplinary efforts of scientific teams of specialists. Therefore it is essential that education and training in toxicogenomics become a continuous, ongoing process that reflects the rapid developments in these new technologies. There is a need to develop education and training programs relevant to toxicogenomic applications to predictive toxicology. Specifically, programs are needed to reach the general public, susceptible subgroups, health professionals, government regulators, attorneys and judges, the media, scientists in training, scientists on the periphery of toxicogenomics, and institutions that participate in toxicogenomic research.

Conclusions

In summary, toxicogenomic technologies present a set of powerful tools for transforming current observation-based approaches into predictive science, thereby enhancing risk assessment and public health decision making. To leverage this potential will require more concerted efforts to generate data, make multiple uses of existing data sources, and develop tools to study data in new ways. Beyond the technical challenges and opportunities, other challenges in the communication, education, ethics, and legal arenas will need to be addressed to ensure that the potential of the field can be realized.

INDEX

solvent susceptibility, 91
Stein, M.A., 308, 309
stem cells, 227
Sullivan, A., 330
Summers, L., 306–7
susceptibility: defining, 123–24;
disease vs. environmental, 111,
117–18; expectations of protection,
5; genetic variability and, 41–43,
116–18; identifying, 29; individual,
correlated to group membership, 314;
nongenetic, 121; predicting, 29–30;
variability in, 116–17, 142, 294–96,
350
susceptibility, genetic: to air pollutants,
evidence for, 120–23; complexity of,
268–69; environmental justice and,
109–12; justice and fairness concerns,
7, 98–100; relevance to standard-
setting, 126; risk and, 103–4; in risk-
assessment models, 156; toxic tort
suits and, 82, 87–92
susceptibility biomarkers, 249
susceptibility genes, 82, 87–92, 111,
117–18
susceptible individuals, 123, 185–88.
See also hypersensitive individuals
susceptible subgroups: defining for
use in standard-setting, 127–28;
differential treatment of, conditions
for, 314–15; duty to compensate,
279; duty to test, 85–86; duty to
warn, 88–89, 190; identifying,
consequences of, 61–62, 134;
inclusion criteria, 123; OSHA
protections for, 185–87; protecting,
210–14, 272–74; regulatory policy
development, 5–7, 18–19, 123–29,
185–88, 269–79, 280–85; risk
assumption, 90; utilitarianism's
concern with, 270–72. See also
hypersensitive subgroups
susceptible subgroups, protecting: under
current law, 61–62; equal protection
from harm principle, 276–79; hybrid
regulatory-compensation proposal
for equality in, 280–85; moral choice
in, 130–31, 258–66, 269–79; needs
assessment, 290–91; obligation to,
without regard for economics or
feasibility, 90, 129–32; responsibility
for, 5–6; social support for, 62;
targeted protections, 132–34

Sutton v. United Air Lines, Inc., 192,
193
Swada, S., 39
Swift, M., 207
syphilis, 311

Takami, K., 39
technology, emergent, 77–78
thimerosal, 89, 301
Thompson, D.K., 224
Thompson, K.M., 293
3M Company, 73
Three Mile Island incident, 84
Title VI, Civil Rights Act, 102, 105, 111
Title VII, Civil Rights Act, 184
tort law: etiological studies importance
in, 81–82; protection of the
vulnerable under, 94, 275–76,
320–21; purpose of, 94, 275
toxicity, mechanisms of, 59, 223, 225,
228–29; testing for, 13–16, 27–28,
49–52, 55
toxicity signatures, 37–38
toxicogenetics, 60–62, 221, 248
toxicogenomic data: adverse
effects reporting, 73–77; areas of
greatest application, 67; database
development by for-profit entities,
54–55; disincentives for open sharing
of, 55; obstacles to using, 53–55,
68–73, 87, 125–26; potential
applications of, 68, 82; regulatory
applications of, 2–5, 55–59, 125–26;
traditional methods of gathering,
advantages over, 48–50
toxicogenomics: barriers to application
of, 52–55, 62, 345–46; challenges
facing, 47–48, 226–27; conceptual
dimensions of, 228–32; conclusion,
21; costs and opportunity costs of,
232–33; defined, 221, 248, 344–45;
development of, 53–59; education
and training in, 353; of exposure and
effect, 224–25; future of, 219–23,
343–48; limitations of, 19–21,
234–36; normative dimensions of,
232–35; peril and promise debate,
308; potential applications of,
223–28; for predictive toxicology,
349–53; regulatory applications of,
11–19, 55–59
toxicological testing, 47–50, 59, 62
toxicology, 12, 37–38, 224, 345, 349–53